INTERNATIONAL LIBRARY OF ETHICS, LAW, AND THE NEW MEDICINE

VOLUME 29

The titles published in this series are listed at the end of this volume.

Ethics and Intersex

Edited by

SHARON E. SYTSMA, PH.D.

Northern Illinois University,
DeKalb, U.S.A.

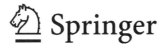 Springer

A C.I.P. Catalogue record for this book is available from the Library of Congress.

ISBN-10 1-4020-4313-9 (HB)
ISBN-13 978-1-4020-4313-0 (HB)
ISBN-10 1-4020-4314-7 (e-book)
ISBN-13 978-1-4020-4314-7 (e-book)

Published by Springer,
P.O. Box 17, 3300 AA Dordrecht, The Netherlands.

www.springer.com

Printed on acid-free paper

Printed in the Netherlands.

TABLE OF CONTENTS

PREFACE

The chief goal of this book is to improve the quality of life for intersexual people. That goal requires not only the improvement of our medical practices, but also an increasing social awareness and understanding of intersexuality and its implications. To this end, I have sought contributions reflecting many different disciplines and contributors from many different countries. The book includes twenty chapters addressing controversial ethical and medical issues concerning infant genital surgery, neglected ethical issues, and the challenges intersexuality raises for both traditional medical practices and traditional cultural and religious views on human sexuality in general.

The book is meant to have an eclectic audience: intersexuals, their families, intersex advocates, urologists, endocrinologists, gynecologists, psychologists, psychiatrists, sexologists, biomedical ethicists, hospital ethics committee members, medical lawyers, medical ethicists, research ethicists, gender theorists, philosophers, theologians, sociologists, and anyone who wants to further their education on human sexuality. Chapters may be more technical than required by some people, and perhaps not as technical and others would want. I asked my authors to aim for clarity for a general readership without sacrificing the quality, accuracy, and creativity of their projects.

The chapters do not represent a single point of view, but instead include quite opposing views that reflect the contentious issues we face today. Readers should not assume that the chapters reflect the opinion of the editor, except of course, the chapters written by her.

ACKNOWLEDGEMENTS

With pleasure I take this opportunity to thank the many people who helped to make this book possible. Thanks to David Buller who first introduced me to the topic, to Cheryl Chase for sending me materials to begin my education on intersexuality, and to Ian Aaronson, for inviting me to serve as Ethics Consultant to the North American Task Force on Intersexuality. It was here that I was introduced to leading medical experts on intersexuality, who treated me with unexpected graciousness and impressed me with their sincerity and dedication to examining and improving the medical management of intersexuality, and some of whom generously agreed to contribute chapters in this book. Thanks also to Gilman Grave for inviting me to participate in the research-planning workshop on intersexuality sponsored by the National Institute of Child Health and Development, a very exciting and wonderful learning experience indeed. I am especially grateful to Heino Meyer-Bahlburg, from whom I learned so much, both from his published works and from some telephone and email conversations.

I also wish to express my thanks to Northern Illinois University for granting me a sabbatical enabling me to conduct my research and plan for this book, and also for helping to support my attendance at national and international bioethics conferences where I presented papers on intersexuality, which eventually worked their way into chapters in this book. Warm appreciation is especially owed to the participants of the annual David Thomasma International Bioethics Retreats, whose comments following my several presentations on intersexuality in 2001, 2003, and 2005, were a source of insight and inspiration. Deep thanks to Thomasine Kushner who pointed me in the right direction, and to David Weisstub for taking an interest in and realizing the urgency of this project.

Going further back, it is unlikely this book would have appeared without the wonderful education in philosophy I had at Loyola University after having been granted the Crown Humanities Fellowship. There I was able to pursue my already strong interest in biomedical ethics, largely under the direction of David Ozar, who later became a fellow traveller in my investigations into intersexuality. Also, the audacity to offer my services as an ethics consultant to the task force was empowered by the fabulous experience of being a Teaching Scholar at the 2-year program on Research Ethics organized by Timothy Murphy, and funded by the National Institute of Health at the University of Illinois/Chicago. Thanks also to Tim for his many comments, constructive and destructive, which helped me to improve my chapter on the use of dexamethasone to reduce virilization of female infants at risk of Congenital Adrenal Hyperplasia. Any remaining flaws are my own responsibility.

Thanks to Peter Nichols and Emily Strom, and especially to Molly Gardner, for providing welcome professional assistance with the editing of several chapters, and to Fritz Schmuhl and Natalie Rieborn for their patience and helpfulness in helping me to properly prepare the manuscript for publication.

NOTES ON CONTRIBUTORS

Hazel G. Beh, MSW (1975), Ph.D. American Studies (1985), JD (1991) is a Professor of Law at the William S. Richardson School of Law, University of Hawaii at Manoa. She is the current chair of Education Law Section and past chair of the Contracts Section of the American Association of Law Schools. Her scholarship often considers legal issues related to higher education, insurance, health, sexuality, and medical research.

Vijayalakshmi Bhatia, M.D. is Additional professor of endocrinology at the Sanjay Gandhi Postgraduate Institute of Medical Sciences in Lucknow, India. Her work and publications are on aspects of pediatric endocrinology relevant to a tropical developing country, such as endemic iodine deficiency cretinism, calcium deficiency rickets, vitamin D deficiency in adolescence and pregnancy, diabetes mellitus, and disorders of sexual differentiation. She has co-edited a clinical handbook of pediatric and adolescent endocrinology.

Peggy T. Cohen-Kettenis is a clinical psychologist and psychotherapist. She is professor of medical psychology at the Department of Medical Psychology of the Vrije Universiteit Medical Center (VUmc), Amsterdam, The Netherlands, and director of the Gender Dysphoria Knowledge Center in this hospital. She has published on gender dysphoria, gender development and the relationship between gender-related behavior/psychopathology and sex hormones. In 2003 she published a book "Transgenderism and Intersexuality in Children and Adolescents: Making Choices" with professor Friedemann Pfäfflin.

Sarah M Creighton, M.D., FRCOG, is Consultant Gynecologist at University College Hospital, London, UK and at Great Ormond Street Hospital, London, UK. She works as part of a multidisciplinary intersex team offering gynecological input for children, adolescents and adults. I have a major research interest in the adult outcomes of intersex and related conditions. I have focused particularly on the gynecological and psychosexual consequences of reconstructive genital surgery and have published widely in peer review journals.

Milton Diamond, Ph.D., Professor in the Department of Anatomy, Biochemistry, Physiology, and Reproductive Biology, and Director of the Pacific Center for Sex and Society at the John A. Burns School of Medicine, University of Hawaii. He has published two books, *Sexual Decisions* and *Sexwatching: Looking into the World of Sexual Behavior,* both reprinted in other languages, edited several others, and has published over 150 articles on scientific, medical and ethical issues related to both animal and human sexuality, several of which are on intersexuality. He is the recipient of the Magnus Hirshfeld Medal for Outstanding Contributions to Sex Research and has earned international recognition in his field. He is one of the key figures to have brought problems with our traditional medical treatment of intersexuality to light, as well with the scientific hypotheses about human sexuality underlying it.

Alice Domurat Dreger, Ph.D., is Visiting Associate Professor of Medical Humanities and Bioethics in the Program in Medical Humanities and Bioethics at the Feinberg School of Medicine, Northwestern University, and Director of Medical Education for the Intersex Society of North America. Her books include *Hermaphrodites and the Medical Invention of Sex* (Harvard University Press, 1998), *Intersex in the Age of Ethics* (University Publishing Group, 1999), and *One of Us: Conjoined Twins and the Future of Normal* (Harvard University Press, 2004).

Julie Greenberg, B.A., J.D., Professor of Law, Thomas Jefferson School of Law. Professor Greenberg is an internationally recognized expert on the legal issues relating to gender, sex, sexual identity and sexual orientation. Her path-breaking work on the legal aspects of gender identity has been cited by a number of state and federal courts, as well as courts in other countries, and has been quoted in more than 100 books and articles.

J. David Hester, Ph.D. is co-founder of the Centre for Rhetorics and Hermeneutics, co-Senior Editor of "Queen: a journal of rhetoric and power". He is a member of the Zentrum für Ethik in den Wissenschaften of the University of Tübingen, and a research fellow of the Alexander von Humboldt Foundation. His doctorate is in rhetorical theory and criticism of the New Testament, from out of which his current research focus has turned upon the questions of the origins of rhetorical strategies of sex, sexuality and sexed identity in the public sphere, including the biblical origins of the heterosexist paradigm and its impact upon culture, law, and medicine.

Edmund Howe, M.D., J.D., is a medical ethicist and Professor in the Department of Psychiatry at the Uniformed Services University of the Health Sciences in

Bethesda, Maryland. He has authored over a hundred articles on biomedical ethics and is Editor-in-Chief of the Journal of Clinical Ethics.

Patricia Beattie Jung, Ph.D., is a Professor of Moral Theology at Loyola University Chicago. Her research focuses on a variety of issues in Christian sexual ethics. Recently she edited with Joseph A. Coray *Sexual Diversity and Catholicism: Toward the Development of Moral Theology* (The Liturgical Press, 2001) and co-edited with Mary E. Hunt and Radhika Balakrishna, *Good Sex: Feminist Wisdom from the Worlds Religions* (Rutgers University Press, 2001).

Stephen F. Kemp, M.D., Ph.D. is Professor of Pediatrics and Medical Humanities at the University of Arkansas for Medical Sciences. He has been at the University of Arkansas for Medical Sciences and Arkansas Children's Hospital since 1984, and was Chief of the Section of Pediatric Endocrinology from 1987-2001. His research interests have been in the field of growth and growth hormone therapy, and he is the author of a number of publications related to this topic. Dr. Kemp is currently President of the Human Growth Foundation.

Lih-Mei Liao, BSc, MSc, PhD is a Consultant Clinical Psychologist & Honorary Senior Lecturer at the Sub-Department of Clinical Health Psychology of the University College in London. She works with women presenting psychological difficulties associated with reproductive and sexuality issues. She has published over 40 papers and chapters in women's health. Her current interests are broadly concerned with female sexuality. She leads a group of clinical psychologists also providing services to obstetrics and gynecology in several hospitals in London.

Iain Morland, MA, Mphil, is a Doctoral Candidate in English Literature at the Royal Holloway, University of London. Author of articles on intersex in publications such as *The Psychologist*, *Continuum*, and *Studies in Law, Politics and Society*, Iain Morland proposes a multidisciplinary approach to intersex that includes the humanities as well as health sciences. His doctoral dissertation examines the ethics of narrative-based intersex treatment. He is also co-editor, with Annabelle Willox, of *Queer Theory* (Palgrave Macmillan, 2005).

Timothy F. Murphy, Ph.D., is Professor of Philosophy in the Biomedical Sciences at the University of Illinois College of Medicine at Chicago. He is the author or editor of eight books, including *Justice and the Human Genome Project* (University of California Press), *Gay Science: The Ethics of Sexual Orientation Research* (Columbia University Press), and *Case Studies in Biomedical Research Ethics* (MIT Press). He has also written extensively on ethical issues in genetic research, human sexuality, transplantation, and assisted reproductive technologies. With grant support from the Department of Defense, he convened one of the first national conferences dealing with the Human Genome Project. He has also had grant support from the National Institutes of Health and has sponsored two national conferences dealing with the ethics of research with human beings. He has also been a Visiting Scholar at the Institute for Ethics of the American Medical Association.

David T. Ozar, Ph.D., is Professor and Co-Director of Graduate Studies in Health Care Ethics in the Department of Philosophy at Loyola University Chicago, and Director of Loyola's Center for Ethics and Social Justice. He has taught at Loyola since 1972 and has been Director of the Center for Ethics and Social Justice since 1994. He has published two books and more than a hundred articles and book chapters on ethical issues in health care, the professions, and other social systems.

Friedemann Pfäfflin, M.D., is Professor of Forensic Psychotherapy and Head of the Forensic Psychotherapy Unit at the University of Ulm, Germany. He is editor of the International Journal of Transgenderism (IJT), President of the International Association for the Treatment of Sexual Offenders (IATSO), past president of the Harry Benjamin International Gender Dysphoria Association (HBIGDA), past president of the International Association for Forensic Psychotherapy (IAFP).

William G. Reiner, M.D. is Director, Psychosexual Development Clinic. Associate Professor, Section of Pediatric Urology, Adjunct Professor, Division of Child and Adolescent Psychiatry, University of Oklahoma Health Sciences Center (Oklahoma, USA). With his training and professional experience in Urology, Psychiatry, and Child and Adolescent Psychiatry, Dr. Reiner conducts research on psychosocial development in children, adolescents, and young adults with major genito-urinary birth anomalies. He has published and spoken internationally on topics of sexual identity and psychosexual development in children with intersex conditions and other disorders of sexual differentiation, children with myelomeningocele, and on children with classical bladder exstrophy.

Justine Schober, M.D., from Erie, Pennsylvania has published dozens of articles on intersexuality in national and international journals since the late 1980's and has lectured on the topic even more extensively in the United States and throughout the world. She was a member of the North American Task Force on Intersexuality, and is a consultant to the Intersex Society of North America.

Herman Stark, Ph.D. He is currently head of the philosophy program and the international honors society at South Suburban College in South Holland, IL. He has received numerous teaching awards. His philosophical novel, *A Fierce Little Tragedy* (2003, 2005), has been nominated for the Society for Phenomenological and Existential Philosophy and American Philosophical Association book awards. He has published articles on Heidegger, Philosophy of Mind, Epistemology, Philosophy of Science, and Logic.

Sharon Sytsma, Ph.D, is an Associate Professor of Philosophy at Northern Illinois University. She has served as Chair of the Ethics Subcommittee of the North American Task Force on Intersexuality and an ethics consultant at a workshop sponsored by the National Institute of Child Health and Human Development. She has published articles on ethical issues pertaining to intersexuality in *Cambridge Quarterly of Health Care Ethics* and *Dialogues in Pediatric Urology,* and a case study and commentary in the *Hastings Center Report*. She has also published articles on other biomedical ethical issues, and in ethical theory.

Garry Warne, MBBS, FRACP, is Senior Endocrinologist and Director, RCH International (RCHI) at the Royal Children's Hospital, Melbourne. His basic and clinical research on aspects of sex differentiation spans 30 years. He has received a Golden Orchid award from the AIS Support Group (UK) and Honorary Life Membership of the AIS Support Group Australia Inc. He has written two widely-used parent and patient information booklets, "Your Child with Congenital Adrenal Hyperplasia" and "Complete Androgen Insensitivity." He visits Asia frequently for the purposes of teaching, research, and project administration.

Kenneth Zucker, Ph.D., C.Psych., is Professor of Psychology and Psychiatry at the University of Toronto and Head of the Gender Identity Service, Child, Youth, and Family Program Centre for Addiction and Mental Health. His clinical and research interests pertain to psychosexual differentiation and its disorders. He is the current President of the International Academy of Sex Research, and Editor of the *Archives of Sexual Behavior.*

SHARON E. SYTSMA

INTRODUCTION

The term "intersexuality," while increasingly more common, is still unfamiliar to most people, and is often misunderstood, so I begin with a simple definition: Intersexuality is the biological condition of being "in between" male and female. There are many different kinds of intersexuality, and many different degrees of each. Sometimes intersexuality can be recognized by a mere visual inspection, such as when it is manifest in ambiguous genitalia. In other cases, genitalia will appear to be typically male or typically female, but will be discordant with the "sex" of the chromosomes, the gonads, or both. Intersex conditions are somewhat rare, though not nearly as rare as one might think. While the percentage of the population affected is difficult to determine, suffice it to say at this point that about 3500 infant genital surgeries take place each year for cosmetic and/or for sex assignment purposes in the United States alone.

To some extent, it is an accident of historical influences that we have been kept in the dark about intersexuality, as Alice Dreger explains in her book *Hermaphrodites and the Medical Invention of Sex* (Harvard University Press, 1998). But it is important to realize that intersexuality is a natural phenomenon occurring in animals as well as in human beings. Some societies have recognized the existence of intersexual individuals and have "made room" for them in their social structure. Others have rejected them, leaving such infants to be exposed to the elements and perish. Yet others have raised them to a status higher than ordinary males and female, or have attributed to them superior qualities or gifts, or have simply thought them to be economically desirable members of a family.

The awareness of human intersexuality has emerged largely as a result of the trauma and harm some intersexuals attribute to its medicalization—that is—to the fact that it has been treated as a kind of pathology in need of medical intervention. The internet has also played a role in bringing intersexuality into the public consciousness, because it has facilitated communication between intersexed people, allowing them to share their experiences (which has been life-saving for some), develop advocacy groups, and gather the confidence, energy, and strength to challenge long-standing, but ultimately unexamined and unsupported medical practices dealing with them. In fairness, these medical practices were grounded in larger unexamined historical and cultural presuppositions. The challenges have raised profound and urgent ethical issues for medicine. Even while motivated by sincere benevolence, there is no doubt that certain aspects of common practices indeed have been unethical, some more forgivable than others.

Already there has been significant progress in the medical management of intersexuality. Physicians treating intersexed children have been sensitized to the psychological damage that has resulted from the use of intersexed children as teaching tools or as curiosities. There have been huge advances in the area of informed consent. In the past, doctors have often made decisions regarding infant genital surgery for normalizing or sex assignment purposes without informing the parents about the child's intersexual condition. They were convinced that it would be too traumatic for parents to know the whole truth, and that withholding information was necessary to ensure both parental bonding with the infant and unambiguous gender-rearing. It was unthinkable that children could grow up with ambiguous genitalia and be well adjusted and stable. Even when some information was provided to parents, the parents were often advised not to inform their children of their intersexed condition or medical history, but to raise them unambiguously in the sex assigned at birth. Intersexuals and others have written extensively about the damage that secrecy has done in compounding the already difficult situation. The importance of full disclosure is a lesson apparently in need of repetition. We have previously made the same mistake regarding the disclosure of terminal diseases to adults and children. We tend to exaggerate the harms of disclosure and underestimate its benefits. If physicians have not been convinced of the beneficence of extending complete disclosure to the parents, at least they now know, or ought to know, that informed consent is a legal obligation. Progress has also been made in helping physicians learn to convey information to parents and to intersexed children in ways that will cause the least amount of pain and trauma. Books and videos are available for these purposes.

Further progress has been made in detailing the information needed in order for parental decisions to be based on informed consent. Specifically, it has been stipulated that parents should be informed that traditional surgical practices have not been based on evidence–that follow-up studies have not been conducted to ensure that medical protocols were really working to increase the quality of life of intersexuals, or that those practices would be better than simply providing psychological counseling to help parents and children deal with the ignorance and prejudices of people under the influence of the "sexual dimorphic" assumption. Physicians now realize that parents should know that not performing surgery is an alternative in most cases.

Other changes in our practices include the reduction of surgeries performed in certain cases. Female sex assignment surgery is not as often performed in cases of XY infants with micropenis due to growing evidence of prenatal hormonal imprinting and the realization that men with micropenises can have satisfactory sexual relations and even father children. Clitorectomy is rarely performed in the United States, although it still is standard procedure in some European and other countries. It has also been reported that parents and physicians are less likely to opt for clitoral recision or reduction in cases of mild virilization of female infants, due to the growing awareness that in these cases, the enlargement of the clitoris becomes less noticeable as the child grows, and also because of concerns about damaging sexual responsiveness.

Still, many difficult and urgent ethical issues raised by intersexuality and by traditional practices are still facing us today: Is it morally permissible to conduct infant genital surgery when we don't know whether allowing children to grow up with ambiguous genitalia is really necessarily damaging, or whether counseling could help them survive the teasing and taunting from their children? Is it morally permissible to perform vaginoplasty when we don't know whether vaginoplasty is more successful if done shortly after birth or when the child is older and able to express a desire for it? When we don't know whether people who complain about surgery do so because of the harms from some other aspect of the treatment, such as by the humiliation of being examined regularly in front of many people, or by secrecy? When we don't know if those who do not complain about effects of their surgery are really satisfied or whether they could have been happier having been raised with ambiguous genitalia with the assistance of psychological counseling? We cannot reliably predict gender identity or sexual orientation. In light of the dearth of long-term studies, what should physicians now recommend? Should they proceed with "business as usual"? Should a moratorium be called? Or should parents have the right to make decisions regarding genital surgery for their children? Is it likely that society can change and be more accepting of intersexuality? Can we judge what will be more important to the intersexed person—genital sensitivity and capacity for pleasure or reproductive capacity?

Clearly, the most urgent issues have to do with whether or not genital surgery should continue to be performed on infants for either sex-assignment or for cosmetic purposes. These issues are addressed by many of the contributors to this book, though not with any unanimous consensus about what is best. These surgical and ethical issues have dominated our attention because intersexuality has been regarded as primarily a *surgical* issue. Intersexuality has been the province of urology, with input from endocrinology, but those focuses need to be informed by other disciplines as well—both medical and non-medical. Only fairly recently has the idea that psychology and psychiatry could have an important role in the clinical management of intersexuality been gaining recognition, yet we are far from the point where psychologists are routinely incorporated into the clinical management team.

Sexuality is a pervasive and important dimension of existence, and intersexuality raises questions that go beyond the surgical, medical, and psychological domains. For this reason, in addition to urologists, endocrinologist, psychiatrists, and psychologists, I have invited members of many other professions to contribute chapters to this book in the hopes of increasing the depth and breadth of our understanding of intersexuality in order to better inform the discussion of our surgical practices. These professions include gynecology, theology, law, history of medicine, medical ethics, and philosophy. I have also sought contributions from experts on intersexuality from many different countries, including Canada, Germany, The Netherlands, England, Australia and India. Indeed, the chief mark of the uniqueness of this book is its attempt to provide a multi-disciplinarian and multi-cultural approach to intersexuality. This global approach is extremely important. International collaboration provides a larger pool of cases, helping to broaden our knowledge of techniques and practices as well. An international focus also would help in developing retrospective and prospective studies needed to fill in for the dearth of evidence supporting surgical practices. Also, noting cultural differences in approach and attitudes will encourage reflection on our own and speed the development of our knowledge and understanding.

Intersexuality isn't just about individuals and conditions that have nothing to do with those who are not intersexed. Rather, becoming educated about intersex is to become educated about important dimensions of what it means to be a human being. Thus, learning about intersexuality leads not only to the understanding of others, but to self-understanding. The fact of intersexuality has implications that have the effect of shaking up our worlds, and demanding a reorientation to our understanding of ourselves as sexual beings. Intersexuality has important implications that impose the need to rethink strongly ingrained beliefs. To borrow from Rawls, the fact of intersexuality upsets the harmony between our set of beliefs, provoking the need to reestablish a "reflective equilibrium" between them. Some will experience this as a daunting task demanding the sacrifice of tenacious beliefs central to their own identity. For others, the experience can be liberating and even life saving.

Let us take as our starting point that intersexuality is *natural*. If intersexuality is natural, then the assumption that all human beings are either wholly male or female, the theory of sexual dimorphism, is false, or at least it is not the whole truth. Because there are so many causes of intersexuality, and because all these causes admit of degrees, the idea of a continuum between male and female emerges as a substitute for the "either/or" model of human sexuality. Given the range we find of femininity in females and masculinity in males, this idea of a continuum between sexes appears to be plausible.

Another implication of the facts and etiologies of intersexuality is that neither chromosomes, nor gene sequences, nor gonads, nor hormones, nor rearing, nor genital appearance alone determine sexuality. Talk about being able to determine the "true sex" of a person by attending to just one of these physical elements is not only arbitrary, but greatly misleading, and even harmful. The truth is: some people are intersexed.

These revelations regarding the complexity of sexuality parallel those regarding sexual orientation. Some people are attracted exclusively to the opposite sex and some exclusively to their same sex, and some to both, in varying degrees. While there is higher incidence of homosexual orientation among intersexed people, sexual orientation cannot be predicted with any kind of certainty either for them or for non-intersexed individuals. Sexual orientation also has been known to shift throughout the course of a lifetime, sometimes as a result of traumatic experiences, and sometimes for no apparent reason at all.

Yet another continuum characterizes gender identity. While most of us, intersexed or not, think of ourselves as having either a masculine or feminine gender identity, some of us feel in between these largely socially-constructed gender categories, or capable of identifying with either in varying degrees. Further, gender identity is even more complicated, as is evidenced by the fact that in some individuals it changes throughout the course of their lives. Children with gender dysphoria (a loaded term) often grow out of it. Tomboys become debutantes.

Most intersexed persons receiving sex assignment surgery at birth do not report feelings of gender dysphoria and do not seek reversals of those surgical procedures. But while most intersexuals "accept" their assigned gender in the sense that they don't seek surgical sex reassignment, we ought not to conclude that they come really to "identify" as members of their assigned sex, or even if they do, that surgical sex assignment is the best response to ambiguous genitalia. It may be that rejecting one's sex assignment received at birth and choosing to live as a member of the opposite gender is associated with too many emotional, social, financial, or physical costs. Or it may be that gender identity is just very flexible, or at least very flexible in some people, just as sexual orientation is more flexible in bisexuals than in people who are strictly heterosexuals. Studies indicating the higher incidence of male sex assignment of intersexed infants in cultures that confer more rights and freedom to males than to females support this hypothesis.

The implications of intersexuality are far-reaching indeed. This is why education about intersexuality is so important today. It is likely that intersexuality can shed light on the variations in the continua of sexual orientation, and gender identity, and gender expression.

For instance, these complexities are relevant to the distinction espoused by some feminist philosophers between the "masculine" and the "feminine" voices in ethics. The attitude towards this distinction is far from univocal—some feminists urging the superiority of the feminine over the masculine voice (care ethics vs. rights approaches to ethics), some urging women to celebrate and hold on to the feminine voice rather than relinquishing it and adopting the masculine voice, and some who urge that both voices can be informed and enlightened through the other, so that each are natural starting points, but can be open to the balancing influence and insights of the other. Intersexuality implies that there are voices other than the merely masculine or the merely feminine, and that intersexuals may have uniquely gifted moral voices because of their interim position. If some men seem to be from Mars, and some women seem to be from Venus, some men and women must come from somewhere in between—in fact from any number of places in between. This observation calls to mind Coleridge's claim that all great minds are androgynous. Virginia Woolf also shared this insight. For the creative mind, she claimed: "It is fatal to be a man or woman pure and simple: one must be a woman manly, or a man womanly."

Intersexuality also has implications for our understanding of homosexuality. While we don't understand all the factors that contribute to the development of homosexuality, it is no surprise that a person with XX chromosomes, but who is born with perfectly normal male genitalia and is raised as a male, would be attracted to women. Note how cumbersome the term "homosexual" is when applied to such people. Furthermore, sometimes a person is born with male chromosomes, but because of the inadequate size of the penis, or because of congenital malformations of the genital area, is surgically assigned to the female sex, but nevertheless develops an orientation to females. This shows that not only are some homosexuals born that way, but some are made that way as a result of human intervention. Surely this should cause those condemning homosexuality to pause and reconsider. In light of these reflections, no longer does the French phrase "Viva la difference!" retain its light-hearted charming quality. A modification, however, is easily substituted: "Mais, vivent *toutes* les differences!"

Rethinking the naturalness and the morality of homosexuality necessitates the rethinking of religious views and biblical interpretation, and the adoption of a more humble stance with regard to them. Yet openness to this rethinking might very well lead to social changes more in keeping with the most profound aspects of religious outlooks. The ideas of radical bifurcations between males and females, the masculine and the feminine, between homosexuals and heterosexuals fall away as the implications of intersexuality are appreciated. Would that the barriers, social prejudices, and condemnation that have arisen out of these bifurcations fall away as easily!

The twenty chapters included in the volume are independent of each other and can be read in any order according to the readers' preferences and needs. There is, however, an underlying logical flow. The first three chapters provide background information on intersexuality. Rather than offering a mere overview, however, they give fresh perspectives on the issues and should be of interest even to those who are well-read on extant literature on intersexuality. Stephen Kemp provides the biological background by identifying and explaining the genetic and hormonal causes of the major forms of interexuality. He includes summaries of the newest scientific discoveries and theories concerning both sexual differentiation and gender identity. Next, David Ozar develops a conceptual scheme that not only aims to uncover presuppositions in and expand the general public's notions of gender differences, but also to do the same for the intersex advocacy movement. That is, he provides a language that contains enough distinctions to capture not only the experience of intersexuals, but also that of transgendered and bigendered individuals. David Hester compares narrative reports from intersexuals with different conditions, and also the narrative responses of those who have had surgery as infants and those who didn't have it. His essay highlights the current controversy between our traditional practices, which have not been subjected to retrospective studies, and those that intersexuals would consider dramatic improvements over them. These narratives have the effect of allowing non-intersexed people insight into the effects of medical practices and social attitudes concerning intersexuality by giving them the "inside view." They are important in that they sensitize non-intersexed people to the plight of intersexuals. Too long have the voices of intersexed people remained unheard.

The three following chapters focus on rights and the law relative to the issue of intersex. Alice Dreger, veteran intersex advocate, calls for immediate reform in our medical practices. She reflects on the reasons why intersex reform has taken so long, and argues that it is because the problems that led to ethical lapses in the treatment of intersexuals are actually endemic to the medical profession generally. She claims that a distinctive feature of the intersex advocacy movement only recently explicitly articulated is that infant genital surgery is a human rights issue. She goes so far as to claim that such surgery is a violation of human rights analogous to those perpetrated in the infamous Tuskegee Syphilis Study.

Julie Greenberg then reviews recent legal developments around the world to address the issue of whether there ought to be a moratorium on infant genital surgery. Not believing that an absolute moratorium would be in the best interest of intersex children, she proposes a protocol that would likely have the effect of greatly reducing the number of such surgeries performed. The protocol respects parental autonomy, but requires that a committee of experts on intersexuality, ideally including adult intersexuals, oversee the process of obtaining their informed consent. Milton Diamond and Hazel Beh appeal to John Stuart Mill's Principle of Liberty to defend the right of individuals to make their own decisions about sex and gender, whether in cases of intersex or of transgender. They argue that infant genital surgery would involve a violation of the right to autonomy, and should be deferred until the intersexed person can make judgments about their own gender identity and participate in the decisions about which medical procedures they desire.

Next, Edmund Howe explains some of the psychological and practical causes of the resistance to change among medical professionals. After identifying questions relevant to the issue about whether infant genital surgery ought to be our response to the birth of an intersexed child, and also identifying the reasons (usually, the lack of empirical knowledge) why these questions are difficult to answer, Howe advances a Rawlsian argument for delaying surgery until the child can participate in the decision. His argument proceeds on the basis of the "maximin principle" that we ought to choose from alternative policies the one that has the least worst consequences for those who are least well off. Timothy Murphy then examines the question of whether developments in research ethics standards since the 1960's might have prevented some of the ethical lapses of John Money's handling of the David Reimer case (perhaps better known as the John/Joan case), in which a twin boy whose penis was accidentally destroyed in an accident during circumcision was surgically assigned and raised as a female. Drawing on the distinction between clinical practice and medical research and pointing out the importance of the freedom of physicians to engage in non-validated treatments, he argues that it is likely that even given contemporary mechanisms such as Institutional Review Boards, it is very likely that experiments in gender sex assignment like that of John Money's John/Joan case could still occur. However, the existence of responsible Institutional Review Boards might have prevented other ethical failings, such as the continuation of such surgeries without informed consent or without follow-up studies on the long-term sequelae of such surgeries.

A series of chapters on scientific studies follow that make clear how deficient our current knowledge is and how far we have to go in our ability to enable sound judgments regarding infant genital surgery. William Reiner presents data from studies of genetic males who because of developmental defects or aberrations were raised as females according to the theory that men without adequate penises would be better off as female. Based on his own studies and the studies of others, Reiner subscribes to the theory of prenatal hormonal imprinting. He concludes with implications for the Standard of Care for certain conditions, and with some ethical prescriptions based on lessons learned from our past errors. Kenneth Zucker, on the other hand, argues that the evidence for prenatal hormonal imprinting is far from conclusive. Not only are there studies that provide conflicting evidence, but even when the sex of rearing does not yield a concordant sexual identity, there are other factors that can explain this discordance, such as the failure of the parents to raise the child unambiguously as male or female. He proposes that we ought not to abandon the hypothesis that sex of rearing determines gender identity on the data available to us at this point. Garry Warne and Vijayalakshmi Bahtia present outcomes of studies conducted in their respective countries, Australia and India, and also in Vietnam, along with interesting descriptions of the cultural influences influencing decision-making for medical treatment. Sarah Creighton discusses the various techniques and their respective problems involved in feminizing surgery, whether clitoral surgery or vaginoplasty. She reviews data regarding outcomes from her own studies and those of other researchers. The news is not good. Clitoral surgery, even when involving techniques less drastic that clitorectomy, compromises adult sexual functions. She reports that vaginoplasty, particularly when performed in early childhood, leads to poor outcomes: it often needs to be repeated later in life, and it is fraught with complications.

Traditionally, psychological care for parents of intersexuals and for intersexuals themselves has been woefully lacking. Of late, there has been more awareness of the need for on-going psychological assistance, both for children receiving genital surgery and for those who don't. The next two chapters address the important need for psychological counseling, and the many ways it can improve outcomes. Friedemann Pfäfflin and Peggy Cohen-Kettenis detail their recommendations for the many ways psychologists can help parents adjust to their children's condition, make responsible decisions regarding treatment based on full disclosure, inform their children in age-appropriate ways, and prepare for dealing with relatives, neighbors and day-care centers. They also show how counseling can help children develop self-esteem, a healthy lifestyle, and later, maneuver the rough roads of puberty, sexual awakening, and intimate relationships. Lih-Mei Liao, focuses her attention on the ways psychological counseling can help bring about more positive quality of life outcomes for women undergoing either vaginoplasty or dilation to increase the size of their vagina. Counseling can help with compliance issues, overcoming psychological barriers to intimacy and the unnecessary preoccupation with vaginal sex. She also discusses the ways that psychologists can help physicians design more accurate and thorough outcome studies, develop better communication skills, and advise their patients more effectively.

Sharon Sytsma introduces two ethical issues that have not received much attention due to the spotlight on infant genital surgery. The first of her articles examines the prevalent use of dexamethasone to treat pregnant women at risk for giving birth to children with Congenital Adrenal Hyperplasia in order to avoid virilization of the genitals, a practice that has been shown to be successful. However, the drug has never been tested for this purpose, and there are an increasing number of studies that suggest that prenatal use of DEX may have negative long-term effects. She argues that prenatal DEX use for this purpose should not be considered the standard of care, should not be recommended or prescribed by physicians outside of clinical studies, and that even continued research with it might not be justified. The second issue is addressed through a very troubling, even haunting, case study. How should we handle cases in which parents from other countries come to ours to have their adolescents receive genital surgery for their intersexed conditions, yet because of cultural norms, insist that their children do not play a deliberative role in choosing surgery, but that the surgery be performed based solely on the parents' (usually the father's) decision? Sytsma addresses the question of the limits of our duty to respect other cultures when requests are made that violate our own ethical norms.

The next two chapters include articles from theological and philosophical viewpoints. Patricia Jung examines the presupposition of sexual dimorphism in Christian thought and shows that an examination of biblical texts does not rule out sexual polymorphism. She points out the important implications of intersexuality not only for Christian ethics, but also for Christian teaching on marriage and parenting, and even for how we think about God. She urges that reasonable biblical interpretation should cohere with sound science and that therefore Christians should come to see intersexuals as "made in the image and likeness of God." Herman Stark illustrates how Heidegger's notion of authenticity provides a way of thinking about existential aspects of the lives of intersexuals. Like David Hester, he draws from autobiographical experiences of intersexuals, and points to both what is universal and what is particular in their experience. He shows how the notion of authenticity can help to illuminate various aspects of the plight of intersexuals who have been sex-assigned at birth or in early childhood—the plight that arises in large part because of the artificial enforcement of a sexually dimorphic paradigm on them. He also argues that intersexuality raises interesting questions about the limits of Heidegger's own construal of authenticity.

In the penultimate chapter, Justine Schober describes new possibilities for the treatment of intersex deriving from stem cell research and tissue engineering. Using autologous totipotent stem cells in vaginoplasty and phalloplasty could avoid problems of rejection, desensitization, and other complications of current treatment modes. Furthermore, these developments may make it easier to delay certain aspects of genitoplasty until the intersexed person can participate in the decisions about the surgery. Further promising research likely to improve genitoplasty concerns the role certain hormones can play in the healing process, suggesting timing considerations for surgery, or the modification of naturally occurring hormonal factors. Finally, Iain Morland undertakes an examination of whether, as Alice Dreger had argued in her epilogue in *Hermaphrodites and the Medical Invention of Sex*, postmodern approaches ensure the optimal treatment of intersexuality. His claim is that all the features of postmodernism identified by Dreger do not unequivocally support the ethical views shared by intersexual advocates, but rather, that they provide only ambiguous guidelines, which could actually work against those views. The issue is an abstract philosophical one that essentially advocates an appeal to the Doctrine of Socratic Ignorance: it is better to know that you don't know, than to think you know and be mistaken. Thus, Morland urges taking up a posture of epistemic humility in order to allow the truth regarding the best medical practices to emerge most effectively. As a philosopher, I find this recommendation to be a most suitable note on which to conclude this volume.

Sharon Sytsma, Associate Professor, Department of Philosophy, Northern Illinois University, DeKalb, Illinois, U.S.A..

STEPHEN F. KEMP

THE ROLE OF GENES AND HORMONES IN SEXUAL DIFFERENTIATION

1. INTRODUCTION

This chapter describes the process of sexual differentiation from a genetic and hormonal point of view. It is useful to view sexual differentiation as having five aspects: genetic (or genotypic) sex, gonadal sex, hormonal sex, phenotypic sex, and psychological sex. In most individuals each of these aspects develops along the same lines, so that they are all male or all female. However, discordance among the different aspects of sexual differentiation occasionally occurs. In older literature the term "hermaphrodite" was used to describe discordance of sexual differentiation. This term is now avoided, primarily because it has a pejorative connotation in popular usage. The term "intersex," is preferred, which refers to a variety of conditions with mixed sexual anatomy (Intersex Society of North America). Sometimes intersex individuals have ambiguous genitalia, but intersexuality may not be evident from an external examination.

2. GENETIC SEX

Genetic sex is described by the karyotype, that is, the collection of chromosomes that an individual possesses. In the human there are usually 22 pairs called autosomal chromosomes, with the additional two sex chromosomes (X and Y). Before it was possible to analyze human chromosomes it was generally believed that the Y chromosome was inert. It is now recognized that the Y chromosome is important for sexual differentiation.

During meiosis (the process of gamete formation) the autosomal chromosomes line up, and exchange of genetic material between the pairs ("recombination") is possible. In the sex chromosomes this process is limited to small regions on the distal ends of the X and the Y, which have been called "pseudoautosomal" regions (see figure 1-2). The existence of these pseudoautosomal regions led Ohno (1967) to propose that the X and Y-chromosomes may originally have been a pair of autosomes. The Y chromosome is thought to have evolved sometime between 170 and 310 million years ago when a sex-determining locus arose on one of the proto-sex chromosomes, resulting in the accumulation of other sex-specific alleles nearby.

1

S.E. Sytsma (Ed.), Ethics and Intersex, 1–16.

This resulted in large parts of the Y chromosome no longer undergoing recombination with the X chromosome, with shrinking of the Y chromosome (Marshall-Graves, 2002). It has been postulated that this shrinking may continue with the ultimate disappearance of the Y chromosome in 5-10 million years (Aitken & Marshall-Graves, 2002), although Vilain (2004) has suggested that the present Y chromosome may be stable at its present size, which is 10-20% the size of the X chromosome. The length of the Y chromosome varies as much as threefold in normal men.

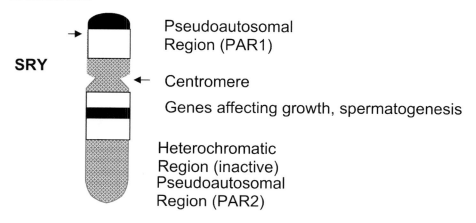

Figure 1. Structure of the Y chromosome

Most human males have 46 chromosomes with an X and a Y chromosome (46XY), and most human females have 46 chromosomes with two X chromosomes (46XX). However, other karyotypes exist. Common examples are 45 chromosomes with only one X (45X) (Turner Syndrome) or 47 chromosomes with two X chromosomes and a Y chromosome (47XXY) (Klinefelter Syndrome). Although Turner Syndrome and Klinefelter Syndrome represent variations in sexual differentiation, they are often not classified as intersex conditions, since there is usually no discordance between elements of sexual differentiation. Very complex karyotypes also exist in which different cells from the same individual have different karyotypes (mosaicism). Examples of such mosaic karyotypes include 45X/46XY (indicating that some cell lines are 45X and others are 46XY) and 45X/47XYY. Individuals with either of these karyotypes may have ambiguous genitalia, and thus, such a mosaic karyotype may be a cause of intersexuality. There are also rare situations in which an individual with a 46XX karyotype has internal genitalia consisting of vas deferens, seminal vesicles, and epididymis and external genitalia with an apparent penis and a completely fused scrotum. Likewise it is possible to have an individual with a 46XY karyotype who has fallopian tubes, a uterus and external genitalia with unfused labia and a small clitoris.

3. PHENOTYPIC SEXUAL DIFFERENTIATION

3.1 Phenotypic Sex: Development of the Internal Genitalia

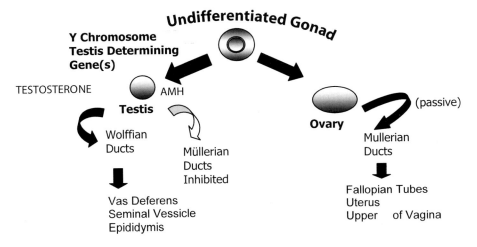

Figure 2. Paradigm of Sexual Differentiation

A paradigm for sexual differentiation of the internal genitalia is shown in figure 1-2; this paradigm is largely based on the investigations of Jost in the 1940's (Jost, 1947). Jost castrated rabbit fetal embryos (both males and females) and reimplanted them into the mother. He discovered that the castrated embryos all developed into females, and he concluded that the ovary was not necessary for female development. Female internal genitalia are derived from embryologic anlage termed "Müllerian" ducts, and ultimately develop into the Fallopian tubes, the uterus, and the upper ⅔ of the vagina. In the presence of a testis, development usually proceeds with male differentiation. Male internal genitalia are derived from anlage termed "Wolffian" structures, which give rise to the epididymis, vas deferens, and seminal vesicles. The fetal testis secretes testosterone, which stimulates development of the Wolffian system; the testis also secretes a glycoprotein, anti-Müllerian Hormone (AMH, also known as Müllerian Inhibitory Hormone (MIH), Müllerian Inhibitory Substance (MIS), or Müllerian Inhibitory Factor (MIF)), which inhibits development of the Müllerian structures. In the presence of full testicular function, there is regression of internal Müllerian structures and stimulation of the development of internal Wolffian structures. The effects of AMH and testosterone are local; that is, limited to the area of that testis. If one testis does not develop (leaving a single testis), there is development of Wolffian structures and regression of Müllerian structures on the side of the testis, but there is no Wolffian development and no Müllerian regression on the side where the testis is absent.

3.2   Phenotypic Sex: Development of the External Genitalia

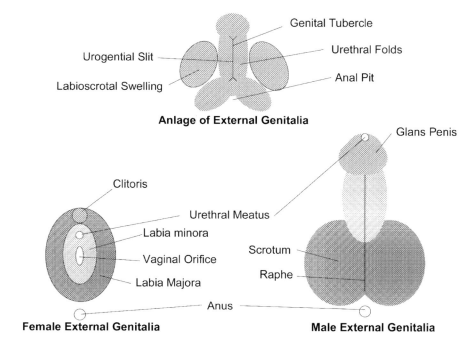

Figure 3. Development of the External Genitalia

Without hormonal stimulation the external genitalia ordinarily develop into female structures. In the male the external structures are virilized by dihydrotestosterone, which is converted from testosterone by 5-α-reductase, an enzyme present in the genital skin tissue. The structures in the male and female come from the same tissues (see figure 1-3). Thus, in the absence of androgen exposure the phallus remains small, and if the individual is presumed to be female, the phallus is referred to as a clitoris. In the presence of androgen stimulation the phallus enlarges, and if the individual is presumed to be male, the phallus is referred to as a penis. In the absence of androgen the urethral opening is below the phallus; with sufficient androgen exposure the urethra opens at the tip of the phallus. In the absence of androgenic stimulation the labioscrotal folds remain separated and are referred to as labiae; when exposed to androgen these same tissues fuse, leading to development of the scrotum. Although the androgen dihydrotestosterone is most potent in virilizing the external genitalia, other androgens in large concentrations (e.g. testosterone or the weaker testosterone precursors androstenedione and dihydroepiandrosterone (DHEA)) can also cause external virilization.

3.3 Development of Intersex

How does this paradigm account for intersex individuals? The first possibility is from discordance between the steps so that one or more steps develop along different lines that the others. The other possible way for intersex to develop is to have a step that is not entirely male or female, but somewhere between.

There are a number of instances in which one step may develop differently than the others. An individual with a 46XY karyotype could have a testis that produces testosterone, but a gene for AMH that is inactive. The result would be an individual with normal male internal genitalia (vas deferens, seminal vesicles, and epididymis) and male-appearing external genitalia, but this individual would also have Fallopian tubes, a uterus, and part of the vagina. Similarly, if there was an individual with a 46XY karyotype with an inactive enzyme needed for one of the steps in the pathway to produce testosterone, the Wolffian system would not develop, the Müllerian system would not develop, and the external genitalia would appear female. Another example is the individual with a 46XY karyotype with complete androgen insensitivity syndrome (CAIS). In this case the androgen receptors do recognize androgen, and the result is the similar to the case in which testosterone cannot be produced.

Another example of intersex that results from a discordance of development is 5-α-reductase deficiency. An individual with a 46XY karyotype and inactive 5-α-reductase will make sufficient testosterone to cause Wolffian development, and the testes produce AMH resulting in Müllerian regression. However, dihydrotestosterone is not produced from testosterone, and the external genitalia are only partially virilized; the penis will be small and the urethral opening is on the shaft of the penis (hypospadias) or on the genital skin below the penis. At puberty the levels of testosterone are high enough to bind to dihydrotestosterone receptors, which causes enlargement of the penis. In the Dominican Republic there are villages in which 5-α-reductase deficiency is not uncommon. Individuals with this condition are often reared as females when young, but establish a male gender identity and a male role at puberty.

Most biological systems operate with a continuum rather than "all-or-nothing" phenomena. Certainly with regard to sexual differentiation most individuals cluster at the male or female ends of the spectrum, but there are individuals who are on the continuum between male and female in one or more aspects. This is especially the case with hormone levels; there may be enough androgen effect to begin virilizing the internal and external genitalia, but not enough effect to entirely virilize the individual. For example, if a child with a karyotype that is 46XX is exposed prenatally to androgen (for example, if the mother took an androgen during pregnancy), this child may have some development of the Wolffian structures, but because testes are not present, this individual would undergo development of Müllerian structures. The androgen exposure may also be sufficient to cause some degree of virilization of the external genitalia, such as enlargement of the phallus and fusion of the labio-scrotal folds. Another situation in which this occurs is with congenital adrenal hyperplasia (CAH). With CAH there is an enzyme in the adrenal pathway to cortisol that has incomplete activity. Metabolic intermediates accumulate, and are converted to androstenedione and dihydroepiandrosterone (DHEA), which are weak androgens. When CAH occurs in an individual with a 46XX karyotype, the prenatal levels of androstenedione and DHEA cause virilization of the external genitalia. The enzyme activity may be partial; the lower the activity of the enzyme, the greater the prenatal concentration of the androgens, and the more complete the virilization. With a large degree of virilization the individual with CAH who has a 46XX karyotype may have the urethral meatus at the end of the phallus, and may be presumed to be a male at birth.

Not all cases of intersex are related to the paradigm. There may be an event that occurs at the time of development of the genitalia, which causes the genitalia to develop incompletely, in much the same way that other congenital malformations occur (e.g., congenital heart defects). An example of this is cloacal exstrophy, in which individuals with a 46XY karyotype do not develop structures in the pelvis, resulting in a small or absent penis.

Intersex is a broad term that encompasses many different situations, all of which have mixed sexual anatomy. Intersex may result from many different events that occur during the steps in the cascade of sexual differentiation, as well as developmental events unrelated to genes or hormones. Because of the many etiologies of intersex, it is not always possible to identify the situation with a specific individual from examination of the external genitalia. Nor is it a simple matter to draw conclusions from one group of intersex individuals and apply those observations to individuals who are intersex because of a different etiology.

How common is intersex? It depends largely on which conditions are described as intersex. The incidence of any malformation of the genitalia is about 1%, but this includes such variations of normal anatomy of the genitalia as enlarged clitoris (clitoromegaly), a small penis (micropenis), an abnormal position of the urethral opening (hypospadias), or undescended testes (cryptorchidism) (Vilain, 2002). By themselves most of these conditions would not be included in the description of intersex. Gondal dysgenesis, in which there is discordance between the karyotype and the internal and external genitalia occurs with an incidence of about 1/20,000 (Vilain, 2002). The condition 21-hydroxylase deficiency is the most common cause of congenital adrenal hyperplasia, and account for most of the cases of intersex in infants who have 46XX karyotypes. The incidence of 21-hydroxylase deficiency varies in different populations, but overall occurs in about 1/5000 to 1/15,000 live births in most western populations (New, 1995) (although the incidence is 1/300 to 1/700 live births among Alaskan Yupic Eskimos (Hirshfield & Fleshman, 1969; Pang et al., 1982)). Complete androgen insensitivity syndrome occurs in about 1/20,000 live male births (Bangsbøll et al., 1992).

4. GONADAL SEX: DEVELOPMENT OF OVARY AND TESTIS

The first step in sexual development appears to be the determination of gonadal sex, that is, differentiation of the bipotential gonad into a testis or an ovary. This dependence on differentiation of the undifferentiated gonad as the first step upon which all other aspects of sexual differentiation depend has been called the "central dogma" of sexual differentiation (Vilain, 2002). Developments in understanding of this process have been recently reviewed (MacGillivray & Mazur, 2003; MacLaughlin & Donahoe, 2004). The bipotential gonads develop along paths that appear to be indistinguishable until the 7th week of gestation, when migration of the primordial germ cells begins. Testicular development starts during the 8th week of gestation and finishes by the 9th week. If there is no signal to stimulate testicular development, the gonad develops into an ovary, which is completed by the 12th week of fetal development. Intersexuality may result at this stage of differentiation; it is possible to have an internal testis on one side and an ovary on the other. It is also possible to have ovarian and testicular tissue present in the same gonad (an "ovotestis").

Germ cells first appear in the outer ectodermal layer of the embryo (the proximal epiblast), and their differentiation appears to be influenced by two genes, Fragilis and Stella, which have been studied in mice (Saitou et al., 2002). Fragilis first appears in the proximal epiblast under the influence of the bone morphogenetic protein 4 (BMP4). Later Stella begins to be expressed, as expression of Fragilis diminishes.

4.1 Testicular Differentiation

It has long been understood that usually the presence of a Y chromosome (regardless of the number of X chromosomes) leads to the development of a testis, and the absence of a Y chromosome leads to development of an ovary. There are, however, clinical situations that appear to contradict this rule. Rarely, there are XX individuals with no obvious Y chromosome who have male internal and external genitalia and develop a testis. There are also XY individuals with female internal and external genitalia who develop ovaries (although these ovaries are often "streaks"). These conditions are given the name "gonadal dysgenesis". The incidence of XX individualsl who have male internal and external genitalia is about 1/20,000 (de la Chapelle, 1981). These individuals also have a male sexual identity. They are similar to men with Klinefelter syndrome (47, XXY), in that they often have some degree of testosterone deficiency, gynecomastia, and small testes with azoospermia (Boucekkine et al., 1994). In 10% of these patients there is hypospadias, in which the urethral opening is not at the tip of the penis. The hypospadias is thought to be caused by a deficiency in fetal testosterone production. In the 1980's Page and de la Chapelle (1984) showed that most men with XX gonadal dysgenesis had one X chromosome from the mother and the second X chromosome from the father. Using *in situ* hybridization, Andersson et al. (1986) demonstrated that probes designed to detect Y chromosome short arm sequences clustered on the distal portion of one of the short arms in the "pseudoautosomal" region of the X chromosomes in these men. This is the portion of the X chromosome that pairs with the Y chromosome during meiosis. These findings suggested that in XX individuals with male internal and external genitalia there must have been acquisition of genetic material from the paired Y chromosome during meiosis. The transferred material must have contained a gene normally on the Y chromosome that directed the determination of the gonad to become a testis. This postulated gene was named "testis determining factor gene" (TDF).

There is also a syndrome termed XY gonadal dysgensis (sometimes called Swyer Syndrome). These individuals are female in terms of internal and external genitalia and sexual identity. They are often tall in stature, and at puberty are found to have ovarian failure with streak gonads. Many of these individuals have been found to have deletions in the Y chromosome, again in the same region as the proposed TDF gene. A search was undertaken to localize the TDF gene by identifying the smallest region of the Y chromosome that was able to induce a male phenotype in an XX individual. By 1989 the region on the Y chromosome was narrowed down to about 35,000 base pairs (Palmer et al., 1989). The next year Sinclair et al. (1990) cloned a gene from this region that was named SRY (Sex-determining Region Y). In the mouse (where the gene is named SRY to distinguish it from the human SRY) this gene is turned on between 1.5 and 12.5 days of gestation, just before the appearance of the differentiated testis. It was possible to produce phenotypic male mice after introduction of the SRY transgene into XX mice (Koopman et al., 1990), further confirming that this gene (at least SRY in the mouse) is the TDF gene. A subgroup of individuals with 46XY karyotypes and pure gonadal dysgenesis have been shown to have mutations in the DNA-binding region of the SRY gene (McElreavey et al., 1992).

What do we know about SRY? We know that in humans it is expressed in the testis and in the brain. The SRY gene product is a protein that is 204 amino acids in length, and it functions as a transcription factor. Transcription factors bind to and bend DNA strands, thus allowing access of the DNA to other transcription factors. The middle one-third of the SRY protein has a DNA-binding domain that was previously known to be present in nuclear high-mobility-group proteins HMG1 and HMG2 (Sinclair et al., 1990), and thus is called an "HMG box protein." It also has homology with a mating-type protein from the fission yeast Schizosaccharomyces pombe, known as Mc. SRY is expressed early in development and then quickly disappears. It induces development of the Sertoli cells (cells involved in spermatogenesis, as well as production of Anti-Müllerian Hormone (AMH)) in the testis, which is followed by the differentiation of seminiferous tubules and the formation of Leydig cells (cells that secrete testosterone).

It is clear that SRY is not the only gene involved in testicular differentiation. SRY alone does not account for all cases of phenotypic females with XY karyotypes; only 25% of 46, XY individuals with streak gonads and a female phenotype have a mutation in SRY. Like SRY, many of the other genes that appear to be important in sexual differentiation are transcription factors (see Table 1). Some non-Y genes have been described which are similar to the SRY HMG box region. They have been termed SOX genes (an abbreviation for SRY-homeobOX-like genes). SOX9 (located on 17q24-25), like SRY is a male determining gene, which is necessary for Sertoli cell differentiation. The importance of this gene in sexual differentiation was discovered in a 46, XY infant with a mutation in SOX9, who presented with campomelic dysplasia (a skeletal disorder) and streak ovarian-like gonads (Koopman, 1999). Tommerup et al. (1993) have reported rearrangements of chromosome 17 involving the SOX9 gene which have been responsible for this syndrome.

Other transcription factor genes have now been described with are also a part of this process. Studies in mice have identified a number of transcription factors necessary for genital development, including empty-spericles homeobox gene 2 (Emx2), GATA-4, Lim 1, and lim homeobox 9 (Lhx9). In humans it appears that there are three genes necessary for gonadal development: 1) the steroidogenic factor 1 (SF-1), 2) Wilms' tumor-suppressor gene (WT1), and 3) DAX1.

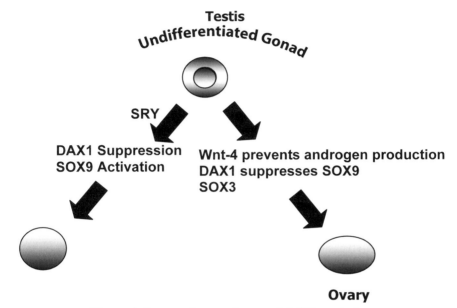

Figure 4. Proposed events in gonadal differentiation

SF1 and WT1 appear to be essential for gonadal development, but they do not seem to be specifically sex determining. Disruption of SF1 results in disruption of both gonadal and renal development. (Luo et al, 1994). A mutation of SF1 has been shown to be responsible for adrenal hypoplasia and sex reversal (female phenotype with a 46, XY karyotype) with gonadal dysgenesis (Achermann et al., 1999). WT-1 is a zinc-finger protein. Zinc fingers are a group of transcription factors that have a region rich in the amino acid cysteine, which binds zinc. The zinc-binding region is involved in binding and bending of DNA strands. There are two syndromes known in humans that indicate that WT-1 is important for development of both gonads and kidneys. In the Frasier syndrome there are streak of gonads along with nephrotic syndrome. If the karyotype is XY there is a female phenotype with retained müllerian ducts. In mice with WT-1 knockout there is maldevelopment of both gonads and kidneys. (MacLaughlin and Donohue, 2004).

The Denys-Drash syndrome involves milder impairment of testicular function. Testicular synthesis of testosterone is impaired, but the testes do produce mullerian inhibitor factor. In addition there is an increased risk of Wilms' tumor. It is thought that the difference in the two syndromes has to do with proximity of the mutation to a region known as KTS, so named because of three amino acids (lysine (K), threonine (T), and serine (S)), which may be deleted or maintained between the third and fourth zinc fingers of the DNA-binding domain of this transcription factor. Patients with the Frasier syndrome who have mutation that inactivates KTS are not susceptible to Wilms' tumor.

Table 1. Genes involved in gonadal differentiation (from Vilain, 2002; MacGillivray & Mazur, 2003; MacLaughlin & Donahoe, 2004)

Gene (Localization)	Gene Family	Function
SRY (Yp11)	High-Motility-Group Protein	Transcription factor
SOX9 (17q24)	High-Motility-Group Protein	Transcription factor
SF-1 (9q33)	Nuclear receptor	Transcription factor
WT1 (11p13)	Zinc finger protein	Transcription factor
DAX1 (Xp21.3)	Nuclear-receptor protein	Transcription regulator
WNT4 (1p35)	WNT (mouse)	Growth factor

The DAX1 gene (located on the X-chromosome) is duplicated in adrenal hypoplasia congenita (Huang, 1999; Parker et al., 1999) and appears to code for a member of the nuclear-receptor family of proteins. In adrenal hypoplasia congenita there is both impaired development of the adrenal cortex and the gonads, resulting in adrenal insufficiency along with gonadal failure due to lack of stimulation from the pituitary gland (the pituitary gland does not secrete LH or FSH, which is called hypogonadotropic hypo-gonadism).

Vilain (2002) has proposed a model for mammalian sexual differentiation in which SRY might antagonize a presumed gene (Z), which would then inhibit male specific genes. This model was developed in order to account for the recessive mode of inheritance of XX males without SRY. Based on the observation of XY females with a duplication of DSS and the antagonistic effects of SRY and DAX1 in mice, Vilain suggests that the gene Z may well be DAX1. During testicular development DAX1 may be suppressed by SRY, thus permitting expression of SOX9 leading to male development (see Figure 1-4).

4.2 Ovarian Differentiation

Ovarian development is less well understood than is testicular development. Ovarian development also appears to depend upon a number of genes and transcription factors. The genes that likely suppress testicular development include DAX1, SOX3, and WNT4. When not suppressed by SRY, DAX1 may inactivate SOX9, blocking testicular development. Wnt4 may prevent androgen production in the developing ovary (by Leydig cell precursors), while also stabilizing oocytes and inducing Müllerian development. The WNT family represents locally acting signals (rather than transcription factors). In a mouse Sertoli cell line, Wnt4 has been shown to up-regulate Dax1 expression (Vilain, 2002). Thus, Wnt4 could act as a molecular link between SRY and DAX1. In the case of XY males who inherit a duplication of DAX1, it has been suggested that SRY is unable to suppress fully the double dose of DAX1, which, in turn, leads to a female phenotype and gonadal dysgenesis (Bardoni et al., 1994; Arn et al., 1994).

5. DEVELOPMENT OF SEXUAL IDENTITY

Psychological sex is a term for sexual identity or gender identity, that is, the sense of oneself as male or female. This aspect of sexual development has proven to be the most enigmatic. In humans anatomical differences exist between the male and the female brain; at least 9 reports of such structural differences have been documented (Gorski, 1999). In the rat brain the nucleus of preoptic area is larger in the male and the anteroventral periventricular nucleus of the preoptic area is larger in the female.

One's sexual identity is generally established between 2½ and 3 years of age (Federman, 2004). It had been thought that human sexual identity was largely derived through internalization of social cues, which led to the idea that sexual identity could be produced by adhering to a sex of rearing in a young child (younger than 2 years of age), even if the sex of rearing was different than the genetic, gonadal, hormonal, or phenotypic sex (Money et al., 1957; Money, 1969). Several observations in humans have cast doubt on this view. The first relates to sexual identity in individuals with cloacal exstrophy, a rare defect of the pelvis and its contents, in which there is severe phallic inadequacy or phallic absence in genetic males. These individuals had 46XY karyotypes and were born with testes, but fourteen out of sixteen were reared as females. The two who were raised as males, remained male. Of the fourteen reared as females, eight later took a male identity (Reiner & Gearhart, 2004). In two disorders of sexual differentiation, 5-α-reductase deficiency (Imperato-McGinley et al., 1975) and 17-ß-hydroxysteroid dehydro-genase deficiency (Farkas & Rosler, 1993), newborns appear female and are often reared as females, but at puberty undergo dramatic virilization, often accompanied by a change to a male sexual identity and role.

These cases seem to suggest that 1) sexual identity is, at least in part, a product of biology, and may not be easily overridden by adherence to a sex of rearing, and 2) there is likely a hormonal and perhaps a direct genetic component to development of sexual identity. Apparently, the male and female human brain not only differ anatomically, but may also be different in terms of sexual identity, either because of direct genetic influence (Arnold, 1996; Vilain & McCabe, 1998) or because of hormonal exposure (Gorski, 1999; Hrabovszky & Hutson, 2002), or some combination of both of these influences. It would be logical to assume that the hormone that masculinizes the brain would most likely be testosterone or its metabolite dihydrotestosterone.

Another approach to understanding the extent of hormonal influence has been to study individuals in which the usual hormonal aspects have been altered during development. One such example is congenital adrenal hyperplasia. This disorder is caused by an enzyme deficiency in the biochemical pathway leading to cortisol, with the result that there are extraordinarily high prenatal levels of the androgens dihydroepiandrosterone (DHEA), androstenedione, and to some extent, testosterone. These hormonal alterations seem to have little effect on the male fetus, but may cause virilization of the female fetus. There may also be significant postnatal androgen exposure. It has been of great interest to examine these individuals for evidence of any alteration in sexual identity. When the karyotype is 46, XX, these individuals are usually given a female sex of rearing, and the majority have female gender identity (Money and Ehrhardt, 1972). Some of these individuals experience gender dysphoria during puberty and a subset of this group change to a male gender identity (Meyer-Bahlburg et al., 1996). It has been recognized that these girls have a tomboyish personality, and tend to play with toys that are usually favored by boys (Ehrhardt & Meyer-Bahlburg, 1981). The degree of masculinization of behavior does not correlate with the degree virilization of the genitals (Slijper, 1984). As adults, these women tend to be sexually attracted to men, but may be more likely to have bisexual or homosexual interest than the general population (Ehrhardt & Meyer-Bahlburg, 1981). The mild masulinization of behavior in these individuals suggests a role for prenatal exposure to androgens. It has also been suggested that there may be a component of parental anxiety related to virilization (i.e., parental doubt and self doubt regarding sexual identity after early genital virilization), which could influence the child's sexual identity and behavior (Slijper, 1984). However, it is just as likely that the behavioral differences are related to androgen effect on the developing brain (Hrabovszky & Hutson, 2002).

Another group that may shed some light on the issue of prenatal androgen exposure are individuals with complete androgen insensitivity syndrome (CAIS). These individuals have a 46, XY karyotype, but they have an ineffective androgen receptor (even though they make adequate amounts of testosterone and dihydrotestosterone, the hormonal signal from these androgens is not recognized). Thus, these individuals should have no effective androgen exposure, but any genetic influences associated with the Y chromosome would be expected to be intact. Individuals with CAIS have normal female external genitalia. Internally they have normal testes that secrete both testosterone and Müllerian inhibitory factor. Thus, they do not have Müllerian structures nor do they have any Wolffian structures because of the inability to respond to testosterone. Individuals with CAIS are virtually always given a female sex of rearing. There have been several recent reports of psychological outcomes and gender-related development in individuals with CAIS (Wisniewski et al., 2000; Hines et al., 2003; Melo et al., 2003). In all of these studies the psychological outcomes in subjects with CAIS were similar to those of other women, suggesting that if there are Y chromosome-related genetic influences, they are not sufficient to cause a male sexual identity in the absence of an androgen effect.

There is also compelling evidence that the hormone that has direct effect in masculizing the brain may actually be estrogen (Gorski, 1999). The enzyme aromatase is responsible for conversion of testosterone to estradiol, and it has been know for some time that this enzyme is localized to several regions of the brain that are known to contain estrogen receptors and are known to be involved in reproductive behavior (McEwen et al., 1977). It is interesting that estrogen, which is a metabolic product of testosterone, has also been recognized as the hormone that causes epiphyseal fusion of the skeleton during puberty in both males and females.

The central dogma of sexual differentiation contends that even sexual differentiation of the brain is first dependent upon differentiation of the gonad into a testis or an ovary, which then influences differentiation of somatic tissue according to the presence of absence of testosterone or its metabolites. Dewing et al. (2003) have challenged the central dogma with the demonstration of sexually dimorphic gene expression in mouse brains that precedes gonadal differentiation.

How does the concept of sexual identity apply to an intersex individual? We live in a culture that abhors sexual ambiguity (Crouch, 1999), which puts pressure on each individual to declare either a male or female gender identity. In spite of this cultural pressure, some intersex individuals claim not to be entirely comfortable declaring that they are male or female. Of the sixteen individuals with cloacal exstrophy studied by Reiner and Gearhart (2004) there were three individuals with unclear sexual identity. These individuals should have experienced the same prenatal genetic and hormonal influences that other males experience, suggesting a role for environmental factors. If gender identity is indeed the product of complex genetic, hormonal, and environmental influences, it is plausible that sexual identity may not be any more "all-or-nothing" than other biological phenomona. There may be a continuum from feeling male to feeling female, which would depend upon the degree of genetic influences, prenatal concentrations of hormones, and the environment in which the individual is raised.

6. CONCLUSION

Human sexual differentiation is the result of a series of genetic and hormonal events that influence the development of the internal and external genitalia. Intersexuality may be the result of biological variability in genetic and hormonal steps in the cascade of sexual differentiation, but may also result from unrelated developmental events. Development of gender identity is less will understood, but also appears to be the result of genetic and hormonal influences, and to some degree, environmental influences. Prenatal exposure of the brain to androgen appears to be important for the development of male gender identity, although there is some evidence that the hormone that most directly influences brain sexual development may be estrogen. Further, there is some evidence that sex specific genetic events may occur in the brain before production of testosterone, indicating that there may be important genetic influences in development of sexual identity independent of hormonal exposure.

Departments of Pediatrics and Medical Humanities, The University of Arkansas for Medical Sciences and Arkansas Children's Hospital, Little Rock, U.S.A.

REFERENCES

Achermann, J. C., M. Ito, M. Ito, P. C. Hindmarsh, and J. L. Jameson. "Mutation in the Gene Encoding Steroidogenic Factor-1 Causes XY Sex Reversal and Adrenal Failure in Humans." *Nat. Gen.* 22 (1999): 125–126.

Aitken, R. J., and J. A. Marshall-Graves. "The Future of Sex." *Nature* 415 (2002): 963.

Andersson, M., D. C. Page, and A. de la Chapelle. "Chromosome Y-Specific DNA is Transferred to the Short Arm of X Chromosome in Human XX Males." *Science* 233 (1986): 786–788.

Arn, P., H. Chen, C. M. Tuck-Miller, C. Mankinen, G. Wachtel, S. Li, C. C. Shen, and S. S. Wachtel. "A Sex Reversing Locus in Xp21.2–p22.11." *Hum. Genet.* 93 (1994) 389–393.

Arnold, A. P. "Genetically Triggered Sexual Differentiation of Brain and Behavior." *Hormones and Behavior* 30 (1996): 495–505.

Bangsbøll, S., I. Qvist, P. E. Lebech, and M. Lewinsky. "Testicular Feminization Syndrome and Associated Gonadal Tumors in Denmark." *Acta Obstet. Gynecol. Scand.* 71 (1992): 63–66.

Bardoni, B., E. Zanaria, S. Guioli, G. Floridia, K. C. Worley, G. Tonini, E. Ferrante, G. Chiumello, E. R. McCabe, M. Fraccaro, et al. "A Dosage-Sensitive Locus at Chromosome Xp21 is Involved in Male to Female Sex Reversal." *Nat. Genet.* 7 (1994): 497–501.

Boucekkine, C., J. E. Toubland, N. Abbas, S. Chaabouni, S. Ouahid S., M. Semrouni, F. Jaubert, M. Toublanc, K. McElreavey, E. Vilain E., et al. "Clinical and Anatomical Spectrum in XX Sex Reversed Patients: Relationship to the presence of Y specific DNA-sequences." *Clin. Endocrinol.* 40 (1994): 733–742.

Crouch, R.A., "The Past and Future of Intersexuality," in *Intersex in the Age of Ethics*, A. D. Dreger, ed., University Publishing Group, Hagerstown, MD, 1999, 29.

De la Chapelle, A. "The Etiology of Maleness in XX Men." *Hum. Genet.* 58 (1981): 105–116.

Dewing P., T. Shi, S. Horvath, and E. Vilain. "Sexually Dimorphic Gene Expression in Mouse Brain Precedes Gonadal Differentiation." *Mol. Brain Res.* 118 (2003): 82–90.

Ehrhardt, A. A., and H. R. Meyer-Bahlburg. "Effects of Prenatal Sex Hormones on Gender-Related Behavior." *Science* 211 (1981): 1312–1318.

Farkas, A., and A. Rosler. "Ten Years Experience with Masculinizing Genitoplasty in Male Pseudohermaphroditism Due to 17 Beta-Hydroxysteroid Dehydrogenase Deficiency." *Eur. J. Pediatr.* 152 (1993): S88–90.

Federman, D. "Three Facets of Sexual Differentiation." *New Engl. J. Med.* 350 (2004): 323–324.

Ferrari, S., V. R. Harley, A. Pontiggia, P. N. Goodfellow, R. Lovell-Badge, and M. E. Bianchi. "SRY, Like HMG1, Recognizes Sharp Angles in DNA." *EMBO Journal* 11 (1992): 4497–4506.

Giese, K., J. Cox, J., and R. Grosschedl. "The HMG Domain of Lymphoid Enhancer Factor 1 Bends DNA and Facilitates Assembly of Functional Nucleoprotein Structures." *Cell* 69 (1992): 185–195.

Gorski, R. "Development of the Cerebral Cortex: XV. Sexual Differentiation of the Central Nervous System." *J. Am. Acad. Child and Adolescent Psychiatry* 38 (1999): 344–346.

Harley, V. R., D. I. Jackson, P. J. Hextall, J. R. Hawkins, G. D. Berkowitz, S. Sockanathan, R. Lovell-Badge, and P. N. Goodfellow. "DNA Binding Activity of Recombinant SRY from Normal Males and XY Females." *Science* 255 (1992): 453–455.

Hines, M., S. F. Ahned, and I. A. Hughes. "Psychological Outcomes and Gender-Related Development in Complete Androgen Insensitivity Syndrome." *Arch. Sexual Behavior* 32 (2003): 93-101.

Hirshfield, A. J., and J. K. Fleshman. "An Unusually High Incidence of Salt-Losing Congenital Adrenal Hyperplasia in the Alaskan Eskimo." *J. Pediatr* 75 (1969): 492–494.

Hrabovszky, Z., and J. M. Hutson. "Androgen Imprinting of the Brain in Animal Models and Humans with Intersex Disorders: Review and Recommendations." *J. Urol.* 168 (2002): 2142–2148.

Huang, B., S. Wang, Y. Ning, A. N. Lamb, and J. Bartley. "Autosomal XX Sex Reversal Caused by Duplication of SOX 9." *Am. J. Med. Gen.* 87 (1999): 349–359.

Imperato-McGinley, J., R. E. Peterson, T. Gautier, and E. Sturla. "Androgens and the Evolution of Male-Gender Identity among Male Pseudohermaphrodites with 5 Alpha-Reductase Deficiency." *N. Engl J. Med.* 300 (1979): 1233–1237.

Intersex Society of North America. http://www.isna.org

Jost, A. Recherches Sur la Differenciation Sexuelle de l'Embryon de Lapin. III. Role des gonades foetales dan la differenciation sexuelle somatique. *Archives d'Anatomie et de Microscopie Morphologique Experimentale* 36: (1947) 271–315.

Koopman, P., A. Munsterberg, B. Capel, N. Vivian, and R. Lovell-Badge. "Expression of a Candidate Sex-Determining Gene During Mouse Testis Differentiation," *Nature* 348 1990: 450–452.

Koopman, P. "Mammalian Testes-Determining Genes," *Cell. Mol. Life Sc.* 55 (1999): 839–856.

Luo, X., Y. Ikeda, and K. L. Parker. A Cell-Specific Nuclear Receptor is Essential for Adrenal and Gonadal Development and Sexual Differentiation, *Cell* 77 (1994): 481–490.

MacGillivray, M. H., and T. Mazu. Management of Infants Born with Ambiguous Genitalia," in: *Pediatric Endocrionlogy: A Practical Clinical Guide*, S. Radovick & M. H. MacGillivray, eds. Totowa, NJ Humana Press, 2003, 429–449.

MacLaughlin, D. T., and P. K. Donahoe. "Mechanisms of Disease: Sex Determination and Differentiation." *New Engl. J. Med.* 350 (2004): 367–378.

McElreavey, K., E. Vilain, N. Abbas, J. M. Costa, N. Souleyreau, K. Kucheria, C. Boucekkine, E. Thibaud, R. Brauner, F. Flamant, and M. Fellous. "XY Sex Reversal Associated with a Deletion 5' to the SRY "HMG Box" in the Testis-Determining Region." *Proc. Natl. Acad. Sci., U. S. A.* 89 (1992): 11016–11020.

McEwen, B. S., I. Lieberburg, C. Chaptal, and L. C. Krey. "Aromatization: Important for Sexual Differentiation of the Neonatal Rat Brain." *Horm. Behav.* (1977): 249–263.

Marshall-Graves, J. A. "The Rise and Fall of SRY." *Trends Genet.* 18 (2002): 259–264.

Melo, K. F. S., B. B. Mendonca, A. E. C. Billerbeck, E. M. F. Costa, M. Inácio, F. A. Q. Silva, A. M. O. Leal, A. C. Latronico, and I. J. P. Arnhold. "Clinical, Hormonal, Behavioral, and Genetic Characteristics of Androgen Insensitivity Syndrome in a Brazilian Cohort: Five Novel Mutations in the Androgen Receptor Gene." *J. Clin. Endocrinol. Metab.* 88 (2003): 3241–3250.

Meyer-Bahlburg H. F., R. S. Gruen, M. I. New, J. J. Bell, Morishima, A., M. Shimshi, Y. Bueno, I. Vargas, and S. W. Baker. "Gender Change from Female to Male in Classical Congenital Adrenal Hyperplasia." *Hormones & Behavior* 30 (1996): 319–32.

Money, J. "Psychologic Counseling: Hermaphroditism," in *Endocrine and Genetic Diseases of Childhood*, L. I. Gardner, ed., Philadelphia: W. B. Saunders Company, 1969, p. 542.

Money, J., and A. A. Ehrhardt. "Gender Dimorphic Behavior and Fetal Sex Hormones." *Rec. Prog. Horm. Res.* 28 (1972): 735–763.

Money, J., J. G. Hampson, and J. L. Hampson. "Imprinting and the Establishment of Gender Role." *AMA Arch. Neurol. Psych.* 77 (1957): 333.

New, M. I. "Steroid 21-Hydroxylase Deficiency (Congenital Adrenal Hyperplasia)." *Am J. Med.* 98 (1995): 2S–8S.

Ohno, S. *Sex Chromosomes and Sex Linked Genes.* New York: Springer-Verlag, 1967.

Page, D. C., and A. de la Chapelle. "The Parental Origin of X Chromosomes in XX Males Determined Using Restriction Fragment Length Polymorphisms." *Am. J. Hum. Genet.* 36 (1984): 565–575.

Pang, S., W. Murphey, L. S. Levine, A. L. Spence, S. LaFranchi, A. S. Surve, and M. I. New. "A Pilot Newborn Screening for Congenital Adrenal Hyperplasia in Alaska." *J Clin. Endocrinol. Metab.* 55 (1982): 413–420.

Parker, K. L., B. P. Schimmer, and A. Sched. "Genes Essential for Early Events in Gonadal Development." *Cell. Mol. Life Sci.* 55 (1999): 831–838.

Palmer, M. S., A. H. Sinclair, P. Berta, N. A. Ellis, P. N. Goodfellow, N. E. Abbas, and M. Fellous. "Genetic Evidence that ZFY is Not the Testis-Determining Factor." *Nature* 342 (1989): 937–939.

Reiner, W. G., and /J. P. Gearhart. "Discordant Sexual Identity in Some Genetic Males with Cloacal Exstrophy Assigned to Female Sex at Birth." *N. Engl. J. Med.* 350 (2004): 333–341.

Saitou M., S. C. Barton, and M. A. Surani. "A Molecular Programme for the Specification of Germ Cell Fate in Mice." *Nature* 418 (2002): 293–300.

Sinclair, A. H., P. Berta, M. S. Palmer, J. R. Hawkins, B. L. Griffiths, M. J. Smith, J. W. Foster, A. M. Frischauf, R. Lovell-Badge, and P. N. Goodfellow. "A Gene from the Human Sex-Determining Region Encodes a Protein with Homology to a Conserved DNA Binding Motif." *Nature* 346 (1990): 240–244.

Slijper, F. M. E. "Androgens and Gender Role Behavior in Girls with Congenital Adrenal Hyperplasia (CAH)," *Prog. Brain. Res.* 61 (1984): 417–422.

Tommerup, N., W. Schempp, P. Mienecke, S. Pedersen, L. Bolund, C. Brandt, C. Goodpasture, P. Guldberg, K. R. Held, H. Reinwein, O. D. Saaugstad, G. Scherer, O. Skjeldal, R. Toder, J. Westvik, C. B. van der Hagen, and U. Wolf. "Assignment of an Autosomal Sex Reversal Locus (SRA1) and Campomelic Dysplasia (CMPD1) to 17q24.3-q25.1." *Nature Genetics* 4 (1993): 170–174.

Vilain, E., E. R. B. McCabe. "Mammalian Sex Determination: From Gonads to Brain." *Molecular Genetics and Metabolism* 65 1998: 74–84.

Vilain, E. "Genetics of Sexual Development." *Ann. Rev. Sex Res.* 1 (2000): 1–25.

Vilain, E. "Dead Chromosome Walking." *Pediatr. Res.* 55 (2004): 539–540.

Vilain, E. "Anomalies of Human Sexual Development: Clinical Aspects and Genetic Analysis," in *The Genetics and Biology of Sex Determination*, R. V. Short, ed. Novartis Foundation Symposium 244, John Wiley & Sons, Chichester, UK, 2002, p. 43–56.

Wisniewski, A. B., C. J. Migeon, H. F. L. Meyer-Bahlburg, J. P. Gearhart, G. D. Berkovitz, T. R. Brown, and J. Money. "Complete Androgen Insensitivity Syndrome: Long-Term Medical, Surgical, and Psychosexual Outcome." *J. Clin. Endocrinol. Metab.* 85 (2000): 2664–2669.

DAVID T. OZAR

TOWARDS A MORE INCLUSIVE CONCEPTION OF GENDER-DIVERSITY FOR INTERSEX ADVOCACY AND ETHICS

1. INTRODUCTION

Intersex advocates urge the families of intersex infants and the professionals who assist those families to assign each child a gender at birth so that the child grows up a gendered person (masculine or feminine, boy or girl) as society requires. However, they stipulate that all involved should consider the assignment provisional. They stress that the family and the child should have counseling, and that the child, in particular, should be educated in age-appropriate ways regarding the provisional nature of his or her gender-assignment. Then, when the young person is able to do so thoughtfully, he or she should select his or her own gender on the basis of his or her experience of gender-identity. Intersex advocates are also well known to urge that surgery designed solely to address gender concerns should not be performed until the intersex person is able to thoughtfully choose or decline it.

In urging this approach to rearing and gendering intersex children, intersex advocates readily acknowledge that a person's experience of his or her gender-identity is not something easily understood or articulated. This is especially true for a person in his or her early teens, ordinarily a time when the awareness of one's gender identity is just becoming strong enough to guide one's conduct and to shape one's choices concerning the future. Even among mature adults, a person's experience of his or her gender-identity is often quite subtle: the experience is complexly constructed out of self-awareness and self-reflection, out of social interaction reviewed inwardly, and out of others' perceptions, communicated to the individual, of the person as gendered. Gender-identity is not something simply given to a person; it is something achieved, and, for intersex persons and many others, achieved only with effort.

The subtlety of these matters and the need for careful education and counseling suggests that the literature of intersex advocacy should be paying serious attention to the conceptions of gender, gender-identity, gender-assignment, and gender-expression that it employs. The alternative is to accept such conceptions as they are

17

S.E. Sytsma (Ed.), Ethics and Intersex, 17–46.
© 2006 *Springer. Printed in the Netherlands.*

perpetuated in the larger community, since it is the larger community that chiefly shapes the conceptions that families of intersex children, most counselors, and most educators bring to the situation. But in fact, the recommendations of intersex advocates presuppose conceptions of gender, gender-identity, gender-assignment, and gender-expression that are profoundly different from the conceptions of these things that are employed in contemporary societies. In short, the intersex advocacy community relies upon a much more inclusive notion of gender-diversity than is accepted, or even available for consideration, in the larger community. Therefore, in order to achieve their goals, intersex advocates must work to articulate the gender-related conceptions on which their positions depend, and they must engage in the systematic re-education of members of their own community and of the larger community, respectively.

The aim of this essay is to address this gap in the intersex literature by proposing an appropriately inclusive conception of gender-diversity. Specifically, this essay will propose conceptions of gender-identity, gender-assignment, and gender-expression that are more informative and more inclusive than those in common use in contemporary societies. My hope is that these concepts will have educational value for all involved, and that these concepts will assist intersex advocates in formulating their recommendations for practice and policy more cogently.

This essay builds on a foundation of conceptual work already begun by members and friends of the transgendered community. More than any other group, the transgendered community has had to, for its own sake, develop creative ways of articulating conceptions of gender-diversity, gender-identity, gender-assignment, and gender-expression. For this reason, the transgendered community and those who support it are currently the most active resource for assisting the intersex community's construction of more inclusive gender-related conceptions and the most natural allies of the intersex community in these efforts. For this reason also, the final section of this essay will call upon the intersex advocacy community to build new relationships with the transgendered community in order to achieve the groups' common goals more effectively.

2. TWO EXTRAORDINARY IDEAS: PROVISIONAL GENDER AND SELF-CHOICE OF GENDER

For most people in today's world, gender-diversity is something of acknowledged importance. It is something that is structurally simple, although very complex in practice. To oversimplify for a moment (a more detailed account will be offered shortly), the larger community's understanding of gender-diversity can be summarized by saying simply that there are two and only two genders and each of us belongs to one of them. Nothing could be structurally simpler than this. What is complex is the different ways that men and women live out this simple division in practice. These are the differences that constitute gender-diversity on the ordinary view.

What makes gender so diverse, on the ordinary view, is that there are no clean lines that fully differentiate the two genders with regard to conduct, appearance, social expectations, and many other things. One reason for diversity in practice is the tremendous variation among individuals belonging to the two genders, including variation in conduct and appearance. A second reason for diversity in practice is that there are fundamental moral convictions, in many parts of the world, about the equal dignity and rights of all human persons; these convictions and the social policies they give rise to require considerable tolerance of differences in practice (though this tolerance is practiced in varying degrees and in many different ways in different parts of the world). As a consequence, except for some of the differences either directly associated with typical biological characteristics of males and females or functionally associated with these biological differences (e.g., differing roles in reproduction), gender-diversity is something acknowledged to be very complex for many of the world's societies in spite of its structural simplicity.

But the challenge that the intersex community, and the transgender community as well, poses to the larger community's understanding of gender-diversity is not primarily directed towards those practices that the larger community considers complex. That is, it does not concern the range of individual variation within the two genders. The intersex community's challenge concerns the aspect of gender-diversity that the larger community considers simple and obvious, namely, what genders there are and how people belong to them to begin with. Comprehending the depth of this challenge and acting and educating accordingly is crucial to the success of the intersex and the transgendered communities' goals within society.

It is, of course, true that the members of the intersex and the transgender community deserve the same respect for their human dignity as every other person. They deserve the same acceptance of their individual differences and the same tolerance of their individual efforts to work out their lives, personally and in relation to others, so long as they do not harm others in the process. In these important respects, which have many implications for practice and policy, intersex and transgendered persons are no different from and deserve to be treated with the same respect as everyone else. But this does not mean that accepting the intersex and the transgender communities' understanding of who they are is therefore a less fundamental challenge to what the larger community considers simple and obvious, i.e., what belonging to a gender means in the first place.

The larger society's understanding of gender-diversity was stated in a deliberately oversimplified form three paragraphs back. However, it is now important to articulate its six principal components. For convenience, this conception of gender and gender-diversity will from this point on be called "the Ordinary View." The Ordinary View, which is the view of most people in the contemporary world, is this:

A)   There are two and only two genders.
B)   Every human being belongs to one and only one of these two genders (that is, no one can properly be said to belong to both genders simultaneously).
C)   Belonging to a gender is a permanent characteristic of a human being.
D)   No one can belong to one gender at one time in life and to another gender at another time. (This may seem to be the same point as C, but there is an important difference that will be clarified below.)

E)   The gender to which a human belongs is determined biologically, specifically as being biologically male or biologically female.

F)   The gender to which a human belongs is not a matter of choice either by the person him- or herself or by any other human.

From this more complete articulation of the larger community's understanding, it should be it clear how very extraordinary—how radically challenging to most people's ordinary ways of thinking—it is for intersex advocates to recommend that an intersex infant be assigned a *provisional* gender at birth and that he or she *self-choose* his or her gender later, when able to do so thoughtfully. The challenges that the intersex community's recommendations pose to the Ordinary View can be more fully detailed in terms of seven distinct claims. For ease of reference, the intersex community's understanding of these matters will henceforth be termed "the Intersex View" (although, like all human groups, the intersex community is not completely monolithic in its understanding of these matters).

2.1 Claim 1: Belonging to a gender is certainly not determined by typical biological characteristics of males and females

Such a view is commonplace in the intersex community despite its distance from the Ordinary View. For if gender is a matter of biology, as the Ordinary View holds, then there must be two and only two biological classifications to match the pairing of biology with gender. But as the experience of intersex people aptly demonstrates, human biology is more diverse and more complex than the Ordinary View acknowledges. Therefore, since it is not the case that everyone is a typical biological male or a typical biological female, it follows that belonging to one gender or the other cannot be a simple matter of having typical male or female characteristics.

2.2 Claim 2: Belonging to a gender has been a matter of human choice

A second view that is also commonplace among the intersex community—and that constitutes a second point of departure from the Ordinary View—concerns how gender was initially determined for intersex persons. It was determined either by medical professionals acting solo or by medical professionals acting in concert with parents (and/or other family members). The fiction of its having been determined by biology has often been maintained for years and, for many intersex persons, by the most secretive and deceptive of means. But the reality for intersex persons is that, in contrast to what the Ordinary View holds, their gender has been determined by human choice, not by biology.

The intersex community concedes that, for infants who are not intersexed, the assignment of gender by medical professionals (and families) correlates so closely with the identification of typical male or female anatomical characteristics that it can certainly *appear* to be simply a matter of biology. But the intersex community would argue that every child's gender is actually determined by human choice, not some bare set of biological facts.

2.3 Claim 3: The appropriate person to choose a person's gender is the person him- or herself

A third claim of the intersex community, a claim that is also at some distance from the Ordinary View, follows directly from the second. This is the position that, since belonging to a gender has already been a matter of choice for intersex persons (i.e., at the time of birth and then in childhood), it is appropriate to ask who ought to be making this important choice, and the best answer is the person him- or herself. Especially within the reigning culture of pediatric medical practice, however, it has seemed obvious for many years that this determination should be made by medical professionals alone or, after the rise of informed consent as a central component of medical ethics in some Western societies, by medical professionals in concert with the child's parents. The reason for this pattern of choice is probably the assumption, already challenged, that gender is a matter of biological characteristics.

But the intersex community has argued strongly that, with the exception of a few medical conditions that pose immediate, significant risk to the life and physical health of the child, the question of determining a child's gender is not a medical matter, and therefore there is no good reason for assigning the determination of a child's gender to medical professionals. Instead, the proper thing to do is to ask: Who ought to make that choice? Until that question is resolved, surgical interventions that are not medically needed and that would have gender assignment as their consequence should not be performed.

But who should determine the intersex infant's gender? The intersex community has argued that the proper person to choose a person's gender is the person him- or herself. This position is supported by convictions about the moral and social importance of self-determination, convictions that are widely accepted in many contemporary societies. Indeed, this position of intersex advocates is highly consistent with mainstream ethics, especially in the United States, even though it addresses a question that the Ordinary View, with its narrow conceptions, cannot even formulate. So the distance between the Intersex View and the Ordinary View here is not in the reasoning supporting self-determination; it is in the rejection of gender as a matter for medical professionals to determine.

It is significant, however, that at the time in question, the intersex person is an infant or young child who is unable to make a thoughtful choice about his or her gender. Therefore, the question faced by intersex advocates is what to do in the interim, until the intersex person is of such age and ability that he or she can make this choice thoughtfully. The intersex community's answer allows for the component of the Ordinary View that requires every person to belong to one of two genders. For the child's protection and acceptance into society, the intersex community urges that a gender be chosen for the child and proposes that this choice be made by the child's parents (with as much advice from medical professionals as the parents choose to seek) because the parents are the persons who will be responsible for rearing and educating the child about his or her situation. But there is an important specification about this choice that the intersex community stresses:

that all involved, including the child (in age-appropriate ways), understand that this belonging to a gender is only *provisional*.

2.4 Claim 4: A person's belonging to a gender can be provisional

What does it mean to say that an intersex child's belonging to a gender is, as the Intersex View urges, *provisional*? It might seem that this is simply a shorthand way of saying that, whatever gender is chosen for the child early on, the child is to be counseled and educated in preparation for his or her making a thoughtful, more permanent decision about his or her gender at an appropriate later time. That is, "provisional," in this context, might seem to mean the same thing as "temporary," because another choice will be made later.

But the intersex community's proposal of provisional gender assignment involves something much more radical, something at a much greater distance from the Ordinary View. For it is important to remember that, during the intersex child's infancy and childhood, the child's provisional gender will *be* its gender. It is not the case that a child who provisionally belongs to a gender really belongs to *no* gender, so that viewing the child in terms of the provisional gender is an error. In fact, it is in terms of the provisional gender that the child will be known to others and will be treated by others, even by close family members and other parties who know the child's complex history. The point is that, in so viewing the child and dealing with the child as one belonging to the provisional gender, these persons will not be making a mistake.

So the position of the Ordinary View that gender is invariably a permanent characteristic of a person is being set aside here. Rather, the Intersex View is that belonging to a gender is in some instances a permanent characteristic of a person and in other instances a provisional characteristic. This is a fundamental reconstruction of the conception of belonging to a gender.

In fact, once this revised conception of belonging to a gender is accepted, it becomes clear that the choice an intersex person might make in his or her early teens, to take just one possible example, might still be provisional in his or her mind. Particularly if the intersex person has been living provisionally within the feminine gender as a child and chooses now to live within the masculine gender, or vice versa, it may be wise for the person to consider this choice about belonging to a gender provisional as well. In fact, it may take some time, especially for a person with limited life experience of any sort, to judge wisely about the fit between gender and who he or she most deeply is and is striving to be over a lifetime.

Another, easily overlooked component of provisionality also deserves mention here. There is embedded in the notion of a provisional choice—whether this is a choice of gender or of anything else—an implication that the provisional condition will come to an end, as provisional, at some appropriate point. That is, what is provisional ought to be temporary, ought to be replaced at some point with what is permanent. So even if an intersex teen or young adult were to view his or her current choice of gender as provisional, it would be a misunderstanding of provisionality to think that a person could live his or her life within a gender chosen only provisionally at all times. This logical fact about provisionality certainly does not imply that intersex persons invariably attain great clarity about which gender to belong to permanently. But the logic of this concept does suggest that the intersex advocacy community's recommendation of a provisional gender for intersex infants and children is not a recommendation of permanent provisionality. If the claim were that belonging to a gender should always be viewed as temporary and changeable, that would constitute an even more radical challenge to the ordinary view; but this does not appear to be what the intersex community is proposing.

2.5 Claim 5: A person can belong to one gender at one time of life and to another gender at another time

Some intersex persons, when they reach the age and maturity level for thoughtfully choosing their own gender, choose the *same* gender that they have been living within provisionally since infancy. The transition that takes place at this point in such a person's life illustrates a point made in the previous section—namely, that there is a profound conceptual distance between belonging to a gender provisionally and belonging to a gender permanently.

By contrast, some intersex persons who have lived provisionally within one gender now thoughtfully choose to live permanently within the other gender. In this case there is a *double* transition: a transition from belonging to one gender to belonging to another, and a transition from a provisional choice of gender to a permanent choice of gender.

It is therefore very important to stress that calling the infant's gender *provisional* does not tell us whether the child, when he or she is ready to choose, will change genders or will remain living within the same gender. This is why it is important to differentiate the Intersex View's fourth claim, *that a person's belonging to a gender can be provisional*, from the Intersex View's fifth claim, *that a person can belong to one gender at one time of life and to another gender at another time.* These are two distinct fundamental challenges to the Ordinary View. This is also the reason why, in the above articulation of the Ordinary View, component C, *that belonging to a gender is a permanent characteristic of a human being*, was formulated separately from component D, *that no one can belong to one gender at one time of life and to another gender at another time.* For these two propositions are now seen to be logically distinct components of the ordinary understanding of gender.

2.6 Claim 6: Belonging to a gender is something that should be determined by self-choice because it comes chiefly from within the person rather than from something external

In the discussion of claim three, an argument for the self-choosing of gender was formulated in terms of the value of self-determination within many contemporary societies. The structure of that argument is that the determination of one's gender is an important matter, and if it is a matter of choice, as the intersex view claims, then the moral and social importance of self-determination clearly entails that this choice be made by the person him- or herself. As was mentioned, the value of self-determination is something about which the Intersex View and the Ordinary View usually agree.

But there is a second argument for the self-choosing of gender that places the Intersex View at a considerable distance from the Ordinary View. For the Ordinary Views sees the basis of one's gender as something public and obvious while the Intersex View sees it as something subtle and personal, a matter of careful inner judgment. The second argument for self-choosing therefore has these two steps: (i) determining one's gender is a matter of seeking a fit between who one is and the genders available in the society, and (ii) gender should be a self-chosen because the person him- or herself is the person most able to evaluate this fit. This position presupposes that humans experience themselves as identifying with, in greater or lesser degrees, the genders available in their societies and that they gradually come to view themselves, as part of their overall understanding of who they are, in terms of such identification. Part Two will formulate this idea as a concept of *gender-identity*.

Without denying the role of others in helping a person understand his or her experience of identifying, in greater or lesser degrees, with one of a society's established genders, the intersex view is that this process can be very subtle and that the person him- or herself is by far the best interpreter of such experience. Therefore, even more important than the argument from the value of self-determination (claim three) is this second argument: that in the choice of one's gender, it is the person him- or herself (with appropriate, voluntarily accepted assistance) who ought to make this choice, once he or she is mature enough to do so thoughtfully, on the basis that he or she is the only person who can do it with an adequate understanding of which gender he or she most fully or deeply identifies with, i.e., of who he or she is (claim six).

This second argument for self-choosing puts the Intersex View at a great conceptual distance from the Ordinary View. It does so, first, because it rejects the notion that gender is a matter of the biological characteristics of typical males and typical females; and second, because it suggests that the determination of a person's gender, when made properly, is a personal matter, indeed a matter of great intimacy to the person, which only the person him- or herself can ultimately sort out and resolve. On this view, a person's gender is not something first and foremost public. The physician's typical announcement at birth—"it's a boy," "it's a girl"—may seem to indicate that gender is something public and obvious. But on the Intersex View, the reality of gender for each person is instead something very personal and very subtle, something that emerges as the best fit between the uniqueness of the person and the genders that the society happens to offer. (This essay assumes the general correctness of the position that the specific manifestations of each gender in a society are socially constructed, hence changeable; and that such manifestations are also fallible in terms of their value to various persons or classes of persons in the society. The present discussion is about persons choosing among the genders a society has already constructed. It is not about the complex social processes by which genders are constructed or change in a society.)

2.7 Claim 7: Gender is something "built into" a person, not something chosen arbitrarily. So when a person determines which gender to belong to, the aim is for that determination to "fit" with what he or she experiences as "built in."

There is an easily missed point of confluence between the Intersex View and the Ordinary View, namely, the notion that gender is something "built in," or is part of who the person is "from the start." The Ordinary View considers gender to be "built in" according to the person's biological characteristics as male or female, and therefore to be publicly determinable at birth. On the other hand, the Intersex View sees the determination of a person's belonging to a gender as a matter of a subtle "fit" between who the person is and his or her society's available genders. This is why the Intersex View holds that this determination needs to be made some years after birth, when the person has had enough experience with gender identification to discern a dependable pattern in such experience. But this difference should not mask the fact the both views see gender as something "built in." In fact, there may be a basis for dialogue here that should not be overlooked.

This point of confluence has two important implications. First, by viewing gender as something "built in," both the Ordinary View and the Intersex View reject the position that gender is something shaped solely by a child's environment, and that gender is therefore completely malleable during a child's first 18 to 24 months of life. Second, by viewing gender as something "built in," both the Ordinary View and the Intersex View necessarily hold that a person's choice of gender (if the Ordinary View could accept the validity of claim two) is not something wide open, a matter of whim or mere taste, but is a search for the best fit between who the person is, i.e., what is "already" built in, and the genders available in the society. The Intersex View already understands the choice in this way (as claim six stresses). The Ordinary View, by conceiving gender to be "built in," would agree with the Intersex View on this point if the Ordinary View were to accept that, as the experience of intersex persons indicates so clearly, biological characteristics of human males and females are not the determinants of gender.

3. A MORE INCLUSIVE CONCEPTUAL FRAMEWORK

The aim of Part One was to clarify the points of contrast between the Intersex View and the Ordinary View in order to motivate the intersex advocacy community to first, articulate more clearly the concepts on which its position depends; and second, educate, accordingly, both its own members and those with whom it is in dialogue. The aim of Part Two is to propose an account of the key concepts that the intersex community needs in order to achieve this. But two preliminary points need attention beforehand.

First, whenever someone offers a detailed account of ideas that, before, were largely implicit in a group's literature and practical initiatives, the exposition needs to be treated initially as a set of hypotheses available for testing, rather than as the last word on how these ideas should be understood. It is in this spirit that the following elucidation of concepts important to the Intersex View is offered. The reader should consider the proposed description of these concepts to be a hypothesis to be tested.

The questions that should be asked to test this hypothesis include the following: Is this a valuable way to conceive of these aspects the experience of gender and related matters? Does this way of conceiving of gender and other matters contribute to self-understanding; to people's efforts at describing their experience to others; to others' understanding of that experience; to a sense of shared experience; to clearer reasoning behind personal actions and proposed policies; to clearer criticisms of others' (or one's own) actions or policies; and to clearer evaluations of experiences and patterns of action in individuals, groups, and whole societies? If the proposed account passes such tests, that will recommend it for use and for further improvement by still more careful exposition.

Second, the material that follows could not have been written if the author had not had the opportunity to work with a transgendered support group on developing a document to be used in the group's educational outreach in local colleges and universities. This project is a product of several years of cooperation between members of the support group and a number of its academic friends in the Chicago area. Almost every theme developed in Part Two has been carefully discussed with members of the drafting team and formulated and reformulated on the basis of their assistance. In terms of giving proper credit, however, it is also important to say that the first rule of the support group is privacy. Many transgendered people who participate in the activities of the support group would face a genuine risk of harm to themselves and/or their families if they were to be identified in their daily lives as transgendered persons. For this reason, this paragraph shall constitute the sole formal acknowledgement here that this material could not have been written without the help of many members of the transgendered community.

3.1 The Genders

In most contemporary societies, there are two and only two *genders.* This essay will use the terms *feminine* and *masculine* to refer to the two genders when an adjective is needed and the terms *women* and *men* to refer to them when a noun is needed (or *boy* and *girl* when the parties are children). In this essay, these words will be used only to refer to categories of gender, never to biological categories. For the sake of clarity, the relevant biological categories will be referred to by the terms *male, female,* and *intersex.* Such stipulated clarity in the use of terms, clarity that is not available in ordinary speech, is essential for clear exposition of the ideas being examined here.

Scholars in many fields have studied gender, and it is beyond the scope of this essay to try to summarize their work. For present purposes the genders will be taken to be complex sets of human characteristics, behaviors, roles, rules, and expectations that are constructed by a culture so its people can more easily describe one another, assign tasks and statuses within the society, have fairly stable expectations of one another, and personally incorporate these sets of characteristics (or parts of them) to a greater or lesser degree in forming their individual identities.

The social construction and reconstruction of the genders by a culture is typically something very gradual. Nevertheless, it is clear that genders can change rapidly enough that, for example, important elements of the genders can be seen to have undergone significant change in American and other Western societies over the last half-century. Some behaviors and tasks that were narrowly associated with only one of the genders sixty years ago—for example, competitiveness for the masculine gender and nurturing for the feminine gender—can today be properly undertaken by individuals in the other gender, at least under certain circumstances. But such adjustments in the behaviors and other characteristics considered appropriate to the genders in these societies has not changed the fact that these societies still have two and only two genders. In fact, the increasing acknowledgement in the public cultures of Western societies in the last two decades that there are people who are properly considered to be *transgendered* is itself evidence that the two genders are culturally distinguishable ways of living and continue to have significant, if not precise, boundaries that transgendered persons are considered to be crossing.

For present purposes, however, further discussion of the general notion of gender is not what is needed, but rather a discussion of three settings or contexts in which persons are categorized in terms of gender. These will be examined here under the headings of Gender Assignment, Gender Identity, and Gender Expression.

3.2 Gender Assignment

3.2.1. What is Gender Assignment?

One of the ways in which people are categorized in terms of gender consists of people being categorized as gendered by others. People typically perceive each another as belonging to one or another of the culture's two genders and then treat each other accordingly. Thus, among the first descriptors a person would typically use to describe another person is a term that assigns that person to one of society's two genders. Indeed, many aspects of people's initial interactions with other persons depend upon Gender Assignment.

Gender Assignment is something done from the observer's perspective. The perspective of each person about his or her own gender will be examined under the heading of Gender Identity in the next section. Gender Assignment is obviously fallible ("I thought it was a little girl, but when I got closer I could see that it was a boy..."), but it is so universally applied and depended on that persistent ambiguity about someone's gender is ordinarily troubling. Thus it is easy to imagine someone saying, "I could not tell if I was dealing with a man or a woman" and expecting sympathy from the listener because of the difficulty of interacting properly with someone whose gender is unknown even after the available evidence has been considered. The speaker of such words might accept responsibility for the ambiguity ("I don't know why, but I just could not figure it out…") or might place blame on the other party ("Why would a person present themselves so strangely that people do not know how to react to them?"). But the importance of assigning gender to others in guiding our interactions with them, especially at the outset of dealing with someone and in the absence of additional data about them, is hard to overstate.

This is also the reason why gender ambiguity is a source of humor. The famous "Pat and Pat" skit was a regular feature of the U.S. comedy show, *Saturday Night Live*, because everyone in the audience understood the protagonist's need to assign one of the two genders to Pat in order to interact properly with her or him. The sophisticated humor of Les Ballets Trockadero de Monte Carlo, a company of professional male dancers performing classical ballet *en travesti*, has been applauded enthusiastically all over the world for thirty years because of their amazing artistry and because of our need to assign gender to people in order to interact with them, even from the back row of the second balcony. There are also many instances of humor at the expense of persons considered to be gender-ambiguous by others, humor full of censure or worse.

Most of our assignments of gender to other persons are informal and unofficial. Taken singly, they have considerably less impact on the person whose gender is assigned official forms of assignment have, as when a newborn is declared to be a boy or a girl, or a person's biology and gender are simultaneously categorized on a driver's license. But considered cumulatively, and because such assigning is universal and constant in daily life, the informal but routine Gender Assignment of everyone by everyone has a powerful impact on those assigned and on all our social interactions as well.

What are the bases of these assignments of gender? The official assignments are typically made on the basis of three mistaken assumptions: (a) an assumption about biology, namely, that every human is either typically male or typically female; (b) an assumption about psychology, namely, that every human is gendered either masculine or feminine (this assumption will be examined in the next section); and (c) another assumption about psychology, namely, that a person's gender identity flows directly from his or her being biologically male or female.

The informal assignments of gender that fill our daily lives are typically thought to derive from the official assignments or from the biological categories on which those assignments are taken to depend. But in fact we rarely know the intimate biology of people we deal with day-in and day-out, and, unless we have done some research, we rarely know with any confidence how they have been officially assigned. Instead, the vast array of informal gender assignments that we make daily and that have such profound impact on the persons so assigned depend on the various kinds of overt evidence that have become culturally connected to the characteristics, behaviors, tasks, etc., of the culture's two genders. We make our ordinary gender assignments for the most part on the basis of how persons express themselves, deliberately or accidentally, in culturally gendered ways. The topic of Gender Expression will be examined in detail shortly.

3.2.2. Gender Assignment and Intersex Persons

The universality of Gender Assignment in human interaction and the reality that so many aspects of people's initial interactions with other people depend upon Gender Assignment are the reasons why it would be a serious mistake the think that an intersex child should live without a gender or, alternatively, should somehow try to live in both genders simultaneously until he or she is sufficiently mature and experienced to thoughtfully choose his or her own gender. Gendered life is just too important a part of human social interaction for us to require any child to live for a number of years with the constant burden of gender ambiguity and the adverse reactions that gender ambiguity elicits in many people.

In addition, the fact that most informal assignments of gender are based on overt evidence of the characteristics, behaviors, traits, etc., associated with the culture's genders, rather than on evidence more closely related to either official or biological matters, means that it will not ordinarily be difficult to arrange that the gender assigned to an intersex child by most of the people the child encounters will be the one assigned to the child by his or her parents shortly after birth. Few people will know or have any reason to know that this gender is only provisional. But there will be special circumstances that need to be foreseen and prepared for, both bureaucratic situations (school registration, athletic competition when the child is a little older, etc.) and social situations like gym classes, swimming parties, etc. But in the vast majority of the child's interactions with others, manipulation of the usual overt forms of evidence, i.e., Gender Expression, will ease the child's life among people by assuring Gender Assignment consistent with the provisional gender chosen by his or her parents.

By the same token, however, the child's interactions with most people will produce nearly constant reinforcement of the child's provisional gender. Therefore, parents and counselors will need to take special care, in age appropriate ways, to help the child understand that this apparent abundance of evidence of the child's gender should not replace the child's own efforts, over time, to determine personally which gender he or she belongs to. The child's eventual choice of gender should be based on his or her own reflections on whether his or her provisionally assigned gender is the one with which he or she most deeply identifies, or if he or she identifies most deeply with the other gender, or if his or her grasp of self as gendered is more complex than this (more on this possibility in a moment). That is, the child's education and counseling must lead the child to understand the difference between Gender Assignment and Gender Identity, which is the topic of the next major section.

3.2.3. Gender Assignment and Diversity

For the last half-century, parents in many Western societies and elsewhere have been encouraging their female children to consider a much broader range of careers, and to develop in themselves a much broader range of personal and social characteristics, than females were encouraged to consider in previous eras. Parents have also encouraged their male children to consider a broader range of approaches to adult male life during this period, to a lesser but still significant extent. The result has been that, as these children have grown to adulthood, the boundaries of the genders in these societies have shifted to create what might be described as more "overlap"; there is also more tolerance of variation within each of the genders than there was in the previous era.

As was explained in Part One, these are the features of contemporary life that constitute *gender diversity* according to the Ordinary View. Thus the Ordinary View routinely interprets the experience of intersex and transgendered persons merely as instances of individual variation within the existing genders as ordinarily conceived. The experiences of intersex and transgendered persons are not recognized as challenging the ordinary view to reconstruct its concepts of Gender Assignment, Gender Identity, and Gender Expression, and thereby to broaden considerably its concept of Gender Diversity.

The intersex advocacy community has offered a powerful argument to say that provisional Gender Assignment is absolutely essential to rearing intersex children in psychologically healthful ways (regardless of the obvious difficulties provisional gender assignment presents in contemporary society). But the current concept of gender diversity does not include persons whose assigned gender is provisional. Therefore, our society's concept of gender diversity needs to be reconstructed to include persons whose Gender Assignment is provisional.

This is not merely an abstract point, a change needed in our society's dictionaries and philosophy departments. If taken seriously, it would impact numerous bureaucratic offices where official gender assignments are made. Persons whose Gender Assignment is provisional would have to be acknowledged, either by instituting a formal category for provisional Gender Assignment or by accepting the routine possibility of a change in Gender Assignment in order to provide appropriate record-keeping for those whose Gender Assignment is provisional. In fact, because this conceptual change also entails a distinction between the biological classification of persons and their Gender Assignment (since biological classification, as ordinarily understood, is life-long and does not change), this conceptual change would also challenge bureaucracies to change existing forms and records in order to take account of that distinction as well.

Nor would the reconstruction of the concept of Gender Assignment to include provisional assignment impact only official modes of Gender Assignment. If this reconstruction of concepts became part of the conceptual vocabulary of a whole society, then it would be routinely understood that any young person might be only provisionally a boy or a girl, and might in fact be carefully pondering which of the society's genders he or she most deeply identifies with. Not only parents and counselors, but caring persons of all sorts would not consider making humor of signs of gender ambiguity in a young person who has eventually to deal with so complex a personal choice; such parties might well offer their support for the child's experimenting with gender behavior. Embedding such a reconstructed concept into daily life would almost certainly mean that being assigned one's gender provisionally would not have to be so routinely hidden and that intersex persons could feel free to share their biological condition with select others without the fear that has ordinarily accompanied such a revelation.

And conversely, because the concepts people routinely accept shape their perceptions and expectations so profoundly, it is far less likely that these changes in behavior and conduct will come to pass without such a conceptual reconstruction.

It is also worth noting that the experience of transsexuals likewise suggests a need for a socially accepted conception of provisional Gender Assignment. As the next section will explain, the term "transsexual" will be used here to refer to persons whose sense of their own Gender Identity leads them choose to live their whole future lives within a gender other than the one to which they were assigned at birth (on the basis of unambiguous biological evidence), within which they were subsequently reared, and within which, ordinarily, they have already lived a significant portion of their adult lives. Such persons need to be able to "try out" the gender within which they believe they want to live. Reconstructing the concept of Gender Assignment to include provisional assignments would provide these persons with clear conceptual room for what they need to do in order for their choice of gender to be based on sound evidence of who they are. Thus, the bureaucratic and other social changes that would eventually accompany reconstruction of our concept of Gender Diversity to include provisional Gender Assignment would benefit the transsexual community in ways similar to the ways it would benefit the intersex community.

3.3 Gender Identity

3.3.1. What is Gender Identity?

A second way in which one can be categorized in terms of gender is by oneself. In a society that clearly has genders—whether two and only two, as in our case, or some other number—and in which everyone is constantly assigning everyone else to one of those genders and treating them accordingly, it is a very important component of a person's conception of self to determine which of the society's genders he or she identifies with, or whether his or her grasp of self as gendered is more complex than that. This component of self-definition or self-categorization is what is meant here by Gender Identity. (The expression "gender identity" has been part of the psychological literature since at least the 1960's, for example, in the work of Robert Stoller, who subsequently claimed to have coined the expression (Stoller, *Presentations*, 6). The definition of gender identity offered by John Money in 1972 is often cited in the literature (Money and Ehrhardt, *Man* 4). But more recent scholars, like Steven Smith, have questioned whether the early researchers sufficiently differentiated between affirmation of one's biological sex and identification with socially constructed genders. The concept of Gender Identity offered here stresses identification with the genders available in one's society.)

As has been indicated, the Intersex View is that determining one's Gender Identity can be a subtle matter and is, in any case, something quite personal, a matter chiefly of internal judgment about oneself, even if others' input is typically valuable in achieving it. Because the Gender Assignment of intersex children is provisional, there is no way that such children will not experience some measure of "distance" between how they are gender-assigned by others and who they understand themselves to be, even if this distance is only enforced by the question of whether they should continue to live within the gender to which they have been assigned. But for some intersex children, this sense of distance may be much greater because, for example, they find they are drawn to identify with the other gender. Clearly they will only be able to resolve their Gender Identity by an extended process of careful personal reflection, ideally aided by knowledgeable and sympathetic others.

Many people have little trouble accepting as their Gender Identity the gender that was officially assigned to them at birth and that others have routinely assigned to them since then. For such persons, there may seem to be little need to even discuss the topic of Gender Identity because Gender Assignment has seemed to be a process so straightforward, so unambiguous, and so public that Gender Identity and Gender Assignment are just two sides of exactly the same coin. But for persons who have experienced some distance between how they are gender-assigned by others and who they know themselves to be as gendered persons—that is, how closely or remotely they personally identify with the gender to which they are currently assigned by others—for such persons the categories of Gender Assignment (by others) and Gender Identity (one's understanding of oneself) are quite distinct.

Imagine, for example, a person whose growing understanding of self includes a strong identification with the feminine gender as it is culturally constructed in our society. Note in this connection that the genders in most contemporary societies are not so narrowly drawn that there is only one way to live acceptably within one or the other of them; it has already been observed that they admit of a wide range of acceptable individual variation. But at the same time, the two genders do have boundaries, and to say that someone identifies with the feminine gender is to say that this person determines that life lived within those boundaries makes the most personal sense, given this person's understanding of who he or she is.

We are imagining someone with a strong feminine gender identity, i.e., a strong identification with the feminine gender as it is constructed in his or her society. But suppose this person happened to be born with typical male biology. There is no guarantee (in spite of the assumptions of the ordinary view) that a male human will strongly identify with the masculine gender in that society and will therefore have a strongly masculine gender identity. Nor is there any guarantee that a female human will strongly identify with the feminine gender and have a strongly feminine Gender Identity. The person in our example, having been born with typical male biology, will have been assigned to the masculine gender at birth ("it's a boy") and the masculine gender will have been assigned to this person again and again, many times each day by other persons, including very important persons like parents and relatives, teachers, friends and playmates, etc. It will also have been affirmed by various other official Gender Assignment processes. Meanwhile, within this person's growing awareness of self will be the strong sense of identification with the society's feminine gender, along with the powerful social lesson from the ordinary view that no one can be a member of both the masculine and the feminine genders at the same time.

The inner lives of such persons are very difficult. The lesson they are learning from their society is that who they are from their own perspective is someone who is not supposed to be. They are not supposed to identify with the other gender and they are not supposed to have characteristics of both categories simultaneously. They are anomalous (an abstract word without much social impact); they are strange, they are weird, they are not to be affirmed as who they are. This is the lesson such a person learns over and over while growing up and while coming to grasp who they are from their own point of view.

Some persons undergoing such experiences may be able to bury this powerful negative about themselves for periods of time, and there may be some who succeed in burying it for life. But for many, whether born biologically typically male and strongly identifying with the society's feminine gender or born biologically typically female and strongly identifying with the society's masculine gender, this powerful negative is one of the most prominent realities of their lives.

Some such persons choose to live with the psychological pain of constantly being aware of the distance between who they are and who they are assigned to be, between their Gender Identity and how they are gender-assigned by others. Others, usually as they grow into adulthood or later, choose to change the way they live in order to live within the gender with which they identify. In order to do this, they know they must set aside the gender to which they have been assigned and within which they have lived all their previous lives. In doing this, because gender and Gender Assignment pervade so many aspects of human life, they may have to set aside many other elements of their previous lives, possibly including very important relationships if those persons cannot incorporate the person's change of gender into their lives. Persons who make such a thorough-going change and take up the other gender for the rest of their lives are now generally called *transsexuals,* whether the changes they make include changing their external genital anatomy or not. (Even into the last decade of the 20th century, the designation "transsexual" was reserved for persons choosing reconstructive surgery to make their genital anatomy correspond to the anatomy socially expected of their chosen gender. But today a significant percentage of both biologically typical males and biologically typical females who choose to live full time, not in the gender to which they were assigned at birth, but in the other gender with which they strongly identify, do not choose genital reconstructive surgery. Therefore the designation "transsexual" is more frequently used to refer to someone living full time in the chosen gender, regardless of the person's interest or lack of interest in genital reconstructive surgery.)

There is a second category of persons who experience a significant distance between who they are as gendered persons and who they are assigned to be. These are persons who will here be designated *bi-gendered.* Imagine someone born with typical male biology whose developing sense of self involves strong identification with *both* the masculine *and* the feminine genders of the society. There is no guarantee (in spite of the assumptions of the ordinary view) that a human child or adult will identify strongly with only one of the society's culturally established genders. In fact, every major city in the United States, Canada, and much of Europe, has a support group for males whom the public would likely designate as "cross-dressers." Informal estimates are that male cross-dressing is at least as frequent as 1 in every 2000 males in these societies. (This informal estimate is from one of the Chicago area support groups. The local support groups have had contact with at least 400 males who regularly cross-dress "fully," i.e., in full feminine attire and appearance. The support groups believe there is good reason to assume, given the profound stigma against males in feminine attire in American society, that "for every one we know of there are five to ten in the closet." Such estimates, combined with the number of males in the Chicago metropolitan area, lead to a conservative estimate of 1 in every 2000 males.)

Of course, not everyone who desires to wear the apparel of the other gender does so because he or she is bi-gendered in the sense employed here. There are people who find the other gender's clothing erotic, and there are people who cross-dress for the fun or the drama of it. In addition, among bi-gendered males, for example, some *strongly* identify with the feminine gender as well as with the masculine gender, others genuinely identify with the feminine gender but not as strongly, and so on. That is, not all bi-gendered persons are "50/50," so to speak; some are "70/30" or "80/20," but identify strongly enough with the feminine gender to express this identification in significant ways from time to time. But for those who do strongly identify with both genders—those in the "60/40" to "40/60" range, so to speak—the challenge of reconciling the experience of oneself as gendered (i.e., bi-gendered) with the rules and expectations of the binary gender system of contemporary societies is very significant.

Like the transsexuals described above, such bi-gendered persons have inner lives that are often very difficult. The lesson that they, too, are learning from their society is that who they are is someone who is not supposed to be. Their sense of themselves as gendered persons, that is, as identifying strongly with *both* of the society's genders, is so distant from accepted ways of living as to be literally inconceivable. There is no room for it in the concepts of the ordinary view.

Some of these persons may be able to bury this powerful negative about themselves for periods of time, and there may be some who succeed in burying it for life. But like transsexuals, many bi-gendered persons find that they eventually need to take action in order to be true to their personal experience of who they are. In one sense, bi-gendered persons have even fewer options than transsexuals because switching genders will not enable them to affirm their reality. There is no place in the ordinary view for someone who is *both* deeply masculine and deeply feminine, both a man and a woman. Given the very real boundaries between the genders in contemporary Western societies, the bi-gendered person must always, at any given time, live in and be assigned by others to one and only one of the genders that the person deeply identifies with. (There are a few bi-gendered persons who have tried to construct a third path, trying to live and be accepted by others in androgyny, that is, in a blending of culturally masculine and culturally feminine modes that aims to affirm both genders and express both simultaneously. But contemporary Western societies do not affirm such a third path, and few people have the resources, the opportunity, or the support of caring persons in their lives to be able to attempt this.)

Therefore, for most bi-gendered persons, taking action to affirm a dual gender identity means finding ways for each aspect of one's personality to be expressed for a period of time by turns, alternately living out the person's identification with one of the society's genders and then the other, the best the person can. For most bi-gendered males, this means living most of the time in the masculine gender (since this is the gender to which a bi-gendered male was assigned at birth and within which he was reared and has lived) and then living for very limited amounts of time in the feminine gender, either wholly in private out of fear of the common societal stigma against males presenting themselves publicly as women, or with occasional, discrete activities in public as a woman. (Aside from the aim of joining together persons dealing with the same challenges, the first aim of the support groups for bi-gendered males is to provide safe opportunities for the members to express themselves as women outside their homes. The existing support groups for bi-gendered persons are organizations for bi-gendered males. While numbers of many biological females who are transitioning permanently into the masculine gender, i.e., who would commonly be designated as "FtoM transsexuals" or "transmen," has grown recently to be comparable to the number of biological males transitioning permanently into the feminine gender, "MtoF transsexuals" or "transwomen," there is no dependable evidence suggesting significant numbers of bi-gendered females nor any pattern of support groups for bi-gendered females comparable to those for bi-gendered males.)

A third category of persons who experience a significant distance between who they are as gendered persons and how they are assigned are those who experience that distance as a deep alienation from both genders as their society has constructed them. There is no way that such people can escape being gender-assigned when they interact with others; therefore their sense of distance and alienation from their society's gender categories is constantly being reinforced. Nor is there any simple way to decline to participate in a society's genders globally, and so persons in this category of Gender Identity may try to express their rejection of their society's genders by selecting among the markers of gender in the society and deliberately "mis-using" them or mixing them across genders in deliberately meaningless combinations, the visual and/or behavioral equivalent of gibberish. Both for those who express themselves in this way, of course, such expressions are not meaningless at all, but deliberately meaningful. Their hope is to communicate their rejection of their society's genders as those genders have been constructed. One expression that some persons who relate to genders in this way use to designate themselves is "genderqueer." These three categories, and any other groups who experience a significant distance between who they are as gendered persons and how they are assigned by others, are often collectively designated by the general term "transgendered."

Two additional points need to be made about Gender Identity before considering the implications of this concept for intersex persons. First, although there is disagreement about the matter within contemporary societies and it is something that has not been systematically studied, there is nevertheless wide agreement among transgendered persons, and among many of those who provide mental health services to the transgendered community (although there is very little data about the genderqueer community) that Gender Identity should be thought of as an *orientation,* in the same sense in which this word is used in regard to sexual orientation. That is, Gender Identity is best described as a deeply embedded characteristic of a human being that (a) is present from his or her earliest awareness of him- or herself as being gender-assigned and as identifying with society's genders, and therefore as needing to incorporate gender into his or her understanding of self; and (b) does not ordinarily change across his or her lifetime.

Second, it is important to note how dependent these kinds of discussions of identity are on the use of the words *he/she, her/him his/her,* etc. In English these words only come in gender-assigned forms: *he/him/himself/his* and *she/her/herself/hers.* In some languages, there are pronouns that mean simply *the person*, without gender-assignment in the very saying of the words. But for speakers of English, whenever a word of this sort is needed, one *cannot avoid assigning* gender to the person referred to. In addition, these same words are used, in ordinary speech, to assign persons to *biological* categories, i.e., *female* and *male.* There would be no problem here, of course, if these aspects of life—biological categorization, gender-assignment of a person, and the person's gender-identity—always matched up perfectly. But they do not always match up perfectly. So the English language and every other language whose pronouns are typically gendered has significant potential for describing people incorrectly.

This fact about the English language is not just a matter of inconvenience for speakers who want to speak accurately when discussing intersex or bi-gendered persons. Much more importantly, it shapes people's thinking in English-speaking and linguistically similar cultures, leading people to believe without noticing it that everyone's Gender Identity *is* either masculine or feminine and that, in regard to *biological* characteristics, everyone *is* either simply male or simply female. These mistaken assumptions of the Ordinary View are taken for granted by, and seem therefore to be supported by, the use of gendered pronouns in English and similar languages.

3.3.2. Gender Identity and Intersex Persons

The fact that gender is such a simple and obvious component of most people's sense of who they are—i.e., because they do not experience significant distance between their Gender Identity and their assigned gender—will make it that much harder for those who raise and counsel intersex children to communicate with them about the provisional nature of their Gender Assignment at birth and about the need for them to reflect carefully in order to determine, in due course, what their Gender Identity is. The existence of transsexuals in the population may make it easier for a young intersex person to understand that his or her provisional gender may not be the one he or she might choose when such choice is called for. Indeed mature and caring transsexuals may make valuable role models for intersex persons considering or facing such a choice.

Similarly, the existence of bi-gendered persons in the population may make it easier for a young intersex person to live with the ambiguity of his or her biological gifts. In a society focused on binary categories, intersex individuals may find it consoling to learn that there is another class of persons besides themselves who experience themselves as "both/and" when society tells them that everyone is "either/or." In fact, given the importance for each intersex child to carefully consider, in age appropriate ways, his or her measure of comfort in living within the other gender role, relationships with the bi-gendered community and an acceptance of persons who move comfortably in and out of the society's two genders may be educationally valuable. At the same time, the extent to which the stigma against males presenting themselves in culturally feminine ways and the fact that this keeps most bi-gendered males in the closet or active only in the safe havens of support groups may mean that bi-gendered males may have little to offer intersex persons hoping for social acceptance of their situation. This is something to be carefully considered until such time as both groups are accepted as valuable members of the human family. On the other hand, there is certainly significant potential for political alliances between the intersex community and the transgendered community.

In addition to these possible practical benefits, there are two important conceptual benefits to the intersex community that a careful consideration the varieties of Gender Identity within the human family reveals. First, the claim of the intersex community that the determination of an intersex person's gender needs to be the result of a thoughtful choice *by that person* is strongly reinforced by the experience of transgendered persons. As indicated in Part One, the reason for this claim is not simply an argument from the value of self-determination. A more important reason is that, for persons who need to choose their gender because it is not obvious to them, gender needs to be chosen on the basis of their own experience of who they are as gendered people—whether that experience suggests to them that they identify with their society's feminine gender, that they identify with their society's masculine gender, that they identify deeply with both, or perhaps that they identify with neither.

Second, reflection on the varieties of Gender Identity in the human community should serve to remind intersex persons and those who counsel them that not everyone will find that he or she identifies solely with one of his or her society's two genders. Some people identify strongly with both of their society's genders, i.e., are bi-gendered, and intersex persons of this sort will need to deal with their situation in much the same way that bi-gendered persons with typical male or typical female biology must do. It is in this case, moreover, that mature bi-gendered persons may serve as valuable role models to intersex persons. Others in the intersex community may determine that they are deeply alienated from both of their society's genders. Even if the number of bi-gendered or genderqueer persons within the intersex community is quite limited, as it seems to be in the general population, it is important for intersex persons and their counselors to remember that some intersex children may discover that this is who they are.

3.3.3. Gender Identity and Diversity

It scarcely needs repeating that diversity in the ordinary view does not include persons whose Gender Identity does not match their biology. And it certainly does not include persons whose sense of their gender is that they are strongly both masculine and feminine—both cultural men and cultural women—even if practical needs press them to express themselves in each gender only by turns. And it does not include persons who strongly reject both genders.

The intersex community obviously needs the concept of Gender Diversity to include persons whose gender does not match their biology, because intersex persons' special biological gifts do not accord with the bipolar categorization of gendered people that the ordinary view proclaims. But the intersex community also needs a concept of Gender Diversity in which Gender Identity is distinct from Gender Assignment, as was stressed in the previous section, and this latter need opens the door to experiences of Gender Identity that are not limited to identification solely with the masculine gender or identification solely with the feminine. But why should the intersex community go the next step? Why include in its reconstruction of Gender Diversity the whole range of experiences of Gender Identity, including possibility of bi-gendered persons and genderqueer persons? In principle, it would seem that the intersex community might be able to get along without this more radical challenge to the ordinary view. So what is to be gained by reconstructing Gender Diversity this much?

There are three reasons why the intersex community's reconstruction of Gender Diversity should include the whole range of experiences of Gender Identity, including a place for bi-gendered persons and genderqueer persons. The first is that some intersex persons will, in the normal course of human development, be bi-gendered or genderqueer. Perhaps the intersex community can exclude bi-gendered and genderqueer intersex persons from its conceptual scheme as effectively over time as the ordinary view has excluded intersex persons hitherto. But ought it to? When the purpose of reconstructing the intersex community's—and eventually the whole community's—conceptual system is to render it more inclusive, does it make sense to knowingly exclude small minorities from the beginning, just because they are, so to speak, even more different than the rest?

The answer to the rhetorical question just posed should be "no." The explanation of that negative answer is the second reason that the intersex community's reconstruction of Gender Diversity should include a place for bi-gendered and genderqueer persons. Namely, consistency makes moral demands on those who argue for more inclusion. It requires that they ask whether there are others besides themselves who are being excluded from the ordinary view. The intersex community should work for the reconstruction of the concept of Gender Diversity so that it includes every type of Gender Identity and every pattern of human biology and every blend of these components of identity within the human family. To do otherwise is to pick and choose among the candidates for inclusion in a way that will not withstand the charge of moral arbitrariness.

The third reason is the important practical and educational benefits that have already been described, benefits which the intersex community will reap from a concept of Gender Diversity that includes the whole range of experiences of Gender Identity. Intersex children with a provisionally assigned gender will need the freedom to imagine themselves living within the other gender and possibly in other ways, and to experiment with such living in age appropriate ways. In order to do this, they will need to understand that persons who live in both genders and who seek to live in neither exist and can be valued members of the human family. In addition, some of them will change genders at the appropriate time. They will therefore need to know that there are persons who change genders in order to live in the gender with which they most deeply identify, even if they must thereby set aside a gender in which they have been assigned for years, and that such persons can also be valued members of the human community.

It might seem that these practical and educational benefits may be available without reconstruction of the relevant concepts. But that would profoundly underestimate the power of the conceptual frameworks that humans employ to make sense of their lives. The only alternative to conceptual reconstruction would be to hope that, if intersex children experience distance (as those whose gender is genuinely understood as provisional are almost certain to), such distance would come to be interpreted as being within the range of normal individual variation between the two existing genders, for such variation is expected and tolerated in the ordinary view. But the intersex community needs much more conceptual room to understand its situation, and its children need much more conceptual room in which to grow and to discover who they are, than this interpretation of their experience can provide.

3.4 Gender Expression

3.4.1. What is Gender Expression?
Gender clearly concerns how we humans express ourselves in action, speech, carriage, dress, ornament, etc. The importance of these and other publicly observable marks of gender are the principal determinants of a person's informal Gender Assignment by others. These expressions of Gender Assignment and/or Gender Identity in action, speech, carriage, dress, ornament, etc., constitute what will here be termed Gender Expression.

Almost everyone engages, with greater self-awareness or less, in connecting his or her self-presentation to the accepted patterns of action, speech, carriage, dress, ornament, etc., associated with his or her society's genders. For most people most of the time, such Gender Expression indicates an affirmative connection with the society's genders; i.e., the person aims to be assigned one of the society's genders and expresses him- or herself accordingly. But there are also circumstances in which a person chooses to "mis-use" some elements of the accepted expressive repertoire in order to challenge either the accepted patterns of expression or to question some other aspect of the boundaries of the existing genders in the society. But both affirmative and challenging forms of expression depend for their communicative impact on there being accepted modes of gendered self-presentation in the society.

Most humans find it very difficult to affirm in themselves something that is not also affirmed by others around them. For this reason, the publicly observable marks of gender are also important symbols to the person of who he or she understands him- or herself to be as a gendered person. Gender Expression is not only important in regard to Gender Assignment, it is also important from the point of view of Gender Identity as well.

One reason for distinguishing Gender Expression from both Gender Assignment and Gender Identity is that a person's expression may not be consistent with his or her Gender Identity. If a person's Gender Identity is at odds with his or her Gender Assignment, the person might engage in expression consistent with the assignment in order to hide the mismatch or avoid the impact of improper expression. But in doing so the person might well experience conflict and psychological pain by reason of the mismatch between his or her Gender Identity and what is expressed. So there is descriptive value in discussing Gender Expression as a separate concept.

There are also situations in which a person's Gender Expression may not be consistent with how he or she is Gender Assigned. For example, expression inconsistent with a person's Gender Assignment is ordinarily considered acceptable at a costume party, as when a woman (a person gender-assigned in the feminine gender) wears the costume of a man (clothing etc. typically associated with the masculine gender), or vice-versa. But in other settings, expression inconsistent with assignment may be severely stigmatized, as has long been the case in the United States for males wearing feminine clothing and makeup unless there are special, excusing circumstances like a costume party.

All three categories of transgendered persons described in the previous section regularly experience a mismatch between identity and expression. Many trans-sexuals, for example, grow up with profound awareness of their being assigned to a gender with which they do not identify, awareness of their identification with the gender to which they are not assigned, and awareness that they therefore cannot easily express. If a person who experiences such a mismatch begins to experiment with living within the other gender, one of the first things he or she will do is begin to employ the expressions associated with the other gender in his or her self-presentation, both to affirm identification with that gender in his or her own self-awareness and, if the person eventually ventures into public, in order to be affirmed in that gender by others.

Bi-gendered persons similarly use the modes of Gender Expression associated with the two genders to "move back and forth," usually living most of their lives within one gender, but changing modes of expression (i.e., "cross-dressing") in order to experience living in the other gender for a time. In fact, in a society with two and only two genders with definite boundaries, bi-gendered persons are not ordinarily able to simultaneously employ the expressions of both of the genders with which they identify. That is why, for want of a better expression, they can be described as "moving back and forth." But they do so only in regard to Gender Expression. From the point of Gender Identity, bi-gendered persons are always identifying strongly with both of the society's two genders. In regard to their sense of who they are, in other words, bi-gendered people are "always cross-dressed," never in a position to express all of their sense of who they are as gendered persons.

Genderqueer persons take advantage of the impossibility of culturally expressing both genders simultaneously in their expression of who they are. They will often deliberately combine mis-matched modes of expression from both genders to express their alienation from and rejection of both.

It should also be clear, from what was said in the previous section, that it would be a serious mistake to think that a transsexual or bi-gendered person's expression of another gender is simply a matter of clothing or other aspects of external appearance, even though bi-gendered persons are often referred to by the term "cross-dresser." But what such a person is doing is something far more personally significant than putting clothes on one's body. This use of gender-typical clothing and ornament is an expression of the person's identity to him- or herself, and it is an expression of her or his Gender Identity to the rest of the human family. (Even if done exclusively in private out of fear of the social stigma, such use of Gender Expression to affirm Gender Identity has an implicit social significance.) For this reason, it is also a mistake to think that transsexuals and bi-gendered persons who cross-dress and engage in other activities of Gender Expression within the gender different from their assigned role are trying to deceive others. What they are expressing in their efforts to participate in the currently chosen gender is an aspect of their own reality that they experience, in fact, as profoundly *true*. Far from being a lie, their actions are for them an effort to live their whole truth.

There remains, of course, a serious potential for conflict if other persons encounter transgendered persons "cross-dressed" and happen to recognize the mismatch between their current mode of Gender Expression and their assigned gender. Observers may "read" the transsexual or the bi-gendered person, perceiving the male "behind" the feminine presentation or the female "behind" the masculine. Such perceptions are extremely fallible. But even when they involve a correct biological judgment, they miss the most important point for the person engaged in presenting him- or herself in this way.

The purpose of these examples is to underline the fact that there are many members of the human family whose experience requires a clear distinction between Gender Expression and both Gender Identity and Gender Assignment. The narrow conceptual framework of the ordinary view leads to the conclusion that, except for the idiosyncrasies of people's individual differences in taste and style, Gender Expression flows simply and obviously from Gender Assignment and Gender Identity, which are never seriously at odds. A more inclusive conceptual framework would provide more room for people of diverse physical and personal characteristics to express their Gender Identity in ways that are personally affirming and likely to lead others to assign to them the gender they identify with and are seeking to express, or to lead others to acknowledge their alienation from both genders.

3.4.2. Gender Expression and Intersex Persons

The activities of Gender Expression are obviously not valuable for their own sake, at least from the point of view of gender. They are means, and because of this they may seem to deserve much less attention than what they are a means to, namely Gender Identity and Gender Assignment. But the role of Gender Expression in human experience is closely analogous to the role of the languages we speak.

Language is, in one sense, "only" a means of communication; but it is not only one of the principal means of communication, but it is so intimate to the process of communication that the particular features of specific languages shape not only what can be communicated, but how the world is perceived and understood by those who speak that language. In a very similar way, Gender Expression is so intimate to the experiences of Gender Assignment and Gender Identity that it significantly shapes how gender is experienced, perceived, and understood. In this respect, mere means though they are, the role of the elements of Gender Expression in the lives of intersex persons should not be underestimated, especially when those persons are young and living chiefly within a provisionally assigned gender, but also during their adolescent and young adult years when identity issues begin to be deeply addressed and experimentation in Gender Expression may be appropriate or even essential to their choosing a gender wisely for themselves.

One particular value of the concept of Gender Expression is its usefulness in explaining intersex persons' situation, both to themselves and to others they consider deserving of an explanation. For it is likely that most intersex persons will experience significant ambiguity in regard to gender. One reason is the Ordinary View's assumption, which intersex persons will find operative all around them, that Gender Assignment and Gender Identity follow necessarily from biological classification as male or female. They will know, in age appropriate ways, that they are different, and they will need concepts to explain this difference to themselves and to certain others. They will also need concepts with which to challenge the negative value judgments that so often accompany the experience of difference.

Distinguishing Gender Assignment and Gender Identity will enable intersex people to articulate the difference between who they are in others' eyes and who they are becoming from their own perspective. But they cannot go through life in their society expressing no gender at all, so they will have attend to Gender Expression, i.e., to take a stance on how to present themselves to others and, unavoidably, on how they will relate these modes of self-expression to the society's two genders. The concept of Gender Expression, taught carefully in age-appropriate ways, will enable to them understand how gender-typical expressions can be used to express their provisionally assigned gender, can be used to test other gender possibilities when that is appropriate, and can later be used to express whichever gender they thoughtfully choose to live in thereafter. Gender Expression is not linked to Gender Assignment by some rigid necessity; it is something chosen by a person in order to be affirmed and accepted (Gender Assignment) and in due course to present oneself to the world as one is (Gender Identity). Giving this concept its conceptual due will enable intersex persons and those who rear and advise them to shape their understanding of these matters in ways far better suited to the experience of intersex persons than the ordinary view.

Giving serious attention to the distinction between Gender Expression, Gender Identity, and Gender Assignment will also help parents and counselors articulate what is being considered when, at an appropriate age, intersex children experiment with gender possibilities. In addition to exercising their imagination about who they might be or become if they were living within the other gender, or both genders, or none, intersex children might also experiment with the elements of Gender

Expression associated with the other gender. It is possible that intersex children may experiment in public in order to experience being assigned the other gender (temporarily and as part of the experiment) by others. The point here is not to presume the merits of these as educational experiences for intersex children, but to point out the value of a clear concept of Gender Expression in describing and evaluating them.

3.4.3. Gender Expression and Diversity

The ordinary view associates all diversity with individual differences of taste and style within the two genders as biologically determined. This fact, plus the reality that Gender Expression is "only" a means of expressing Gender Assignment and Gender Identity, can suggest that accepting diversity in people's expression of their gender is simply a matter of greater open-mindedness and not something deserving of significant intellectual effort. All that should be needed, it might seem, is more flexibility on everyone's part and, for those who find this hard, words of persuasion to assist them. But the point of this essay is that profound changes in the concepts our society uses are needed if we are to take serious account of the experience of intersex persons, as well as transsexuals and bi-gendered persons and the rest of the transgendered community.

Now that Gender Expression has been carefully examined, it is possible to gather these separate thoughts together and explain more clearly just how profound a change in the conceptual framework is being proposed. For the diversity that is needed is not just the diversity of including some people who have previously been left out and thereby broadening of the range of gender appropriate assignments and identities that this would necessitate. It is not, even, the broader diversity of including persons with provisional assignments, and therefore including the very possibility of provisional assignments themselves. Nor is it even the broader diversity of including persons whose Gender Identity is understood in terms of deep identification with both genders—i.e., those who "move back and forth" between the two genders at different times, and who thus forge conceptual room for intersex persons who experiment with living in the two genders or who are bi-gendered themselves (or who determine that they identify with neither of the society's genders). Rather, the diversity needed to make conceptual room for intersex persons also requires a conceptual change in how we understand Gender Expression.

For the people we are talking about are people for whom Gender Expression is something deliberately undertaken, not something that, as the ordinary view sees it, flows automatically from one's Gender Assignment and the Gender Identity that necessarily flows from that. Gender Expression, as described here, is always in some sense an experiment, always a testing of personal and social experience in search of identity. Even when an intersex person has thoughtfully chosen a gender to live within, even when that choice has been confirmed over and over for many years, that way of living will always be a choice, never anything automatically set by biology. And the evidence for that choice is chiefly the evidence of the person's own deepest experience, experience that affirms how he or she is living, presenting him or herself to the world, and being received and affirmed (or not) by others. Because that evidence is always continually coming in, because it could conceivably change tomorrow, because who I am as a gendered person has been experienced radically by the intersex person as something contingent, not fixed (as it has by the transgendered person as well), it follows that the concept of Gender Diversity that is needed is one in which all Gender Expression is itself optional, changeable, a matter of choice.

Finally, it is worth noting that nothing fundamental would be lost to those who are not intersex if this broadened concept of Gender Expression were adopted throughout contemporary societies. All those whose gender and gender experience is currently well described by the common view will be included just as adequately in the broadened conception of Gender Diversity here advocated. Indeed it is possible that this broadened understanding of Gender Expression would enhance everyone's understanding of their own gender and of the meaning of Gender Assignment, Gender Identity, and Gender Expression in their lives. But making that case is a task for another time.

4. CONCLUSION: ON ALLIANCES

The point was made earlier that much of the work of formulating the conceptions of Gender Assignment, Gender Identity, and Gender Expression offered here has been done in close collaboration with the transgendered community. For obvious reasons, transgendered persons need to challenge many of the same the assumptions of the ordinary view that the intersex community challenges. This suggests is that there are strong reasons for a much closer alliance between the intersex advocacy community and the transgendered community than has developed up to the present.

The intersex advocacy community has focused its strategic efforts, for understand-able reasons, on providing education and better support for intersex persons and for the parents of intersex children, and on changing the medical community's views about how intersex infants should be treated by physicians in their infancy and their early years. The evidence presented by adult intersex persons whose medical treatment as children has produced significant suffering for them, and the absence of long-term evidence to support the claim that the standard modes of medical intervention for intersex infants produce dependable long-term benefits for those treated, are matters that the intersex advocacy community justly focuses on as it seeks to change how physicians think and respond to intersex persons.

But such efforts have an inherent practical limit unless they also include addressing the conceptual differences that separate the Ordinary View from what has here been called the Intersex View. At some point it will occur either to parties in the medical community or to others in the larger society that the practical changes in treatment, education, and mental health care being advocated by the intersex community presuppose a profound shift in the conceptual framework. The clearer this shift becomes, the more politically powerful will be the absence of a clearly articulated alternative for the intersex community. The Intersex View needs to be carefully formulated, using the account offered here or some other account as a starting point. To be sure, the system of concepts articulated in this essay may need significant adjustment before a conceptual framework is found that fully expresses what the intersex community presupposes about gender, Gender Assignment, Gender Identity, and Gender Expression. But an adequate set of concepts about these things is not only an intellectual need—for clearer education, support, and evaluation of practical initiatives—but also a strategic need for the long run.

Therefore, in closing, it seems important to urge the intersex community to seek alliances with others to whom these concepts are similarly crucial. And the first such group that comes to mind is the same group whose work to date has served as a starting point for this essay, the transgendered community. It may be understandable if the intersex community consciously held back from association with the transgendered community when it began its strategic dialogue with the medical community. Strategic decisions need to be made in terms of political impact, especially when resources are scarce. Thus it has been possible for intersex advocates to talk to medical professionals often in very scientific terms about the harm that surgical interventions in infancy have done to some and about the absence of long-term evidence that such interventions are dependably beneficial to intersex persons over the course of their lives. But the position of the intersex community, even in these efforts, presupposes profoundly different views of gender, Gender Assignment, Gender Identity, and Gender Expression from the views of those whose practice they are seeking to change. While it may be strategically useful to temporarily mute the discussion of such fundamental differences, these differences will come out in time.

It is therefore proposed that the intersex community begin an active discussion of the conceptual framework about gender and Gender Diversity that lies behind their practical initiatives and, in doing so, that it work for closer alliances with those in the transgendered community who are engaged in similar efforts. The immediate beneficiaries, in a variety of ways, will be the members of the intersex and transgendered communities. But eventually such efforts will bring us closer to a set of concepts about gender and diversity that will make it more likely that all people, whatever their biological and gender differences, are accepted as respected members of one human family.

David Ozar, Department of Philosophy and Center for Ethics, Loyola University, Chicago, IL, U. S. A.

REFERENCES

Boylan, Jennifer Finney. *She's Not There: A Life in Two Genders*. New York: Broadway Books, 2002.

Brown, Mildred L. *True Selves: Understanding Transsexualism–For Families, Friends, Coworkers, and Helping Professionals*. San Francisco: Jossey-Bass, 1996.

Bullough, Vern L., and Bonnie Bullough. *Cross Dressing, Sex, and Gender*. Philadelphia:University of Pennsylvania Press, 1993.

Colapinto, John. *As Nature Made Him: The Boy Who Was Raised As a Girl*. New York:Harper Collins, 2000.

David, Fred. *Fashion, Culture, and Identity*. Chicago: University of Chicago Press, 1992.

Doctor, Richard F. *Transvestites and Transsexuals: Toward a Theory of Cross-Gender Behavior*. New York: Plenum Press, 1988.

Dreger, Alice Domurat. *Hermaphrodites and the Medical Invention of Sex*. Cambridge MA: Harvard University Press, 1998.

Dreger, Alice Domurat, editor. *Intersex in the Age of Ethics*. Hagerstown MD: University Publishing Group, 1999.

Ettner, Randi. *Gender Loving Care: A Guide to Counseling Gender-Variant Clients*. New York: W. W. Norton, 1999.

Herdt, Gilbert H. "Mistaken Gender: 5-alpha Reductase Hermaphroditism and Biological Reductionism in Sexual Identity Reconsidered." *American Anthropologist* 92: 433-446.

Herdt, Gilbert H. *Third Sex, Third Gender: Beyond Sexual Dimorphism in Culture and History*. New York: Zone Books, 1994.

Intersex Society of North America. *Redefining Sex: A Half Hour Documentary on theMedical Management of Children with Ambiguous Sex Anatomy*. Videorecording. Rohnert Park CA, 2000.

Intersex Society of North America. *Total Patient Care: The Child with an IntersexCondition*. Video-recording. Rohnert Park CA, 2002.

Intersex Society of North America. Website at: www.isna.org

Kessler, Suaznna J. *Lessons from the Interesexed*. New Brunswick NJ: Rutgers University Press, 1998.

Les Ballets Trockadero de Monte Carlo. Website at: www.trockadero.org

Margolis, Diane Rothbard. *The Fabric of Self: A Theory of Ethics and Emotions*. New Haven: Yale University Press, 1998.

Money, John, and A. A. Ehrhardt. *Man & Woman Boy & Girl*. Baltimore: Johns Hopkins University Press, 1972.

Ozar, David. "Harming by Exclusion: On the Standard Concepts of Sexual Orientation, Sex, and Gender" in *Sexual Diversity and Catholicism: Toward the Development of Moral Theology*. Collegeville MN The Liturgical Press, 2001.

Roughgarden, Joan. *Evolution's Rainbow: Diversity, Gender, and Sexuality in Nature And People*. Berkeley CA: University of California Press, 2004.

Smith, Steven G. *Gender Thinking*. Philadelphia PA: Temple University Press, 1992.

Stoller, Robert J. "A Contribution to the Study of Gender Identity." *International Journal of Psychoanalysis* 49 (1964): 364-368.

Stoller, Robert J. *Presentations of Gender*. New Haven: Yale University Press, 1985.

J. DAVID HESTER

INTERSEX AND THE RHETORICS OF HEALING

What constitutes femaleness? It is my considered position that femaleness is conferred by the final pair of XX chromosomes. Otherwise I don't know what it is…I would not agree with you therefore that CAIS individuals are women, i.e., female...

–Germaine Greer, Letter to Father of Complete Androgen Insensitivity Syndrome (CAIS) daughter

1. INTRODUCTION

Intersex children are born into a state of liminality,[1] a state wherein their "deviation" from physiological norms is understood, in social, legal, religio-ethical, and medical terms, as "illness." The naturalized assumption of an exclusively binary sex system (male/female), informed in the West by a biblically derived view of heterosexual marriage as God-ordained in creation, continues to play itself out in other institutions. Western legal systems, with their roots in property and family law, deny the legal status of intersex[2] by requiring the individual to be identified either as male or female[3] according to chromosomal gender.[4] Christian moral responses to intersex are framed within context of sexual ethics that views intersexuality as a result of the "fallen" state of humankind; such responses often discuss intersexuality in relation to moral issues concerning homosexuality.[5] Even counter-culture critics such as feminists and queer theorists have responded to the liminal state of intersex by shoring up their own agendas: Feminists like Germain Greer respond with a reactionary rejection of intersex people as "not real women";[6] transgender and gender theorists respond by subsuming intersex to another political agenda.[7] To be neither clearly male nor clearly female is to elicit a profoundly powerful reaction from our society that does not know what to do with sexed "deviations" that undermine fundamental assumptions upon which major social, legal and moral systems have been based.

Intersex people begin their lives in liminality, and are threatened with social and legal sanction if they do not conform to the gender binary of the dominant society. Accordingly, the dominant values of the community take supremacy in medical

S.E. Sytsma (Ed.), Ethics and Intersex, 47–71.

decision-making, placing the physician in a context that predisposes certain medical responses: to view the body of the intersex person as a "problem" in need of fixing, as a psychosocial emergency in need of medical intervention, a "disease" in need of a cure. The medical-industrial complex, which includes not only hospitals and clinics, but also professional societies, medical technology manufacturers, pharmaceutical companies, textbook and standard reference publishers, institutions of learning, and even insurance companies,[8] is dedicated (in the industrial North) to providing services for "correcting" the indices of gender ambiguity in order to render the body "normal," often through surgical intervention and hormone therapy.[9] But it is through this sculpting that pathology of the body arises: Liminality is not erased by this intervention, but is reinforced through a pathology of medical practices that renders the body of the intersexed unnatural and suspicious, even after intervention.

What are the responses available to the intersexed when confronted by these (and other) overwhelming forces of "illness"? What are the rhetorics of healing they employ to create for themselves a community of safety wherein they can choose to develop their own identities and find support? What lessons can we learn about the pitfalls and struggles of healing that confront those whose bodies do not conform to the binary heterosexist paradigm? Answers to these questions will bring us new insights into the rhetorics and strategies of "healing" and the relationship of "curing" to "healing."

2. FRAMEWORKS OF HEALING

Strategies to confront the issue of the liminal position of the intersexed have taken two major forms. The first is the creation of a rhetorical space (i.e., a performative-diagnostic space generated most often through the rhetoric of the attending physicians) wherein an intersex condition is not recognized as a pathology or developmental deviation, or if recognized as such, is nevertheless accepted without recourse to immediate medical intervention. This was historically the predominant, if also at times not unproblematic, response by those attending births up through the late 19th century in Europe and America. This approach is still taken today, to an ever-decreasing extent, in mostly non-urban and non-Western settings. Sometimes the rhetorical space is the result of a lack of knowledge or recognition of intersex conditions by those in attendance. Sometimes it occurs through the happenstance of the birth and registration of the infant outside the medical system. It can also be the result of the parents' direct rejection of physicians' attempts to create an alternative rhetorical space, namely, a space of trauma and pathology. Regardless of its origins, the result is the minimization of the pathological experience of liminality by means of a rhetorical space of "acceptance" of people for who and what they are, and not for what they ought to become. A process of naturalization generates processes wherein "healing" is not "healing from," but living comfortably and healthily with oneself as intersex.

Alternatively, marginalization is overcome through direct confrontation of forces of social and medical management seeking to eradicate difference. This usually results from the experiences of those who, at birth, were identified as intersex and for whom medical management and surgical intervention were agreed upon (by both parents and physicians) and enacted. In reaction, intersexed individuals come together to create a rhetorical space of "healing" that is "healing from." However, the circumstances in respect to which the "healing" takes place are not the individuals' intersex identities, but the medical practices whose intentions are to bring them into conformity with the binary gender system. By addressing the strategies that have fostered illness, many intersex people develop counter-strategies of healing that include confronting silence and isolation by seeking out and/ or creating communities of support. Marginalization is eradicated through the rhetorical strategies of outreach, education, and fashioning new facets of identity. Rhetorics of healing emphasize truth-telling, seek to overcome isolation, and reject pathological labels and practices that have dominated the discourse.

In what follows, we will explore several examples of the rhetorics of healing. Drawing from resources made available through the advent of Internet technology,[10] we will turn to the many first-person stories of intersexed individuals and parents of intersexed children, as well as to the discussion-forums hosted by new communities of intersexed identities. Due directly to the advent of this new form of communication, individuals and groups have developed an unprecedented level of outreach, education and advocacy previously unavailable to them. As we consider examples of these developments, we will apply the broad framework outlined above, a framework consisting of non-pathological identity on one hand and anti-pathological identity on the other.

3. RHETORICS OF HEALING: NON-PATHOLOGICAL IDENTITIES

There is very little direct evidence for or against the success of the psychosocial paradigm of the medical management of intersex. Long-term studies of the effects of the current medical practices of rapid gender assignment, surgical intervention, and routine non-disclosure are only just beginning to be proposed. Evidence for or against the long-term effectiveness of early medical and surgical interventions, despite 50 years in which such interventions have been widely practiced, is simply incomplete or non-existent.

On the one hand, this lack of evidence suggests the necessarily tentative and experimental nature of current medical management practices, and it raises a host of ethical and legal questions concerning how physicians represent the results of their interventions. On the other hand, what little follow-up evidence has been published, both directly related to the results of the protocol upon the intersexed and indirectly reflecting it by reference to the long-term effects of the surgical procedures, suggests some very real risks for those who are under the management of doctors dedicated to the interventionist paradigm.

This situation has led to the current state of intersex research and medical practice, a state characterized by a dawning cultural awareness that has been fostered by the patient-advocacy groups first established with the advent of the Internet.

Advocates are beginning to question the medical, theoretical, and ethical soundness of the last 50 years of the dominant modern medical paradigm.

Physicians, however, when confronted with arguments for the rejection of the paradigm, often counter with two arguments of their own: First, they employ an argument from silence as evidence of positive surgical and psychosocial outcomes. Since they have not received negative feedback from the vast majority of their patients, these patients must be doing well. Those from whom they have received complaints must therefore represent a vocal minority.

Second, they suggest that doing nothing with the infants would wreak social and psychological damage for both the patients and their families. While the first argument is currently being addressed by the several long-term studies finally underway in the United States and elsewhere, it is the latter assertion that concerns us here.

The claim that non-medical and non-surgical intervention would result in social and psychological damage is, at its heart, a value judgment premised upon several naturalized presumptions. These include the presumption that the binary sex-gender system is self-evident, that variations therefrom are pathological deviations in need of repair, that physiological variability of the genitals results in psychosocial stigmatization that patients cannot overcome without medical help, and that it is the role of the physician to ensure psychosocial adjustment through medical and surgical intervention. These presumptions lend their support to the hierarchy of express values that govern medical practice: Namely, values that direct physicians and medical practices to offer means by which "diseased" patients are to be "cured." The confusion that arises in the case of intersex patients and their families is one that views "illness" (social stigmatization) as "disease," and therefore puts the physician in a place wherein "curing" presumes "healing." In other words, a type of category error can occur when the physician proclaims the birth of an intersexed child as a "psychosocial emergency" and then sets about working upon the patient through medical-surgical means.

Much of the reasoning behind this approach to the issue of intersexuality is the result of certain histories of medical practices, as well as the history of medicine and its social and juridical place in late-modern society.[11] Rather than exploring their historical roots here, I would like to test the presumptions themselves. Taken together, they suggest that those intersexed children upon whom no medical intervention was practiced would suffer severe psychosocial hardships due to their stigmatized status as gender "deviations." This is a claim whose virtue is its testability: Is it in fact the case that intersexed people suffer from their condition without medical intervention?

This question has been recently addressed in two key reports, whose conclusions seem to directly contradict this claim and thereby undermine the presumptions supporting it. The first report is an analysis of over eighty examples (published since 1950) of adolescents and adults who grew up with visibly anomalous genitalia.[12] In at least 37 cases, surgical intervention occurred at the request of the adolescent or adult. In all other cases, surgery was not pursued. When surgical intervention did occur, it was not until well after birth. Only two out of 33 cases of those raised as males were reassigned, both voluntarily. Only seven cases out of 51 cases of those raised as female wished to be reassigned as male. In all but one case, the summaries report that individuals developed into functioning adults, "many of whom have active and apparently satisfactory sex lives."[13] This suggests that immediate surgical intervention upon the birth of the child is neither necessary for successful gender identity development, nor that its absence condemns the individual to a life of difficult psychosocial adjustment.

This conclusion is supported ironically by the research done by John Money, the founder of the current medical paradigm, in his 1952 dissertation at Harvard University on "hermaphroditism" exploring the lives of intersexed individuals who did not undergo surgery. His work was further supported by his research with John and Jane Hampson at Johns Hopkins. By 1961 the Hampsons published the data collected on over 250 postadolescent "hermaphrodites" and concluded, "The *surprise* is that so many ambiguous-looking patients were able, *appearance notwithstanding*, to grow up and achieve a rating of psychologically healthy, or perhaps only mildly non-healthy."[14] Contrary to the expectations of the report's authors, intersexed individuals grew up comfortable with their genital ambiguity.

These findings are supported by additional evidence from India,[15] Saudi Arabia,[16] South Africa,[17] and Turkey,[18] as well as anthropological evidence from the Dominican Republic[19] and elsewhere.[20] In these cultures, researchers have found varying social responses to intersex, including noteworthy differences that cultural values play in assigning gender to these children. However, the studies share a common conclusion: The lack of surgical intervention upon the genitals does not seem to have the negative social effects anticipated by and justifying the modern medical paradigm adopted in the West.

Anecdotal evidence from the intersexed themselves confirms these reports. Such first-hand accounts are infrequent and difficult to find.[21] Nevertheless, when discovered, they all reflect certain similar features of experience: All relate some degree of awareness of difference with their peers, but no traumatological relationship to their own bodies:[22]

> But of course it bothered me that the periods had never started. I just told myself that it would never happen now and hey what the hell I didn't care…I was saving a ton of $$ on pads and tampons and being "sick" once a month like so many girls. Besides, I was just going to stay single and I still didn't want kids anyhow. I truly felt 'blessed' by not having this monthly curse and thought of myself as a very unique special girl. And I had just accepted the fact that in my mind I just never developed "downstairs" and my insides there were still like a little girls, OK so what I can live with that![23]

A curiosity about this difference usually leads individuals to a revelation (through television, Internet searches, and an eventual medical diagnosis) of their intersex status. This in turn leads to a confirmation of intuitive experiences, and offers them an identity that upholds their own sense of uniqueness. As one put it, after reading a newspaper article on intersexes (a term she had never heard before):

> I just remember being like…Oh my God, I think this is me. I was overjoyed to know what I was.[24]

When asked if they would pursue surgical interventions upon their genitalia, the majority of them reject the idea.[25]

> Of course I was teased about my body when I was growing up, as is the experience of most children, but that is no reason to alter one's body. A couple of my lovers have teased me tenderly about my androgynous body, and I used to be embarrassed about the way my clitoris stuck out – it didn't hid behind my labia like I thought it should – but again that is no reason to surgically alter it. As an adult I have grown to like my body the way it is. I like the fact that we are each unique individuals, which necessitates a wide variety of body shapes, sizes, and colors. I certainly don't feel the medical establishment has the right to determine which of our bodies are socially acceptable.[26]

Unquestioning acceptance of intersexed bodies as normal and natural seems to be a powerful means of "healing." As these examples indicate, intersex people whose bodies diverge from the gender ideal nevertheless find "health" through integration into the community and acceptance of their own bodies simply as individual variations on sex-gender. They share an important perception: They are "healthy" with respect to their sense of gendered/sexed selves. Their distance from a rhetoric of pathology, as initiated by medical practitioners under the modern medical paradigm and reinforced through medical intervention, avoids the creation of a space from out of which the intersexed "must" be "healed." Psychosocial liminality is neither rhetorically generated nor reinforced through the institutional imposition of gender categories by medical means. Rather, the intersexed find identity and place within community, and may or may not choose to turn to medicine in order to address specific features of their individual bodies.

4. RHETORICS OF HEALING: COUNTER-CULTURAL COMMUNITIES OF IDENTITY

Those who have undergone treatment under the "optimal gender" policy have taken another route toward the development of a context of healing. In contrast to those whose intersexuality was not discovered or, for whatever reason, was not surgically addressed, those who have undergone treatment are placed in a context that requires them to "heal from." Some suggestive lessons regarding the development of rhetorics of healing arise from this different context.

On one hand, it is certainly the case that each condition generates a unique context with respect to which the intersexed patient seeks to "heal." This is due to both the nature of the condition and the ways in which the condition is typically and traditionally treated by the medical community. On the other hand, the many first-person accounts now available to the researcher describe several strategies of healing in common among the various conditions. Foremost among them, as we shall see, is the participation in newly-formed communities of shared experience and valuing-practices that provide the intersexed with a space through which they overcome their isolation, in which they begin to validate experiences, and from which they seek to reach out to others.

The narratives of patients with Androgen Insensitivity Syndrome (AIS, which causes people born XY chromosomes to develop a typically "female" phenotype because their cells cannot "read" testosterone) share a similar structural pattern of medical intervention, familial response, and patient experience:[27] At a young age a patient is brought to the doctor and undergoes a series of tests, the results of which are not communicated. "Hernia" operations are then scheduled for the removal of "faulty ovaries" or sometimes the "appendix."

> I had a complete hysterectomy in 1977 at the age of 24, but was not told before the surgery that I was having one, as I went in for another form of surgery, and it took years for me to find out what had been done and why. I was only told my "ovaries" were pre-cancerous. I discovered MANY years later that what had been removed was undeveloped male gonadal tissue.[28]

> I was taken to the doctor and within days surgery was scheduled for what I was told [would be] a hernia repair. When I awoke from surgery, my parents were standing next to the bed. I lifted up the sheet and saw two identical incisions, one on the left, one on the right. I said to my parents, "Why do I have two scars?" My mother, without missing a beat, said, "They also removed your appendix." I didn't know it at the time, but 32 years of lies and shame had just begun.[29]

In some cases, the intervention is prompted by amenorrhea; in other cases, intersex conditions are "discovered" early through a series of accidental or not-so-accidental factors.

> I first learned about my condition, Androgen Insensitivity Syndrome or AIS, in a college classroom, where, as an 18-year-old freshman, I performed a karyotype on the specimen of cells taken from inside my mouth.[30]

> At about 26 I went to see my doctor about some totally unrelated problem and thought I'd ask her one of the questions that had been niggling at me—whether I should be having smears…To this she replied, "No you have no womb, therefore no cervix. You were born with testes but it was decided as you had normal external female genitalia that you would grow up as a girl." She must have seen the mortified look on my face then and she added, "Yes, you are one of them."[31]

With the approach of puberty, the patient is put on hormone replacement therapy (HRT) and is told about not being able to have children (adoption as an option is usually mentioned). The patients feel odd due to the obvious differences in their bodies from those of their peers and/or siblings (taller body, no body hair, and for post-operative Complete-AIS individuals, secondary sex characteristics developing only as a result of HRT). They are rarely told the truth about their condition, and even more rarely given referrals to support groups or counseling.

> After meeting with my sister's doctor, it was decided that I should see a "specialist" in the field of gynecology, so off to the "big" city of Portland I went with my Mom. Not once did anyone take the time to explain to me exactly what everything meant, and I was never presented with the opportunity to talk with a counselor.[32]

> There was really no support from my family at all when I was told I would never have kids (happened in a cold hospital room one late summer day in my 16th year). Dr. blurted out the news to me and walked out. No counseling, no after care, just the bare facts. No diagnosis either, or at least none that was ever told me.[33]

Many patients recount episodes of photographic sessions or display to interns and other doctors.

> The biggest humiliation was when we were shown into a hall that was full of doctors, and bombarded with personal questions.[34]

> I was then placed on a table in a paper gown, feet in stirrups, probed and prodded with God knows what in my genital area, breasts examined, finger up my rectum, with three other interns and a nurse watching, asking questions as if I wasn't even there. Each intern touched my genitals. They took pictures. I was crying and nobody cared or stopped what they were doing. I begged them to stop and they just said "Oh that doesn't hurt that much" and "We'll be done in a minute honey."[35]

> I hated being poked and peered at, lots of strange eyes. Once my sister and I were photographed for medical purposes and once I found "Interesting case" written in block capitals on my medical records folder and I felt completely objectified.[36]

> I spent many years going in and out of hospitals, not the privacy of a one-on-one consultation, but with groups of interested individuals. I often wished my parents said NO—but it was the era of doctor knows best, and they just went with the flow, and I knew no better.[37]

Periods of depression and symptoms of trauma related to these experiences of display are often described. Isolation, deflection, and secrecy take their toll.

> Although the doctors has claimed that knowing the truth would make me self-destructive, it was not knowing what had been done to me—and why—that made me want to die.[38]

> The lies and deception that have occurred throughout my life have taken their toll on me, making me very insecure and unwilling to trust people especially those close to me.[39]

> ...I spent years and years abusing drugs and alcohol. I did everything I could to kill myself, but nothing worked. Eventually I got addicted to crack cocaine, and went into rehab...It wasn't until I got sick in 1997 that I found out that I was intersex.[40]

The AIS narratives that are available for review are usually part of a community of support that has published information on the Internet. As with all other groups we will be considering here, the similarity of the rhetorics of healing can perhaps be explained by the constraints of the context. Nevertheless, it is interesting to note that virtually all narratives describe a remarkably similar process of revelation and healing that is cathartic for the AIS individual. This process usually takes two steps. First is the individual's uncompromised discovery of the truth about the condition, a discovery that reveals the extent to which secrecy and isolation have been intentionally practiced by both parents and physicians. Second is the individual's relief at the discovery of not being alone, neither in condition, nor in experience. As one person put it,

> Three days ago and as part of my ongoing search for the truth about me (my condition) a miracle happened to me: I found the support group and a place with loads of information. No more *pieces* of information. I felt as if I was finally given the permission after 29 years of darkness to step out of my prison to the light. Writing my

story today made me realize that, after all, AIS did not defeat me, and in many ways it
made me a better person.[41]

The result is a rhetoric that underscores the importance of truth for these patients
who have been surrounded by secrecy and paternalism, as well as the need for
community.

Interestingly, few AIS patients, in their narratives, directly question the wisdom
of surgical intervention *per se*; the narratives do not often reflect a motive for
addressing this particular aspect of the medical management paradigm, despite
patients' difficulties finding optimal HRT dosages, and despite their discovering that
only two to five percent of undescended testicles in cases of CAIS patients can
become cancerous. More often come expressions of sadness about childlessness,
reflections of difficult relationships with parents[42] as a result of the fallout of
discovering the truth, and disappointment in, if not outright confusion about and
even outrage at, the paternalism of physicians. It is also clear that parents have a
profound influence on the depth of the "illness" experienced. (In cases of total and
continuing parental denial, such "illness" can be quite overwhelming, but in the case
of parents who are supportive and forthright, the confidence and strength to heal
becomes significantly enhanced.) Influential, as well, are the supportive lovers and
friends who validate the identity and value of the AIS person. In general, what is at
stake in most, if not all of the narratives available, is a rhetoric of truth-telling that
seeks to undo the implicit pathology of the condition, a pathology that has been
orchestrated by silence and paternalism. As one very succinctly put it:

> I think the most vital thing a parent can do for a child with AIS is to be open and not
> pass on their terror of discovery. Children deserve the truth because it is their truth and
> it can be revealed in sensible and caring ways. Parents ought to defend their children
> against the doctors, too, and be assertive. It is very hard to forget being let down by
> your parents.[43]

This truth-telling becomes a shared communal value whose consequences extend to
the sharing of life experiences in an effort to reach out to others just discovering
their condition.

It is the nature of Congenital Adrenal Hyperplasia (CAH) as a potentially deadly
endocrinological condition that discussions available to the researcher are dominated
by parents of children with CAH.[44] (The bodies of patients with CAH cannot
properly treat cortisone. As a result, the adrenal glands produce cortisone in
quantities high enough to cause "virilization" of the body; CAH is also often
accompanied by a salt-wasting propensity that can be deadly.) Given this nature, the
rhetorics of healing that arise out of and give shape to the discussions are primarily
didactic: Parents tend to discuss all the issues necessary for understanding the
condition of their children, including the type of CAH, the results of tests, the
advantages and disadvantages of various treatment options including growth
hormones, the types and dosages of drugs (hydrocortisone, fludrocortisone,
prednisone, dexamethasone, sodium supplements), and how to handle and prepare
for adrenal crises. Sometimes it is clear from the discussion that a parent has been
upset by the ways in which a specific endocrinologist or pediatrician has handled a

child's case, and that the parent is seeking to obtain information, share experiences, seek recommendations, or generally find comfort in identifying with others going through similar circumstances. The following letter, posted on a website forum, is highly representative:

> Hello, I am new to this MB and I am so thankful for all of your responses. Thank you to each and every one of you. You will probably see a couple of messages from me as I become more familiar with CAH. I have been so worried about my little girl. She was diagnosed a couple of months ago. I have a couple of questions: Does anyone know of an endocrinologist that is considered the best in the USA? I don't care where I have to go to get my daughter looked at. We live in the West, but I don't mind going anywhere, even to just confirm my current doctor. I think he is good, but since I know so little about this, I would like a second or third opinion. Another question: My daughter doesn't have the SW or SL kind of CAH. Her tests showed okay. What does that mean? What does she have then? Non-classical? Does she still need meds? My Dr. put her on hydrocortisone. How is it that she got this? I have late onset, I believe, I developed symptoms at age 19. I am not on any meds, and until my daughter was diagnosed I didn't know what was wrong with me. I went to many doctors with my symptoms, and they told me to see a psychiatrist and take anti-depressants. Any input would be helpful.[45]

Under these and similar circumstances, the rhetoric of parental forums assumes a close connection between "healing" and curative procedures, supported by a community-building effort to reach out to and be available to other parents with CAH children.

Interestingly, it appears that a majority of parents seem to accept the necessity of surgical intervention to reconstruct the genitals. This issue has come increasingly under fire from a number of different quarters, including adult CAH individuals and those with clitoromegaly ("enlargement" of the clitoris).[46] Depending upon the context of the particular forum and its discussion history, it appears that parents are aware of the terms of the current debate, and it is often clear that physicians have discussed surgical options with the parents, who then choose to go ahead with the procedure.

> What words would you or have you used to explain to a little girl about the surgery she had performed at eight months old? There are books to help Mommies know how to help guard their children against any kind of abuse. There are books to explain how to explain about where babies come from, as well how to explain most anything about their past, but I have found nothing to help me find the words to explain why her vagina looks different than lots of other girls. Which brings up another question—do girls— most girls? all girls? who have this surgery, which is called corrective, still look different than most other girls? I had a great opportunity for the discussion a couple of nights ago, but the words wouldn't come. No matter how much I try to learn about her condition and this surgery, I need help and good words that have worked to help explain. She **will** be asking before too long. Won't she?[47]

Because CAH is essentially an endocrinological syndrome, it is not immediately clear why CAH "females" require genital surgery—but that they do is nevertheless presumed among the physician community. It should therefore come as no surprise that initial discussions about surgical options are predetermined by the rhetoric of the physicians. Parents tend to accept the physician's assessment that surgery is necessary, and once surgery is found to be necessary, parents tend to agree with the physician regarding the need for early intervention. At those early stages, the parents embrace the physician's assurances that techniques in clitoral recession will result in a "normal" child.

> At the age of two, Dr. Gonzalez recommended that we have her genitalia surgically repaired, although hers was not extremely severe. He referred us to a Pediatric Urologist at Children's, Dr. David Ewalt. He was wonderful, and the surgery was very successful. He performed a clitoral reduction and also made sure her bladder and other internal organs were in the correct places. Kendall did great, and we were home in just a few days! She now looks like a perfect little girl![48]

Once the surgical option is questioned, the opponents of surgery struggle to overcome two clear presumptions at work in the medical-rhetorical context of the debate. The first is the presumption that the parents, along with the physician, have the right to make medical choices on behalf of the infant, even in such cases as clitoroplastic reduction, a permanent surgery premised upon aesthetic considerations of how large a clitoris "ought" to be.

> If you go to see a surgeon with just about any issue, you will leave having been told it can be fixed with surgery. Before any parent reaches that point however, I would encourage them to meet with an endo who isn't so quick to see your baby's genitals as a problem in need of fixing. There are many who don't see it that way. If you need the name of them, send me an email and I will send you their names. Sean, are you within driving distance of Ann Arbor? There's a good one there who actually used to refer patients to surgeons and no longer does.

> Another major bone of contention we have with surgeons is the lack of follow-up. Very rarely do they ever make an effort to follow-up with infants they cut when they become adults. This lack of follow-up is nothing short of unethical because it shouldn't be just about genitals that look good enough for the child to "pass," it should be 100% about whether they function when the child becomes a sexually active adult. That may not happen for decades. One of the reasons the surgeons will tell you that they don't have follow-up studies is because they change the method every few years. By doing that, they effectively render any follow-up studies useless because they say that method is no longer being done and it causes a lack of control group protocols necessary in good research.[49]

The second, and for our study the more important presumption they must confront is an unquestioned connection between "curing" and "healing," namely, the assumption that medical intervention ("curing") must necessarily work towards a "healing" outcome. This presumption is at work in every physician-patient encounter, the idea and hope being that through medicine, one finds a means of overcoming the challenges presented by "disease" and "illness." If and when CAH "females" talk about their surgery experiences, however, their comments reflect experiences that undermine this presumption. More often than not, adult CAH "females" speak of their experience of medical intervention as traumatizing. Often their comments suggest the possibility that *confrontation* with medical practices plays a much more important part in the move toward healing.

CAH narratives, like AIS narratives, relate experiences of secrecy and shame:

> It was never talked about while I was growing up. I guess my parents expected me to deal with my ambiguous genitals on my own. I also suppose I fell within the mark of what a clit can look like before it is chopped. In any case, I was totally left to my own

devices to "understand" my differences and therefore I developed a lot of shame around my genitals and sexuality in general. It wasn't until recently that I could talk with anyone about being IS and then I confronted my dad about it. He finally admitted that he always knew that I was larger "down there" (his words) but just figured that "my mother" would have talked to me about "it." Of course my mom never said anything when I asked her as a child about my genitals. I always felt that if nobody was talking about it that it must be really bad that I had a big clit. Don't get me wrong, I'm not sorry for what god gave me. What I am upset about was the silence and secrecy that both my parents and the doctors fostered around my IS. As you and others probably know, it creates a lot of shame for the child. It would have been so much more healthy for me if there was honest communication around this topic from an early age.[50]

However, for those who underwent surgery, the trauma of the procedure and its aftermath figures much larger than for AIS patients. The reasons for this are simple: the object of surgical intervention is typically the phallus, an object whose sole function is sexual stimulation, and those sharing their stories do so because their surgeries have been a dismal failure. They question the necessity of the surgical intervention, they question the standards upon which to judge surgical outcomes, they express anger at the loss of sensation or the presence of pain, and they express betrayal at the loss of control over their bodies due to the involuntary act of intervention.

I have had nine genital surgeries, which I consider failures but my surgeons deemed a success. The surgeries started when I was an infant...Most of these surgeries had caused scar tissue in the vagina. With every surgery on the urethra it was shortened and has caused other problems. The placement of my urethra by my surgeons has led to a placement that most doctors are not used to, so needless to say any type of exam is painful, because of that and other reasons.

My vagina is about the size of a pencil, which surgeons had been trying to "fix" since birth. I was also born with an enlarged clitoris, which seemed to bother all around me. The surgeons had talked my mother into letting them reduce the size of the clitoris. They reduced the size once but it continued to grow because throughout my life I refused to take my medicine. I had my final surgery, which removed my clitoris at the age of seventeen. That was back in 1987 when you would think that these barbaric surgeries would not have been performed. I knew that this surgery was going to happen all my life and I knew when. This lead to apprehension on every birthday since I was one year closer to my surgery.

Common sense tells me that if with every time a surgery was preformed to remove scar tissue or to "fix" any other problem and it caused more scar tissue then maybe surgeries should have been stopped. I guess that the doctors knew better than anyone but me and I say that what they did was wrong and damaging. After my last surgery I now have pain when aroused or while having sex. I have what I can only describe as many red-hot needles sticking me where my clitoris was and where my stitches were. I also get this feeling anytime day or night, sitting, standing, walking, or just anytime it decides to come. The pain comes and goes and lasts anywhere between 10—30 seconds at any given time. This pain can be enough for me to want to double over but not to be able to because I might be in a public place or at work. I have learned through the years to just act like nothing is happening and keep on going. That is to say, I still feel all the pain, but [have learned] not to draw attention to myself. I act like I am fine.

I had learned a long time ago that my parents and health care professionals did not want to hear what I had to say or thought. I cannot tell you how many times I had heard phrases like these when I would protest any kind of treatment. I would be told "We are doing this to save your life" or "We are doing this to make you normal." These phrases are not reassuring or comforting. These phrases tend to tell a child that you do not care what they think and [that] what others want to do to your body is right. [51]

The rhetoric of healing that arises among CAH patients—particularly CAH "females"—prioritizes truth-telling about the fallout of early genital surgeries. Such a rhetoric is primarily characterized by the catharsis of discovering a community of people with similar experiences. However, it is also often characterized by express commitments to confront the medical community, to increase outreach, and to provide the parents of CAH children with counsel that might undermine the presumption of the need for genital surgery.

> The belief that early surgery fixes the problems of intersexed people is wrong. It only makes the problem disappear in the eyes of the parents and the doctors and shifts the entire burden onto the child. The child knows something is not right but no one is willing to say anything. As one women posted on a CAH (congenital adrenal hyperplasia) message board, "It's as if there was an elephant in the living room but no one would talk about it." Everyone concerned with the care and treatment of an intersexed child needs education and counseling to help them to provide the psychological support that the child will need regardless of whether or not surgery is performed.

> I hope I have made you understand why it is important that the current treatment protocol for the intersexed that is centered on surgery needs to be changed to a patient-centered approach that stresses education, emotional support and counseling for everyone involved. [52]

CAH patients who have undergone surgery embrace a rhetoric of truth-telling in a context that seeks to find a perspective counter to the pathologizing tendencies of medical approaches.

Patients with hypospadias (in which the meatus of the "penis" is located somewhere other than on the tip of the glans) and chordee (in which there is downward curvature of the "penis," sometimes accompanied by twisting) express a much broader range of experiences with the medical and broader communities. [53] This is due, in no small part, to two important factors: First, the frequency of surgeries that a hypospadic male undergoes, typically extending into adulthood, gives him opportunities to interact with the medical profession, particularly urologists. [54] As adults, hypospadic males are far more prone to discussing surgical options from a patient-centered perspective and to evaluating surgical outcomes soberly.

Secondly, the cultural importance ascribed to the penis places patients under a sense of incredible pressure either to seek out solutions to perceived problems with their genitals, or to determinedly accept their differences as natural variations. Under the circumstances of social pressure, hypospadic males tend to suffer greatly from embarrassment about their genitals, especially in the locker room (60.3% Hypospadic Males [HM] v. 24.1% Control Group [CG]), with physicians, (37.8% HM v. 13.7% CG) and with partners (41.0% HM v. 7.0% CG). [55] They tend to fear public bathrooms, and they mention frequently their difficulties urinating, employing the standard "standing to pee" as a goal. Fear of intimacy (35.3% HM

v. 6.5% CG), disgust with penis (23.7% HM v. 4.9% CG) and depression (36.5% HM v. 8.9% CG) are also frequently mentioned. In most cases, these fears and embarrassments are only exacerbated by surgery, the negative outcomes of which tend eventually to bring the hypospadic male to the point of accepting his current status, if not to the point of actively avoiding further surgeries for fear of worsening results.[56]

Nevertheless, discussions tend to be nuanced. In cases of mild hypospadias, surgery is undertaken less than 50 percent of the time. When outcomes are shared, they frequently include frank discussions of failures (fistulae, strictures, hair growth from graft, loss of sensation, multiple repairs, shortening of the shaft), careful consideration of the value of early surgery vs. later, and possible long-term psychological effects.

> The slit is on the underside of my penis starting near the top of the head and is about an inch long and about of an inch below the slit is a small hole making it look like an exclamation mark (!) I urinate from the larger hole but if I squeeze the larger hole together while I pee, the smaller hole lets drips of urine come out (I was curious to see how it worked). At seventeen I had my mom take me to a urologist because I wanted to have a more "normal" looking penis. The doctor told me I needed to have some scar tissue removed and to make my erections less tight. I never had any pain or problems with erections and I told the doctor this but he seemed to think it was a problem so I had this corrective surgery. Honestly I don't notice much of a difference. My penis has never pointed straight out and still doesn't (it leans to my left). I don't recall the reason why but I never went back to the doctor for any more surgeries or even follow-ups.[57]

> I underwent four surgeries as a child to repair the problem, and they seemed to work well for about 12 years. My penis was shaped normally, could achieve erection, and appeared "normal" as compared to others. As I reached sexual maturity, the growth of my penis caused the surgically repaired skin of the base of my penis to tear, revealing several fistulae, or holes, from the base of the penis into a free urethral opening. Although I had a "real" urethral opening at the tip of my penis, I also had several openings on the base. This caused me to leak urine as I urinated and it would get on my pants. This embarrassment caused me to have to urinate sitting down. I was embarrassed to tell my parents, and went until 17 years old avoiding women, because if I was ever in a situation of ejaculation, some semen would shoot out the bottom as well as the tip. I felt women would feel I was a freak. After many years of humiliation, I finally set up an appointment with a urologist. He performed surgery on me in order to repair the shaft leakage. This involved removing skin from my scrotum and surgically attaching it to my penis. Anyway, it held for a year and then the skin died and I am now back at stage one.[58]

In general, very little regret is expressed about the decision to undergo surgery, but outcomes are described with far greater candor and sober assessment than one typically sees, e.g., among adults making choices for their children. As one forum member put it,

> All in all I have been very pleased with the end result although you might not guess it. I would never trade what I have now for what I started out with. I would even endure the pain again if necessary. Perhaps it sounds inconsistent, but I still occasionally have insecurities about how my penis looks in spite of many sex partners telling me it's PERFECTLY ALRIGHT. I have often still doubted them…Why I feel the need to measure up to some other standard is beyond me, but it is what it is. The insecurity issue has been a roller coaster ride…sometimes I'm alright with it…sometimes I'm not.[59]

Moderate and severe cases of hypospadias are much more frequently operated on, with far fewer positive physical, sexual, emotional outcomes. These cases tend toward greater levels of depression (47% Moderate/Severe [M/S] v. 32.5% Mild [Mi]), poor self-esteem [57.5% M/S v. 41.4% Mi] and poor experience with medical intervention (61% report M/S dissatisfaction with penile appearance after surgery vs. 39.3% Mi). In either and both cases, however, adults talking about adult decisions have a different perspective than adults talking about decisions made for them in childhood. The latter, like AIS and CAH patients, mention trauma—particularly shame, powerlessness, isolation, and humiliation—much of it due to a lack of forthright discussion with parents and physicians. This is particularly the case for hypospadic individuals operated upon as pre-teen children. As another poster summed up his experience,

> Surgery at age six was traumatic. Fortunately, much of the detail has faded from my memory, but I remember extreme embarrassment about the entire ordeal. I'm sure that much of the embarrassment stems from the way my parents handled things (though they meant no harm, they had little information from small-town doctors and therefore did not make the wisest decisions). I remember my parents privately telling my teacher about the surgery and encouraging the teacher to lie to the class and say I was having surgery on my arm. Obviously, the full truth would not have been appropriate, but it sent a signal to me that it was something of which to be ashamed. I also remember lying in bed in the hospital after surgery (I was in the hospital for several days) on my back with my legs propped up in some sort of contraption so I couldn't damage the sutures. I was completely naked underneath, except for a blanket draped over the contraption, exposed to nurses, relatives or anyone who walked into the room. I felt vulnerable and somewhat violated in that position. I also remember the catheter and my refusal to obey the nurse and just "let it go" and pee while I was lying in bed. Primarily, I remember the DRAMATIC change in appearance once I finally got the see the finished product after surgery (I can imagine the surgeon could have said something like, "it ain't pretty, but it works"). That caused a sense of confusion, shame, and even a sense of loss for what I no longer had. To a large extent, those feelings remain with me 20 years later.[60]

The discussion among parents reflects concerns about surgery, recovery, and post-surgical care; desires to find others to consult with; and questions about the causes of this congenital condition—topics one would expect to find from those whose children might enter into the surgical unit. A characteristic of these discussions not often found in other forums of parents with intersexed children is the number of postings and discussions related to the high frequency of surgeries that the children undergo in order to repair previous surgeries.

> I am so sad, after going through [surgery 3 times], my son will still look different.[61]

> We haven't had any problems with the scrotum being sewn together and the hypo repair. We did have a complication, but it was because the hole at the tip of the penis closed a bit too much, and a pouch of urethra formed behind it because of too much pressure. We had that fixed six months after hypo surgery, and we haven't had any problems in over a year. We do have a problem with buried penis right now, since his penis is small to begin with and rearrangement of skin has aggravated that, but it will be fixed when he gets a bit bigger.[62]

> [M]y little boy is 5 years old and has had 6 operations. The first one to repair what is considered a mild case. The last 5 operations have been to repair a fistula. (I think where

the original hole that he peed thru). The last operation was about 6 months ago and again it did not fix the problem. Obviously this has been quite stressful, not only for him but for us as well.[63]

[A]fter all the failed operations Hayden has been through, I have found it really hard [to] say anything positive in the group [to] others that [are] looking [for] a bit of hope. And the fact that every time I read the mail in the group and think about what my son has been through in the 4 years of his life brings me [to] tears every time.[64]

His surgery began at 5 months, we were told that it had successfully been corrected with a single stage op that took close to 4 hours. Things looked good for a couple of weeks, but unfortunately a fistula occurred and surgery was rescheduled for another 5 months down the track. The procedure was repeated and again the result not good. We have since had another 5 ops to no avail, we have had full hypospadias surgery 3 times, a repair to the urethra, due to him being born with a double urethra which they didn't pick up until op no. 5, dilations of the urethra. [H]e recently had a supra pubic catheter in for just over 2 months, following surgery on the 2nd Feb, this year. We are at our wits ends not knowing how many more ops are needed as the surgeon is unable to give us an explanation as to why the surgery has been so unsuccessful. Maybe they will get it right next time, let's hope so anyway.[65]

We were told the same thing about 2 months ago after my 11 year-old son's 6th operation. All I could think about is why did we let him go thru all the operations for the end result like this. My son's father and I have decided no more operations. Enough is enough.[66]

Parents facing these circumstances describe frustration, worry, and confusion at the frequency of repairs. They often seek out resources that can direct them to surgeons, they discuss upcoming stages, and they describe their own versions of "case studies" of physicians and physician rhetoric. They rarely employ a rhetoric of "healing from," but rather express trauma about the failures of medical intervention.

Hypospadic males, like other individuals we have considered, report the healing experience of discovering that they are not alone and feeling no longer isolated by confusion and shame about their genitals. Partners who accept these individuals and parents who offer support and candor tend to play a very important role in hypospadic males' self-esteem and healing.

What you need is an open honest relationship with a partner where you explain to them exactly what you have before or as any serious relationship starts. Then it will not be a shock to that person when it is seen for the first time. In fact you can learn to enjoy the difference in exploring your capabilities together. Now, there will always be a proportion of women who will then run away from you too embarrassed to discuss it. That's their problem, not yours. It is better to find that out before you commit to a marriage with the embarrassment deferred to the wedding night. I told my future wife about it very early in our relationship (after about 4 weeks) and although she was mildly interested, it made no difference to our relationship and we have been married for over thirty years.[67]

Here are some thoughts that were stimulated by the hypospadias information on the-penis.com. This was the most complete explanation I'd ever seen, about the way I'm built, and it answered some questions I've had for many years. I've worried off and on about a cock that is different than it was "supposed to be," but once I became sexually active as a gay man in my early 30's I realized that the differences weren't particularly important to me or my partners.[68]

> Since the hypospadias is an important part of my life, I always have to live with the impression of being different. So I have educated myself by reading in various websites and clubs about hypospadias and circumcision on the Internet. It's a relief to hear that I'm not the only one. I also discovered that it's a hard experience to adapt to having this condition.[69]

Eventually, also, some begin to speak of a coming to terms with their difference (often through counseling, but not always), even going so far as to actively downplay the importance ascribed to the penis in the culture, especially with respect to their whole person. When hypospadic males employ a rhetoric of healing, their "healing from" includes overcoming social stigma, recounting numerous surgeries and their repairs, coming to terms with their relationship to their hypospadias, and making a commitment to candor about sexual and medical experiences.

Other intersex conditions facing quite distinct symptomatologies and origins nevertheless share a similar rhetoric in their narratives: insofar as the medical community provides information and support for the families and patients to identify and understand their respective conditions, the individual finds healing *through* medical knowledge and options.[70] This is the case both with Klinefelter "boys," whose symptoms often do not become recognizable until adolescence, and with Turner "girls," whose condition can more often be recognized at birth, though almost half are not diagnosed until later.[71] Full disclosure to and active participation of these patients in the management of the symptoms of their condition allow them and their families the chance to gain a sense of control and insight.

As with all other groups we have looked at, isolation has a profound impact on Turner "girls" and Klinefelter "boys," both before and after their status is revealed. Coming into contact with communities of support provides individuals with a sense of belonging and understanding.

> In the spring of '89 there was a Turner's Syndrome Conference in Ottawa Ontario. These conferences are held so that families who are dealing with the Syndrome can share thoughts, and get some feedback and information on what's happening medically. My Mom and I decided it was time for us to learn more, and create a support system. It was an excellent experience, and one I'll have for a long time. I learned that this wasn't only happening to me.[72]

> I am glad to meet you guys. It is good to talk. [T]here is also another [c]lub, Hypogonadism and Klinefelters. You might like to check it out. There is a lot of info there. You are NOT alone. [T]here are others of us.[73]

For members of both groups, the difficulty can be with reconciling their experiences and senses of difference with the expectations of those around them. Surgeries (including operations on ears or webbed shoulders) and growth hormones to render Turner children more "normal" and mastectomies and HRT to help Klinefelter adolescents develop a more masculine appearance are frequently proposed. The potential pathological implications of "normalizing" approaches can have their negative effects:

> Adult individuals with Klinefelter variations often report undesirable psychological side effects from HRT. Over time, many untreated persons with Klinefelter accommodate themselves to the reality of their unique body structure and mourn the loss of their

feminine identity. For those who decide to have either the mastectomy, HRT, or both, psychological counseling is highly desirable, but typically is not offered. The removal of breast tissue in males can be as traumatic as the loss of a breast is to females, yet the mastectomy is typically treated as no more than cosmetic surgery and no more significant than a haircut. Often what seems desirable to make the body conform to a typical male appearance is deeply regretted later.[74]

For both groups, the knowledge (or discovery) of the condition, the responsibility shared in the medical decision-making processes, and the sharing of experiences in order to break out of the sense of isolation help create a rhetoric of healing. Such a rhetoric can equip individuals with a powerful acceptance of the uniqueness of their experiences and identities. As one Klinefelter post stated,

> I also have come to grips with the term INTERSEXUAL. At first I resented it. Now, I am proud of who I am, where I have been, and what I am doing. I am now a successful businessman, self-employed, and loving it.[75]

5. HEALING, CURING AND NEW APPROACHES

These examples do not represent all intersexes' experiences and discussions. Indeed, given the wide variety of forms intersexuality takes, including those forms that we did not specifically address (5-alpha reductase deficiency, vaginal agenesis, and gonadal disgenesis, among many others), it should not be surprising that each condition would shape unique rhetorical worlds, values, experiences and group dynamics. Nevertheless, despite these differences, the rhetorics of healing share common themes.

Through the stories shared by intersex people it becomes clear that their respective conditions become subjects of discovery that bring them together with others sharing similar experiences. Relief from a sense of isolation often gives way to the joy that occurs when patients discover others similar to them. This discovery leads to community-building exercises, such as the sharing of individual histories, the creation of a community of identity, and often the explicit or implied commitment to outreach in an effort to find others undergoing similar experiences.

In certain cases, the values developed through the process of community-building include outreach to others. A commitment to outreach and education can often develop into an advocacy that embraces a program of change directed at public perception and medical practices. Whether or not a specific community formation develops along such lines, all of the communities seek to support their members by developing non-pathologized identities for them and by offering shared space from out of which the members can confront, educate, or simply recover from the isolation experienced in relation to dominant and pathologizing community norms.

The initial research provided here is not definitive, but it provides an introduction to an approach that highlights and considers the healing strategies used by intersex people. For some, "healing" is a mundane affair, the result of simply living at peace with oneself, when oneself was never problematized to begin with. Distinctions and differences were noted, but not pathologized and marked for necessary "corrective" intervention. For others, "healing" takes place through recovery from social and medical rhetorics of pathology and their resultant practices. Bodies were seen as in need of correction, and procedures were implemented to "normalize" them; recovery is sought from these very procedures. Sometimes what the individual recovers from is a whole rhetorical world of practices and procedures imposed without consent, procedures left unexplained, or discussions that did not tell the whole truth. Sometimes what is recovered from is simply the fallout from the practices themselves, whether wanted or unwanted. Regardless of the object of recovery, the means of recovery is the community of individuals with whom one can share common experiences, validate shared values, explore and expand upon common visions, and practice truth-telling unprecedented in members' lives: The creation of communities of identity marks the most significant catalyst for healing in the rhetorics of these individuals.

What can we learn from these examples about the nature of "healing" and the relationship between "healing" and "curing"? Among many lessons that may be derived, I would like to offer the following for consideration that may have the greatest relevance for the medical treatment of intersex people. In certain cases and conditions of intersexuality, doctors do *not* provide the means for healing. When they do, it is mainly in cases where the intersex patient comes to them as an adult to work with the doctors as partners in determining causes and discussing desired outcomes. In cases of Turner and Klinefelter individuals, physicians can clearly help patients to understand their conditions and to successfully navigate their medical circumstances. Adult hypospadias patients, while frequently critical of outcomes, may also approach the physician as a potential partner in seeking out healing solutions under circumstances when such decisions are in the patient's own hands.

But for other groups, including people with CAH and clitoromegaly, AIS, and adult hypospadias, whose operations were undertaken involuntarily as children, the physician-patient relationship is often reported as compromised through the pathologization of the intersexed body and the medical attention upon the genitalia. For these patients, "healing" takes place in spite of, indeed in recovery from, medical intervention. Here we see how the presumed nexus of "curing" and "healing" is disrupted for the patient; medical intervention does *not* entail healing. Rather, it creates and exacerbates "illness."

All patients speak of an "aha!" experience upon discovering others like themselves. Isolation and liminality are described as having been ever-present, in varying degrees of intensity, while intersex individuals were growing up. It is only upon recognition that they are not alone that relief is expressed and healing can begin to take place.

This suggests that the role of liminality and its relationship to medical decision-making must be more directly addressed. The phenomenon of patient experiences of marginalization and social liminality as a result of *disease* has already and often been discussed. When a healthy person becomes sick, and thereby risks certain social status or position through isolation, it is the physician who seeks to bring about a state of health. The physician provides a cure for the disease, thereby addressing individual needs despite, or even in confrontation with, broader socio-communal reactions to the individual. However, in the case of intersex patients whose very existence results in ostracization and social liminality, the community demands from the physician that these individuals be altered to conform to communal norms. "Medicine does not usually accept the views of society if they are in conflict with the needs of the individual. But we seem to need a categorical statement about a person's sexuality."[76]   The experiences we have described and summarized here give evidence of the results of this kind of approach: By viewing social marginalization as a "disease" in need of "curing," doctors have created rhetorical worlds around patients that can reinforce their "illness" and prevent "healing."[77]

It is only by people's recognizing the validity of difference, accepting the variability of genitals, and demanding the right to bodily integrity and subject autonomy that these particular communities of healing have been formed. They have been formed through the pain intersex people experience at the hands of the community, family, and physicians. Members seek to recover through a rhetorics of healing that brings them together to share, learn, create and support new identities to confront the forces of liminality and isolation on the one hand, and the forces of conformity demanding their erasure on the other.

Setting aside the question of the "success" or "failure" of medical and surgical intervention upon intersexed minors, not to mention the question of developing standards upon which these may be determined, what becomes clear is that a deeper issue is at stake: If alternative strategies of "healing" can be shown to exist, strategies that question and critique the presumed connection between "curing" and "healing," then physicians and parents are obliged to reconsider the medical practices in response to which these strategies arise. This obligation is not due to the quality of being "alternative," but to the insights they raise concerning what, precisely, the people who use these strategies are "healing from"—the current practice of medical intervention itself. These alternative strategies create instead spaces of freedom and safety that allow for a context within which *all* parties can work together to view the *responses to* intersexuality, and not the condition itself, as pathological.

David Hester, Interfakultäres Zentrum für Ethik in den Wissenschaften, Eberhard Karls Universität Tübingen, Tübingen, Germany

NOTES

[1]   Cf. an approach via Turner to bodily liminality that the intersex(es) represent to the physician, who is mandated through this liminality to give this undefined, declassified, "non-existent" body a place within the social sphere. See R. Crouch, "Betwixt and Between: The Past and Future of Intersexuality." *Journal of Clinical Ethics* 9.4 (Winter 1998): 372-384.

[2]   *Michel Reiter v. AG München* 722 URIII 302.22 (September 2002); *Wilma Wood v. C.G. Studios, Inc.* (USDC Penn. Civ. A. No. 86-2563).

3   *In re Estate of Gardiner* 42 P.3d 120 (Kan. 2002), finding that the law contemplates "a biological man and a biological woman" for a valid marriage, therewith overturning court of appeals ruling found in 22 P. 3d 1086 (Kan. Ct. App. 2001).

4   *Littleton v. Prange,* Texas 4th Court of Appeals validated a marriage between two women, one a male-to-female transsexual, on the basis of their inferred chromosomes. Cf., for more information on the legal status of intersex(es), J. Greenberg, "Defining Male and Female: Intersexuality and the Collisions Between Law And Biology." *Arizona Law Review* 41 (1999): 265-328.

5   Cf., e.g., "Intersexuality Fails to Support Homosexuality." *Gospel Gazette* 4.10 (October 2002): 10, available at <http://www.gospelgazette.com/gazette/2002/oct/page10.htm>; Wisconsin Evangelical Lutheran Synod <http://www.wels.net/sab/qa/behav-sex-07.html>; C. Colson, "Blurred Biology: How Many Sexes Are There?" *Breakpoint Online* 61016 (October 16, 1996).

6   S. Schröter, *FeMale: Über Grenzverläufe zwischen den Geschlechtern.* Frankfurt-a-M: Fischer Taschenbuch Verlag, 2002. See also G. Greer, *The Whole Woman.* New York: Anchor Books, 2000.

7   Cf. <www.transfeminism.org/is-survey/survey-summary.txt>.

    Cf. H. F. L. Meyer-Bahlburg, "Gender Identity Development in Intersex Patients." *Child and Adolescent Psychiatric Clinic North America* 2 (1993): 501-512; HFL Meyer-Bahlburg, "Gender Assignment in Intersexuality." *Journal of the Psychology of Human Sex* 10 (1998): 1-21; and American Academy of Pediatrics RE9958," Evaluation of the Newborn With Developmental Anomalies of the External Genitalia." *Policy Statement* 106.1 (July 2000); J. Money, J.G. Hampson, and J. L. Hampson, "Hermaphroditism: Recommendations Concerning Assignment of Sex, Change of Sex, and Psychological Management." *Bulletin of Johns Hopkins Hospital* 97 (1955): 284-300; J. Money, J. G. Hampson, and J. L. Hampson, "Imprinting and the Establishment of Gender Role." *Archives of Neurology and Psychiatry* 77 (1957): 333-336. See also J. Money, *Sex Errors of the Body and Related Syndromes: A Guide to Counseling Children, Adolescents, and Their Families,* 2nd ed. Baltimore, MD: Paul H. Brookes Publishing, 1994; J. Money and A. Ehrhardt, *Man & Woman, Boy & Girl* Baltimore: The Johns Hopkins University Press, 1972; C. Migeon, A. Wisniewski, and J. Gearhart, *Syndromes of Abnormal Sex Differentiation: A Guide for Patients and Their Families.* Baltimore, MD: The Johns Hopkins Children's Center, 2001; J. Hutcheson, "Ambiguous Genitalia and Intersexuality." *eMedicine.com* under "Pediatrics/Urology," available at <http://author.emedicine.com/PED/topic1492.htm>.

9   For views opposing the dominant medical management paradigm, cf. K. Kipnis and M. Diamond,"Pediatric Ethics and the Surgical Assignment of Sex." *Journal of Clinical Ethics* 9.4 (Winter1998): 398-410; A. Dreger, *Intersex in the Age of Ethics.* Hagerstown, MD: University PressGroup, 1999; S. Kessler, *Lessons from the Intersexed.* New Brunswick, N.J.: Rutgers University Press,1998; A. Fausto-Sterling, *Sexing the Body: Gender Politics and the Construction of Sexuality.* New York: Basic Books, 2000. See also S. Creighton and C. Minto, "Editorial: Managing Intersex." *British Journal of Medicine* 323 (1 December 2001): 1264-1265 and "Draft Statement of the British Association of Paediatric Surgeons Working Group on the Surgical Management of Children Born with Ambiguous Genitalia." (July, 2001), available at <http://www.baps.org.uk/documents/Intersex%20statement.htm>. See also the Intersexed Society of North America at <http://www.isna.org>.

10 Among those whose information has been helpful for this study, in addition to those mentioned in the references given below, are the following: Intersexed Society of North America <http://www.isna.org>, The UK Intersex Association <http://www.ukia.co.uk>, Intersex Society of South Africa <isosa@netactive.co.za>, Adrenal Hyperplasia Network <http://www.anh.org.uk>, Cares Foundation <http://www.caresfoundation.org>, The Magic Foundation <http://www.magicfoundation.org>, CAH Support Group of Australia <http://www.vicnet.net.au/%7Ecahsga/>, Bodies Like Ours <http://www.bodieslikeours.org>, Riksföreningen för Adrenogenitalt Syndrom <http://home.bip.net/rf-ags>, Intersex Support Group International <http://www.isgi.org>, MRKH Foundation <http://www.mrkh.net>, The Turner Society <http://www.tss.org.uk>, Mixed Gonadal Dysgenesis Support Group <http://www.xyxo.org>, Klinefelter Syndrome and Associates <http://www.genetic.org/ks>, Hypospadias Support Group <http:// www.hypospadias.co.uk>.

11 Cf. the often-cited work of A. Dreger, *Hermaphrodites and the Medical Invention of Sex.* Cambridge, MA: Harvard University Press, 1998.

[12] A. Fausto-Sterling, *Sexing the Body: Gender Politics and the Construction of Sexuality* New York: Basic Books, 2001, Table 4.3 (pp. 96-100) and Table 4.4 (pp. 102-106).

[13] A. Fausto-Sterling, *Sexing the Body*, 95.

[14] J. L. Hampson and J. G. Hampson, "The Ontogenesis of Sexual Behavior in Man." in: *Sex and Internal Secretions*, W. Young and G. Corner, eds. Baltimore: Williams and Wilkins, 1961: 1401-1432: 1428-1429. J. Money's dissertation was never published, but is reported on by J. Colapinto, *As Nature Made Him: The Boy Who Was Raised as a Girl*. New York: HarperCollins, 2001, and can be obtained under the title "Hermaphroditism: An Inquiry into the Nature of a Human Paradox." *Social Sciences*. PhD Dissertation; Cambridge, MA: Harvard University, 1952.

[15] G. R. Sridhar, "Socio-psychological Aspects of Artificial Sex Change." *Journal of the Association of Physicians of India* 47 (1999): 1217-8. G. R. Sridhar, "Intersex Experience with Indian Endocrinologists." *British Journal of Medicine* (22 December 2001): e5, available at <http://bmj.com/cgi/eletters/323/7324/1264>.

[16] S. Taha, "Male Pseudohermaphroditism: Factors Determining the Gender of Rearing in Saudi Arabia." *Urology* 43 (1994): 370-374. See also H. Al-Attia, "Gender Identity and Role in a Pedigree of Arabs with Intersex due to 5Alpha Reductase-2 Deficiency." *Psychoneuroendocrinology* 21 (1996): 651-657.

[17] I. Aaronson, "True Hermaphroditism. A Review of 41 Cases with Observations on Testicular Histology and Function." *British Journal of Urology* 57.6 (December 1985): 775-9.

[18] G. Ölzer et al, "Evaluation of Patients with Congenital Adrenal Hyperplasia" *Annals of Medical Sciences* 9.3 (September 2000), also available at <http://ams.cu.edu.tr/September2000Vol9No3/guler.html>.

[19] J. Imperato-McGinley, L. Guerrero, T. Gautier, R. E. Petersen, "Steroid 5alpha-reductase Deficiency in Man: An Inherited Form of Male Pseudohermaphroditism." *Science* 186.4170 (27 December 1974): 1213-1215; J. Imperato-McGinley and R. E. Peterson, "Male Pseudohermaphroditism: The Complexities of Male Phenotypic Development." *American Journal of Medicine* 61.2 (1977): 251-272; J. Imperato-McGinley, T. Gautier, R.E. Petersen, and E. Sturla, "Androgens and the Evolution of Male-Gender Identity Among Male Pseudohermaphrodites with 5alpha-reductase Deficiency." *New England Journal of Medicine* 300.22 (31 May 1979): 1233-1237.

[20] G. Herdt, *Third Sex, Third Gender: Beyond Sexual Dimorphism in Culture and History*. New York: Zone Books, 1996.

[21] Among those I have been able to identify and access are included: "Bobby-Jo." <http://www.medhelp.org/www/ais/stories/bobby_jo.htm>, "Tony." <http://home.vicnet.net.au/~aissg/Tony.htm>, "A Berdache's Odyssey." <http://members.tripod.com/~Berdache_Two/>, "Swati's Story." <http://www.medhelp.org/www/ais/stories/swati.htm>, "Intersex Babies: Controversy Over Operating to Change Ambiguous Genitalia." *ABC News* (19 April 2002): <http://abcnews.go.com/sections/2020DailyNews/2020_intersex_020419.html>.See also the following essays in the collection edited by Dreger, *Intersex in the Age of Ethics*: A. Dreger and C. Chase, "A Mother's Care: An Interview with 'Sue' and 'Margaret' by Alice Domurat Dreger and Cheryl Chase," 83-89; D. Cameron, "Caught Between: An Esssay on Intersexuality," 90-96; Kim, "As Is," 99-100. The following quotations taken from the Internet have been slightly redacted for grammar.

[22] All reported teasing from peers and negative reactions by others (from rejection by potential lovers to incestual rape), but none of them reflect a traumatology of their own body and person stemming from their genital ambiguity.

[23] "Bobby Jo's Story," an autobiography of and adult CAIS "female," available at <http://www.medhelp.org/www/ais/stories/bobby_jo.htm>.

[24] Viloria, quoted in "Intersex Babies." *ABC News: 20/20.*

[25] "Bobby-Jo" (CAIS "female") eventually accepted surgery to remove her undescended testicles, "Tony" (PAIS "male") opted to undergo a mastectomy, abdominoplasty and phalloplasty,

[26] Kim, "As Is," 100.

[27] The following analysis is based upon a collection of 71 first-person accounts in English and German culled from the material made available from the following websites: Androgen Insensitivity Syndrome Support Group<http://www.medhelp.org/www/ais>, AIS Support Group Australia Inc. <http://home.vicnet.net.au/~aissg/>, XY-Frauen <http://www.xy-frauen.de/>, Arbeitsgruppe Gegen

Gewalt in der Paediatrie und Gynaekologie <http://www.postgender.de/>. Additional accounts can be found in articles addressing the question of the medical management of intersex(es), for example at <http://mosaic.echonyc.com/~onissues/su98coventry.html>, <http://www.qis.net/~triea/diane.html> and <http://www.nerve.com/dispatches/levay/intersex/intersex.asp>. The lowest reported age of the group of authors was reported to be 18, the highest over 65, with an average age of between 30-35, and a median age of between 35-40.

[28] "April's Story." e1-2: e1, available at <http://www.medhelp.org/www/ais/stories/april.htm>.

[29] "Renee." e1-e4: e1, available at <http://home.vicnet.net.au/~aissg/renee.htm>.

[30] "Jan's Story." e1-2: e1, available at <http://www.medhelp.org/www/ais/stories/jan.htm>.

[31] "Elaine's Story." e1-e2: e1, available at <http://www.medhelp.org/www/ais/stories/elaine.htm>.

[32] "Jan's Story." e1-2: e1, available at <http://www.medhelp.org/www/ais/stories/jan.htm>.

[33] "Carmel's Story." e1, available at <http://www.medhelp.org/www/ais/stories/carmel.htm>.

[34] "Sue." e1-2: e1, available at <http://home.vicnet.net.au/~aissg/sue.htm>.

[35] "Jeanne's Story." e1, available at <http://www.medhelp.org/www/ais/stories/jeanne.htm>.

[36] "Ann's Story." e1-2: e1, available at <http://www.medhelp.org/www/ais/stories/ann.htm>.

[37] "Jay's Story." e1, available at <http://www.medhelp.org/www/ais/stories/jay.htm>.

[38] "Angela." quoted in M. Coventry, "The Tyranny of the Esthetic: Surgery's Most Intimate Violation." *OTI Online*, available at <http://mosaic.echonyc.com/~onissues/su98coventry.html>.

[39] Graham, "My Story." e1-e7: e1, available at <http://home.vicnet.net.au/~aissg/Graham.htm>.

[40] "My Story." e1-e3: e1, available at <http://mypages.blackvoices.com/intersex/aboutus/>.

[41] "Angel's Story." e1-e2, e2, available at <http://www.medhelp.org/www/ais/stories/angel.htm>.

[42] Few stories from the perspective of the parents of AIS children are available. Among those available on-line which are easily located can be found at MedHelp.org <http://www.medhelp.org/www/ais/stories/> and include: "Toni's Story" …/toni.htm, "Virginia's Story" …/Virginia.htm, "Veronica's Story" …/veronica.htm, "Trust Me – I'm a Patient" …/WAVE.HTM, "Niel's Story" …/neil.htm, "Deb's Story" …/deb.htm, and "Gayle's Story" …/gayle.htm.

[43] "Ann's Story" e1-e2: e2, available at <http://www.medhelp.org/www/ais/stories/ann.htm>.

[44] The resources available to the researcher tend for CAH to be dominated by the genre of discussion forums, due primarily to the emergent nature of the condition. Unlike AIS, the parents of CAH patients also tend to dominate the discussion boards. There are very few first-person narrative accounts by those with CAH. Such stories can be found at: CAH Our Voices Our Stories <http://cahourstories.net> (may no longer be serviceable), ISNA "Presented at Robert Wood Johnson Medical School" <http://www.isna.org/library/whelanjan2002.html>, "Kira" (one of the earliest posted first-person narratives on the Internet) <http://www.qis.net/~triea/kira.html>, CAH Support Group <http://www.cah.org.uk> under "CAH Stories," Adrenal Hyperplasia Network "Becky Roche's Experience of CAH" <http://www.ahn.org.uk> under "Personal Stories", and the CAH Organization of Texas <http://www.tdh.state.tx.us/newborn/Cahoot.htm>. Extensive discussions of over 2200 combined postings by parents, patients, and even young adults with CAH (as of February 2003) can be found in forums sponsored by Congenital Adrenal Hyperplasia.org <http://www.congenitaladrenalhyperplasia.org>, Bodies Like Ours <http://www.bodieslikeours.org>, CAH Support Group under "Messages", and Yahoo! Groups "Congenital Adrenal Hyperplasia <http://groups.yahoo.com/group/adrenal_hyperplasia>.

[45] Linda, S, "Some Important Questions." February 1, 2003, available at <http://www.congenitaladrenalhyperplasia.com/mb/index.php?msg=0253830918&forum=main>.

[46] The most widely published and broadly adopted proposal concerning surgical management originated with the Intersexed Society of North America. Cf. "ISNA's Recommendations for Treatment" at <http://www.isna.org/library/recommendations.html>.

[47] April, "Advice on Explaining Surgery to a Child." January 30, 2003, available at <http://www.congenitaladrenalhyperplasia.com/mb/index.php?msg=0009710082&forum=controversy>.

[48] A. Thompson, "Kendall's Story." *The Cahoot* 3. Winter 2002, available at <http://www.tdh.state.tx.us/newborn/Cahoot3.htm#Kendall's%20Story>.

[49] B. Driver, founder of *Bodies Like Ours,* an outreach group dedicated to halting genital surgery upon infants, posting a response to a father who was about to take his 8-month-old daughter to a pediatric

urologist; "My Latest Essay (It's Exceptionally Long This Time)." November 20, 2002. http://www.congenitaladrenalhyperplasia.com/mb/index.php?msg=0008930076&forum=controversy.

[50] Victoria, "I Heard That." August 21, 2002, available at <http://www.bodieslikeours.org/forums/showthread.php?s=6c4474060c5052df793debf2b1e2e3d3&thread id=100>.

[51] "Danette's Story," e1-e4: e1-e2, available at <http://www.cahourstories.net/danette.html>.

[52] J. Whelan, "Presented at Robert Wood Johnson Medical School." *Intersex Panel for Sex Week* (January 2002): e1-4: e4, available at <http://www.isna.org/library/shelanjan2002.html>.

[53] The following discussion is based on 11 first-person narratives (including one by a parent) located at <http://www.hypospadias.net>, 11 first-person narratives (2 of which are duplicates of hypospadias.net) at <http://www.the-penis.com/hypospadias>, 56 original postings and their responses by the first internet forum on hypospadias now archived at <http://www.the-penis.com/hypomessages>, 3500+ postings on Mums With Hypospadias Kids (481 members as of February 2003) located at <http://egroups.yahoo.com/>, 2600+ messages at the Hypospadias Support Group for Parents and Patients (398 members as of February 2003) also located at <http://egroups.yahoo.com/>. Cf. also http://www.hypospadiashelp.fsnet.co.uk for more personal stories and responses.

[54] Johns Hopkins reports from a follow up study that 39 hypospadias 46,XY patients show a statistical mean of 5.8 surgeries. Cf. C Migeon et al, "Ambiguous Genitalia with Perineoscrotal Hypospadias in 46,XY Individuals: Long-Term Medical, Surgical, and Psychosexual Outcome." *Pediatrics* 110.3 (September 2002): e31.

[55] These conclusions are based upon the results of the second of two major surveys of hypospadac males who were members of the Hypospadic Association of America Internet forums. It took place between July and August 2001. 183 men with hypospadias responded, and results were compared to a control group of 1890 males from the general population. Available at <http://www.hypospadias.net>.

[56] 89% of those with "mild" hypospadias (urethral opening at upper 1/3 of the shaft) responding to the survey said they were not planning to have further surgery. 34% of these gave the reason that they were happy with the result, while 31% said they were afraid more surgery would make matters worse. 80% of those with "moderate/severe" hypospadias (middle/lower 2/3 of the shaft) responding to the survey said they were not planning to have further surgery. Of this group, 16% said they were happy with the results, while 51% feared further surgery would make it worse. Only 24.1% of "mild" hypospadias respondents underwent surgery, with an average of 2.2 surgeries performed. In contrast, 85.7% of "moderate/severe" hypospadias respondents underwent surgery, with an average of 3.1 surgeries for "moderate" cases and 5.1 surgeries for "severe" cases.

[57] David, "Living with Hypospdias: a Personal Account," available at <http://www.hypsopadias.net/stories/david.htm>.

[58] No Name, "Another Personal Account," available at <http://www.the-penis.com/hypospadias>, under "Personal accounts of hypospadias from visitors to this site."

[59] No Name, "A Personal Account of the Experience of Hypospadias," available at <http://www.the-penis.com/hypospadias>, under "Personal accounts of hypospadias from visitors to this site."

[60] No Name, "My Story," available at <http://www.hypospadias.net/stories/anonymous1.htm>.

[61] Message 3451, *mumswithhypospadiaskids eGroup,* available at <http://egroups.yahoo.com/groups/ mumswithhypospadiaskids>.

[62] Message 3472, *mumswithhypospadiaskids eGroup,* available at <http://egroups.yahoo.com/groups/ mumswithhypospadiaskids>.

[63] Message 3478, *mumswithhypospadiaskids eGroup,* available at <http://egroups.yahoo.com/groups/ mumswithhypospadiaskids>.

[64] Message 2495, *mumswithhypospadiaskids eGroup,* available at <http://egroups.yahoo.com/groups/ mumswithhypospadiaskids>.

[65] Message 48, *mumswithhypospadiaskids eGroup,* available at <http://egroups.yahoo.com/groups/ mumswithhypospadiaskids>.

[66] Message 3004, *mumswithhypospadiaskids eGroup,* available at <http://egroups.yahoo.com/groups/ mumswithhypospadiaskids>.

[67] No Name, "Living with Hypospadias – My Story," available at <http://www.the-penis.com/hypospadias.html>, under "Personal accounts of hypospadias from visitors to this site."

[68] No Name, "From a Gay Man," available at <http://www.the-penis.com/hypospadias.html>, under "Personal accounts of hypospadias from visitors to this site."

[69] Jehanjh, "Jehanjh," available at <http://www.hypospadias.net/stories/jehanj.htm>.

[70] Among the first-person accounts available, the following were used for the ensuing discussion: D. Brager, "I'm Not Fat, I'm Deformed: Klinefelter's Syndrome & Me" (1997) <http://www.geocities.com/WestHollywood/Castro/4998/klinefl.htm>, Anonymous, "Klinefelter's Syndrome: A Personal Reflection" at <http://www.isgi.org/isgi/Klinefelter.html>, S. Poirier, "My Story" at <http://host.cnwl.igs.net/~destined/page3.html>, "Living with Klinefelters'" at <http://klinefeltersyndrome.org/stefan.htm>. The Turner Syndrome Forum (280 members, 4000+ postings) at http://egroups.yahoo.com/group/turnersydromeforum and the AAKIS Forum (212 members, 10,000+ postings as of February 2003) at http://egroups.yahoo.com/group/AAKSIS were also used.

[71] For more information, visit the Turner Syndrome Society webpage at <http://www.turner-syndrome-us.org>, Turner Syndrome Support Society webpage at <http://www.turner.org.uk>, The Turner Center of the Psychiatric Hospital Aahrus in Denmark <http://www.aaa.dk/TURNER/ENGELSK/INDEX.HTM>, and Deutsche Ulrich-Turner-Syndrom Vereinigung e.V at <http://www.turner-syndrom.de>. See also the very helpful personal page "Tim's Turner Syndrome Page" at <http://www.iland.net/~tdluke/trnrs.html>.

[72] S. Poirier, "Biography." e1-e7: e3, available at <http://host.cnwl.igs.net/~destined/page 3.html>.

[73] Message 6, *livingwithklinefelter eGroup.*

[74] No Name, "Klinefelter's – A Personal Reflection," available at <http://www.isgi.org/isgi/Klinefleter.html>.

[75] Message 8, *livingwithklinefelter eGroup*

[76] C. Toomey, "Hidden Genders." *The Weekend Australian* (8-9 December 2001): e1-5: e3. Reprinted at <http://home.vicnet.net.au/~aissg/hidden_genders.htm>.

[77] See J. David Hester (Amador), "Rhetoric of the Management of Intersexed Children: New Insights into 'Disease', 'Illness', 'Curing' and 'Healing'." *Genders* 38 <www.genders.org> for an incisive critique on the *necessarily* damaging impact of medical intervention upon intersexuality arising from the medical pathologizing of the natural body of the intersex and the artificial construction of "normal" sexuality.

ALICE DOMURAT DREGER

INTERSEX AND HUMAN RIGHTS:

The Long View

1. INTRODUCTION

This is an essay about how an article I published in 1998 was wrong. I hope the reader will bear with me and see this is not an exercise in narcissism or self-flagellation. It is, rather, an attempt to explain why changing the treatment of intersex has turned out to be a much harder job than those of us in the early intersex reform movement imagined it would be.

Probably because we had so few allied doctors back then, in 1998 those of us agitating for intersex treatment reform were naïve about the way medical practice works.[1] Today we know that the standard of care for intersex wasn't the simple anomaly we thought it was. As a consequence, though we started out thinking that to improve the care of people with intersex conditions we would just need to move the care of intersex into line with the rest of medicine, we now know there are some basic problems generalized in the institution of medical practice that contribute to the poor treatment of families dealing with intersex. Fixing the treatment of intersex isn't, therefore, like trying to get one surly elephant to line up in a parade of otherwise well-behaved elephants. It's like trying to push a whole parade of stubborn elephants—and trying to do this with soap on your feet.

I want to suggest, though, that this heavy lifting—or heavy pushing—is worth it. That yes, it is very hard to change intersex practice, because it's very hard to change any entrenched practice that continues to run on the energy of its own inertia. But changing the practice of intersex is going to have (and indeed already has started to have) critically useful effects for many other realms of medical care—for example, the care of gay and lesbian patients, and of children born with various anomalies and disabilities.

This is because—though until recently this has not been well articulated—the intersex reform movement has been essentially a human rights movement.[2] That is—like the civil rights movement against racism, and the women's rights movement against sexism—it has been and is founded on the assumption that people with intersex should not be oppressed simply because their bodies do not rank at the top of the social hierarchy.[3] As a consequence, doctors who have "gotten" intersex as a human rights issue find themselves realizing what it could mean to get beyond the

S.E. Sytsma (Ed.), Ethics and Intersex, 73–86.
© 2006 *Springer. Printed in the Netherlands.*

presumption that Western healthcare "standards of care" are necessarily respectful of human rights. In other words, the intersex reform movement is helping to push the question of what humane healthcare really means.

2. CONCEALING INTERSEX

The theoretical basis for the standard of care for intersex as it existed in the early 1990s grew, historically speaking, out of an interdisciplinary team operating at Johns Hopkins. That group developed what came to be known as the "optimum gender of rearing" model of care, a model that centered on the belief that you could (and should) try to make intersex children as convincing boys or girls as possible, though surgical and medical technologies, and through counseling. The Hopkins team favored the idea that, in terms of gender identity and sexual orientation, children are born as blank slates; they develop a gender identity and a sexual orientation based upon social interactions with the people around them. If you made a child *look* like a girl, and made others *believe* that she was a girl, then she would also *think* she was a girl, and thus would *become* a girl—preferably a straight girl. Because the team believed genitals were the most important aspect of sex and gender identity, and because they believed it was easier to construct good-looking girl genitals than good-looking boy genitals, most intersex patients were made into girls.

Though, in their early writings, members of the team (including the famous John Money) said that patients should be informed of their medical histories in age-appropriate ways, in practice few were.[4] Indeed, many were actively deceived by medical practitioners who thought that the truth would be counter-productive. As a consequence, my colleague Cheryl Chase and I have termed the late-twentieth-century standard of care, as it came to be, the "concealment approach."[5] The goal of this model was, after all, to make intersex disappear—to obscure any appearance of intersex and also most personal and social knowledge of intersex.[6]

I was not at all the first person to criticize the concealment approach. In fact, by 1998 several clinicians had implicitly questioned it through peer-reviewed research articles that showed, for example, the successful rearing of micropenis boys as boys[7], the high frequency of penises fitting the American urological establishment's definition of penile "abnormality,"[8] and the persistence of male gender identity in a boy who had been surgically sex re-assigned in infancy.[9] Meanwhile, criticisms had also started coming from science studies scholars[10] and were flowing like water from an open main from many people with intersex, especially those who had experienced at first-hand the concealment model.[11]

So there was a disparate but clear groundswell already in place when, in 1998, I published in the *Hastings Center Report* an article exploring in detail the concealment model's many ethical problems.[12] As was probably clear to readers of the article, by then I thought it was obvious that the standard treatment of intersex was so morally outrageous that, once exposed, it would quickly change. I was particular struck by three components of intersex treatment that seemed extraordinary for medicine:

In cases of intersex clinicians were intentionally *withholding and misrepresenting critical medical information*. This prevented parents of minors and major patients from making informed choices, from doing their own research on their situations, and from finding others in the same position.

Otherwise healthy children were being subjected to procedures that risked or sometimes negated sexual sensation, fertility, continence, health, and life *simply because their bodies did not fit social norms*. Not only were these children being treated differently from non-intersex children, within intersex clinics they were also being treated in a literally sexist way: "for example, physicians appear[ed] to do far more to preserve the reproductive potential of children born with ovaries than that of children born with testes...Similarly, surgeons seem[ed] to demand far more for a penis to count as 'successful' than for a vagina to count as such."[13] Doctors were equating—or at least conflating—statistical difference and disease, treating healthy-but-funny-looking genitals as surgical emergencies.[14] And, although nearly all clinicians agreed that intersex was primarily a *psychosocial* problem (a problem of norms), very few provided professional or peer psycho-social support to parents and patients.

The final ethical problem was the *near total lack of evidence*—indeed, a near-total lack of *interest* in evidence—that the concealment system was producing the good results intended. The goal of all this work was supposed to be psychosocial health, but the few follow-up studies that existed looked instead at what the surgeon thought of the cosmetic outcome. Not only did clinicians ignore evidence that gender identity was less plastic than Money claimed, not only did they ignore evidence that micropenis boys could do well as boys, not only did they ignore well-known sexological studies that showed how important the shaft of the clitoris is to men and women's sexual pleasure, they used clinical standards for phallic appearance that were so arbitrary as to sound like a bad joke to outsiders.[15] Parents, though, were not told the experimental nature of this treatment system.

Given all this, I ended that 1998 article by arguing that the treatment of intersex was unlike anything else in modern-day medicine. In fact, I said that doctors seemed to be employing for intersex what ethicist George Annas had termed "the monster approach".[16] In other words, children with intersex were being treated as "so grotesque, so pathetic, any medical procedure aimed at normalizing them would be morally justified."[17] In short, they were being treated as non-humans—or at least not fully human—in the sense that they were being subjected to a system of treatment that would have been considered inhumane had it been applied to others.

After I published this article and the related book, many academic ethicists, journalists, and activists readily agreed that the concealment model of intersex treatment was fundamentally flawed and needed changing.[18] But the reaction among the medical establishment (at least the elites at the top of their fields) has been notably slower. And I think that the reason for that must be because, in spite of what we in the intersex reform movement thought in 1998, the treatment of intersex actually looks a lot like other realms of modern medicine. Those three enumerated core components of the treatment of intersex didn't—and don't—shock most of the folks treating intersex because they are in fact pretty familiar to them and their colleagues from other realms of care.

3. SEX, LIES, AND PEDIATRICIANS

Dig a little into the experiences of intersex clinicians and patients, and you soon find that intersex is a hotbed of deception. And in a weird sort of way, the medical profession has been rather honest about that deception. In other words, they talk openly about it—while at the same time lying to individual patients. For instance, in 1995 the Canadian Medical Association awarded a medical student a prize for an article arguing that practitioners had an ethical *duty* to deceive patients with Androgen Insensitivity Syndrome (AIS—an intersex condition) about the nature of their conditions.[19] The logic was that the patients would needlessly suffer from knowing the truth. More recently, the North American Task Force on Intersex (NATFI) found its quest for follow-up data stymied by clinicians who insisted they couldn't possibly tell their patients the truth about what had happened and been done to them. And in a 2000 issue of Discover magazine, in an article entitled "The Curse of the Garcias," a physician wrote—*for popular entertainment purposes*—about how he has been lying for years to one of his patients, a woman with AIS.[20]

In most of medicine today practitioners would never think it their ethical duty to consistently and repeatedly lie and withhold critical medical information; indeed most would see their duty as the opposite. But I've come to realize that, at least in pediatric care of serious medical conditions, it is still often the case that practitioners do withhold critical information from patients and parents under the guise of bearing the burden of knowledge for them.[21] In other words, what happens in intersex treatment is different in degree, but not different in kind, from what happens elsewhere in medicine, especially tertiary pediatric medicine.

Now, because they are experts, doctors almost always know a lot more about a particular condition than they tell their patients. But sometimes doctors choose to reveal *much* less than any reasonable outsider would think they ought, either because they are made uncomfortable by discussing issues or are worried about undermining their authority and heroic images. This seems to be especially true in pediatrics, where parents and patients are often patronized (ex., called "Mom" and "Dad" by team members) and treated with greater than the usual amount of paternalism.[22] The excuse I've heard for this is that there is no point in making the parents or patients "unnecessarily" feel uncertain, but uncertainty about one's life (or one's child's life) is part of the prognosis of that life, and so should be shared, not withheld or glossed over. Yet too often uncertainty becomes an excuse for medical paternalism when it ought to function as a critique of it.

In intersex, as is other situations, sometimes the information withheld by doctors is about well-established and well-respected patient advocacy groups who would provide an alternative perspective on treatment options (often available at rival institutions), sometimes the information is about how little is known about outcomes for recommended options, and sometimes it is about how much difference it makes which surgeon you engage for a particular procedure.[23] Many physicians feel this sort of information is either not relevant or too political to reveal. Yet it seems to me—from conversations I've had with parents and with persons born with atypical anatomies—that this information is exquisitely relevant to making informed decisions.

One response to the observation that intersex isn't the only realm of medicine where information is misrepresented or withheld is to throw up one's hands and say deception is "normal" medical practice in certain arenas—that there's nothing you can do about it. But I think this is the wrong approach. Paul Farmer, a Harvard-based international infectious-disease specialist, suggests that when we see two groups of people being treated differently in medicine for social (and not metabolic) reasons, we should not make that observation the end of the conversation.[24] It should rather begin a conversation that inquires into what would happen if you treat both groups as equally human.

If we decline the "monster approach" and consider persons with intersex as fully enfranchised human beings—as I think we should—we realize that they and their parents have the right to know at least as much as their doctor is willing to tell his or her colleagues, no less the one million readers of *Discover* magazine. Indeed, all over medicine physicians need to realize that informed consent means more than giving the usual disclaimers about, say, anesthetic risks; it ought to mean educating patients (and parents, if applicable) about the specific medical condition at issue, handing over without reservation copies of everything in the chart, explaining what is known and unknown and what is under serious debate.

What I'm suggesting is that we reject the idea that (a) intersex is so freakish it calls for extraordinary behavior on the part of clinicians, or (b) clinicians' treatment of intersex is appropriate because it looks like behaviors we find in other realms of medicine, and instead adopt the notion that (c) the treatment of families with intersex has often been very poor indeed—so poor that, like a lens, it helps us see what other parts of medicine might also need immediate revision to effect humane care.

3. NORMAL MEDICINE?

What, then, about this issue of changing otherwise-healthy children to fit social norms? Isn't that unusual in medicine?

Hardly. It happens during most circumcisions, during non-emergent conjoined twin separation surgeries, and when children who are just short are put on growth hormones.[25] Increasingly, all over medicine, children are subject to drugs, surgeries, and intensive behavioural therapies specifically aimed at making them fall into the boundaries of an idealized norm.

But whereas I used to think that this push to "normalize" signaled a rejection of the "abnormal" child, I am now more inclined to think that those pushing see it (paradoxically) as loving acceptance of the child. Since becoming a parent in 2000, I've realized how much I underestimated the parental (and sometimes pediatric-paternalist) desire to "normalize" children, a desire that is clearly a manifestation of the visceral—almost savage—desire to protect children. The parent (and pediatric surgeon) sees the child as essentially perfect, and wants the often-cloddish and boorish world to see the same, so she "reconstructs" the child to "normality." In

1998, when, thanks to sociologist Arthur Frank's work,[26] I recognized the mythology of calling intersex surgeries "reconstructive" I think I failed to understand how much parents and surgeons *believed* in the restitution narrative they spoke. They really think they are *restoring* the child to the normality they've come to see within that child.

In that sense, I think I failed also to see what social scientist Adrienne Asch does in "Distracted by Disability,"[27] namely the conflicted position of the physician approaching the congenitally or chronically "disabled" patient. How is it the surgeon can truly accept the whole child born with an unusual anatomy—including the supposedly "deformed" anatomy which will very likely form a critical aspect of that person's identity—and also seek to "rescue" her from it? In 1998 I thought doctors treating intersex had put themselves in an awkward position—wanting to help patients while unintentionally hurting them. Now I realize what I am calling them to is a much more awkward position. I'm asking them to put down their tools of "correction" when in their minds that would signal abandoning the child, rather than accepting her.

More generally put, I think I misunderstood to what extent medical and surgical intervention is the primary means of demonstrating *caring* for many clinicians, patients, and family members. This is especially true as non-intervention gets represented almost always as cheapskate HMO-type behavior, or as racist, sexist, or classist (which it sometimes is). Doctors see something as abnormal—anatomically or behaviourally—and think the way to help is to change what they see as the primary problem. The child is subjected to procedures aimed at changing their body or behaviour, and no one questions whether the norm itself might need correction.

But again, what I want to suggest here is that we reject the idea that (a) intersex is so freakish it calls for extraordinary behaviour on the part of clinicians, or (b) clinicians' treatment of intersex is appropriate because it looks like behaviours we find in other realms of medicine, and instead adopt the notion that (c) the treatment of people with intersex has been problematic enough that it helps us see what other parts of medicine might also need immediate revision to effect truly humane care.

In this case, I think what we can learn from the history of intersex experience is that there are other ways to care for people (especially children) who are "abnormal"—i.e., different from the social norms—than to throw medicines and surgeries at them. In fact—aside from the underlying metabolic dangers such as salt imbalance, adrenal crisis, or cancers that sometimes attend intersex conditions, all of which everyone agrees you should treat thoughtfully—the challenges families with intersex face are *social* challenges. Like racism and sexism, they are social challenges, even if they do arise—as some sociobiologists and surgeons will claim—from "hardwired" fear of difference.[28] When doctors see a clash between a child's body and the social body and they choose to address that clash by changing the child, they are in effect saying the social body cannot, will not, or should not be changed. But to consider this as a matter of human rights—that is, to consider people with intersex as we would other humans—means considering the possibility that the child is not the wound that needs healing. It is, for example, to consider that the correct response to oppressive racism is to work against racism, not to eliminate racial differences in infancy (or during gestation). And the correct response to the

dehumanization" within the study's internals records and its published reports—that is, language that made the researchers sound like passive tools of medical science, language that made the subjects sound like mere sites of disease, and language that "highlight[ed] a relatively minor difference (skin color) between groups of subjects as it obscure[d] their more numerous and significant resemblances."[38] Language that made it sound like the subjects were something other than humans.

It seems to me, given how things are going socially and clinically, that most people a few decades from now will view today's treatment of intersex like people today view the Tuskegee Syphilis Study. There will be a myth that the people who carried on, for decades, with the concealment approach and its derivatives were bad, hateful, overtly sexist people. There will be a myth that the whole thing happened because it was hidden from view. But as in the case of the Tuskegee Syphilis Study, none of that will be true. The truth will be that what kept the unethical intersex system going was institutional inertia, the desire to maintain professional reputations and careers, the use of language and pictures that dehumanized patients and posed them as if they were mere sites of localized disease, and the subsequent harm that arose from accidentally treating subjects as exempt from the rights accorded others. The lesson of the Tuskegee Syphilis Study and the treatment of intersex ought to be the same: Being well-meaning is not enough.

Is it hard to change practice? Yes. Especially when insurance companies and government agencies don't want to pay for long-term psycho-social services, when there doesn't seem to be anyone to provide those services, when parents seem more grateful for confident assurances than honest uncertainty, and when changing means admitting your field's heroes or your mentors (or you) were wrong. But you know what I would tell those practicing today? The old-time clinicians have learned the hard way that kids with intersex do grow up, and become quite obviously human. Whether they end up as men or women, straight or gay, they end up as quite obviously human. And they become quite articulate about how they wish they had always been treated that way. Start assuming that outcome now.

Alice Domurat Dreger, Visiting Professor, Medical Humanities and Bioethics Program, Northwestern University Feinberg School of Medicine, Chicago, Illinois, U.S.A.

NOTES

[1] On early intersex reform work and relations with the medical profession, see Cheryl Chase, "Hermaphrodites with Attitude: Mapping the Emergence of Intersex Political Activism," GLQ: A Journal of Gay and Lesbian Studies, 4(2)(1998):189-211; and see Alice Domurat Dreger, "Cultural History and Social Activism: Scholarship, Identities, and the Intersex Rights Movement," in *Locating Medical History: The Stories and Their Meanings*, ed Frank Huisman and John Harley Warner (Baltimore: Johns Hopkins University Press, 2004), pp. 390-409.

[2]   The San Francisco Human Rights Commission and the South African Human Rights Commission are the leaders in this realm. See Marcus de Maria Arana, *A Human Rights Investigation into the Medical "Normalization" of Intersex People: A Report of a Public Hearing by the Human Rights Commission* (City and County of San Francisco, 2005); Wendell Roelf, "Intersex Children Must Be Protected from Temptation of Parents to 'Fix' Them Socially," Cape Times, December 1, 2004, available at http://www.capetimes.co.za/index.php?fSectionId=271&fArticleId=2329017.

[3]   Alice Domurat Dreger, *One of Us: Conjoined Twins and the Future of Normal* (Harvard University Press, 2004), chap. 5.

[4]   See, for example, John Money, Joan G. Hampson, and John L. Hampson, "Hermaphroditism: Recommendations Concerning Assignment of Sex, Chang of Sex, and Psychologic Management," *Bulletin of Johns Hopkins Hospital*, vol. 97, no. 4 (1955): 284-300.

[5]   Alice Dreger, "Shifting the Paradigm of Intersex Treatment," available at www.isna.org/drupal/compare.

[6]   Cheryl Chase, "Affronting Reason," in *Looking Queer: Body Image and Identity in Lesbian, Bisexual, Gay, and Transgender Communities*, edited by Dawn Atkins (Haworth Press, 1998), pp. 205-220.

[7]   Justine M. Reilly and C. R. J. Woodhouse, "Small Penis and the Male Sexual Role," *Journal of Urology*, vol. 142 (1989): 569-571.

[8]   Jan Fichtner et al., "Analysis of Meatal Location in 500 Men: Wide Variation Questions Need for Meatal Advancement in All Pediatric Anterior Hypospadias Cases," *Journal of Urology*, vol. 154 (1995): 833-834.

[9]   See Milton Diamond and H. K. Sigmundson, "Sex Reassignment at Birth: A Long Term Review and Clinical Implications," *Archives of Pediatrics and Adolescent Medicine*, vol. 150 (1997): 298-304; Natalie Angier, "Sexual Identity Not Pliable After All, Report Says," *New York Times*, 14 March 1997, p. 1; John Colapinto, "The True Story of John/Joan," *Rolling Stone*, 11 December 1997, pp. 54-73, 92-97.

[10] See Suzanne Kessler, "The Medical Construction of Gender: Case Management of Intersex Infants," *Signs: Journal of Women in Culture*, vol. 16, no. 1 (1990): 3-26; Anne Fausto-Sterling, "The Five Sexes: Why Male and Female Are Not Enough," 1993, *The Sciences* 33 (2): 20-25.

[11] See, for example, Cheryl Chase, Letters from Readers, *The Sciences*, July/August 1993, p. 3; Cheryl Chase, "'Corrective' Surgery Unnecessary" (letter), Johns Hopkins Magazine (February 1994), pp. 6-7; Cheryl Chase, "Intersex Society of North America: Intersexuals Advocate for Change," *American Medical Student Association Task Force Quarterly*, Fall 1994, pp. 30-31; Cheryl Chase, "Re: Measurement of Evoked Potentials during Feminizing Genitoplasty: Techniques and Applications" (letter), *Journal of Urology*, vol. 156, no. 3 (1996):1139-1140; Cheryl Chase, "Stop Medically Unnecessary Surgery" (letter), San Francisco Bay Times, 28 November 1996, p. 17; Cheryl Chase, "Re: Measurement of Pudendal Evoked Potentials during Feminizing Genitoplasty: Techniques and Applications" (letter), *Journal of Urology*, vol. 156, no. 3 (1996):1139-1140; Cheryl Chase and Martha Coventry, Special Issue on Intersexuality, *Chrysalis: The Journal of Transgressive Gender Identities*, Fall/Winter 1997; Cheryl Chase, "Phallocentric Criteria" (letter), *Clinical Psychiatry News*, September 1997; Cheryl Chase, "Spare the Knife, Study the Child" (letter), *Ob.Gyn. News*, 1 October 1997, pp. 14-15; Cheryl Chase, director, *Hermaphrodites Speak! San Francisco: Intersex Society of North America*, video tape (30 minutes), 1997, available from www.isna.org; Anonymous, "Be Open and Honest with Sufferers," *BMJ*, vol. 308 (1994): 1041-1042; B. Diane Kemp, letter to the editor, *Canadian Medical Association Journal*, vol. 154 (1996), p. 1829; Sherri A. Groveman, letter to the editor, *Canadian Medical Association Journal*, vol. 154 (1996): 1829 and 1832. By 1998 there were also many autobiographical accounts and first-hand former-patient critiques available on the web through, for example, the now-defunct "Intersex Voices" website created by Kiira Triea.

[12] Alice Domurat Dreger, "'Ambiguous Sex' – or Ambivalent Medicine? Ethical Problems in the Treatment of Intersexuality," *The Hastings Center Report*, vol. 28, no. 3, May/June 1998, pp. 24-35.

[13] Ibid., pp. 28-29.

[14] See, for example, the discussion of to what extent "ambiguous genitalia" constitute a "medical and social emergency," in Richard H. Hurwitz, H. Applebaum, and S. Muenchow, *Surgical Reconstruction of Ambiguous Genitalia in Female Children*, videotape, 1990; available from Cine-Med at www.cine-med.com. In this training film, Dr. Hurwitz claims that, "In most cases it is better to wait until the child is six months old when the anesthetic risks are minimized. If the clitoris is very large, however, it may need to be taken care of earlier for social reasons." In other words, social

distress on the part of surrounding adults is sufficient reason to risk a child's life in a "normalization" procedure.

[15] ISNA found it useful to lampoon clinical standards for phallus length by producing and distributing "phall-o-meters"—little plastic measuring sticks that showed who was a good girl and who was a bad boy according to leading American pediatric urologists. These trinkets proved very popular—I'm still asked for them, years after ISNA stopped producing them—but they didn't accomplish much in terms of changing clinical practice. A point relevant to this article's thesis: the Smithsonian Institution now possesses an ISNA phall-o-meter as part of a special collection on the intersex rights movement.

[16] George J. Annas, "Siamese Twins: Killing One to Save the Other," *Hastings Center Report* 17 (April, 1987): 27-29. Annas used the term in relation to the treatment of conjoined twinning; he did not advocate the approach.

[17] Dreger, "'Ambiguous Sex'," p. 33.

[18] Alice Domurat Dreger, *Hermaphrodites and the Medical Invention of Sex* (Harvard University Press, 1998).

[19] Anita Natarajan, "Medical Ethics and Truth Telling in the Case of Androgen Insensitivity Syndrome," *Canadian Medical Association Journal*, vol. 154 (1996): 568-570. For responses to this article from women with AIS, *see Canadian Medical Association Journal*, vol. 154 (1996): 1829-1833. Dr. Natarajan retracted her remarks to some extent in an online follow-up statement, available at http://www.happinessonline.org/CommonSenseMoralCode/p3.htm.

[20] Robert Marion, "The Curse of the Garcias," Discover, December 2000, 42. See also response to this from Sherri A. Groveman, "Lifting the Curse," *Discover*, March 2001.

[21] On this point, see Dreger, *One of Us*, chap. 2.

[22] This is developed more fully in Alice Domurat Dreger, "What to Expect When You Have the Child You Weren't Expecting," in *Surgically Shaping Children*, edited by Erik Parens (Washington, Georgetown University Press, 2005).

[23] See Dreger, One of Us, pp. 80-81.

[24] Paul Farmer, "Pathologies of Power: Rethinking Health and Human Rights in the Global Era," public lecture delivered at Calvin College, Grand Rapids, Michigan, January 10, 2005.

[25] Alice Dreger, "When Medicine Goes Too Far in Pursuit of Normality," New York Times, July 28, 1998, p. B-10; reprinted in *Health Ethics Today*, vol. 10, no. 1, August, 1999, pp. 2-5.

[26] Arthur W. Frank, *The Wounded Storyteller: Body, Illness, and Ethics* (University of Chicago Press, 1995), chap. 4.

[27] Adrienne Asch, "Distracted by Disability," *Cambridge Quarterly of Healthcare Ethics*, 7 (1998): 77-87.

[28] I discuss this attitude—that discrimination and bullying is hardwired and therefore inevitable—in Alice Domurat Dreger, "Etiologies of Revulsion" (essay review of Margrit Shildrick's *Embodying the Monster: Encounters with the Vulnerable Self*), in *Health: An Interdisciplinary Journal for the Social Study of Health, Illness, and Medicine*, vol. 9, no. 1 (2005): 113-116.

[29] This point is more fully developed in Alice Dreger and Bruce Wilson, Commentary on "Culture Clash Involving Intersex," *The Hastings Center Report*, vol. 33, no. 4 (July/August 2003), pp. 12-14.

[30] For a history of debates surrounding mastectomies and reconstructive surgeries, see Barron H. Lerner, *The Breast Cancer Wars: Hope, Fear, and the Pursuit of a Cure in Twentieth-Century America* (Oxford University Press, 2001).

[31] For references to this issue, see http://www.lpaonline.org/resources_faq.html, website resource of *Little People of America*.

[32] See, for example, Catherine Minto, Lih-Mei Liao, Christopher R. J. Woodhouse, Philip G. Ramsley, and Sarah M. Creighton, "The Effects of Clitoral Surgery on Sexual Outcome in Individuals Who Have Intersex Conditions with Ambiguous Genitalia: A Cross Sectional Study," *Lancet*, vol. 361, no. 9365 (April 2003): 1252-1257; Thomas Mazur, David E. Sandberg, M.A. Perrin, J. A. Gallagher, and M. H. MacGillivray, "Male Pseudohermaphroditism: Long-Term Quality of Life Outcome in Five 46,XY Individuals Reared Female," *Journal of Pediatric Endocrinology and Metabolism*, vol. 17, no. 6 (June 2004): 809-823.

[33] H. F. L. Meyer-Bahlburg, C. J. Migeon, G. D. Berkovitz, J. P. Gearhart, C. Dolezal, and A. B. Wisniewski, "Attitudes of Adult 46,XY Intersex Persons to Clinical Management Policies," *Journal of Urology*, vol. 171 (April 2004): 1615-1619.

[34] For evidence people with intersex have survived psychologically and socially without early surgical "correction," see John Money, *Hermaphroditism: An Inquiry into the Nature of a Human Paradox* (Doctoral Dissertation, Harvard University, 1952); Dreger, *Hermaphrodites and the Medical Invention of Sex*; Hida Viloria in Chase, *Hermaphrodites Speak!*; Alice Domurat Dreger and Cheryl Chase, "A Mother's Care" (interview with woman with intersex and her mother), in *Intersex in the Age of Ethics*, edited by Alice Domurat Dreger (Hagerstown, Maryland: University Publishing Group, 1999): 83-89; Hale Hawbecker, "Who Did This to You?," ibid., 111-113; Intersex Society of North America, "What evidence is there that you can grow up psychologically healthy with intersex genitals (without 'normalizing' surgeries?", http://www.isna.org/faq/healthy.

[35] Allan M. Brandt, "Racism and Research: The Case of the Tuskegee Syphilis Experiment," *Hastings Center Report*, vol. 8, Dec. 1978, pp. 21-29.

[36] See the letter of Irwin J. Schatz to Donald H. Rockwell, 11 June 1965, and the annotation accompanying it ("This is the first letter of this type we have received. I do not plan to answer this letter") reprinted on pp. 103-104 in Susan M. Reverby, editor, *Tuskegee's Truths: Rethinking the Tuskegee Syphilis Study* (Chapel Hill: University of North Carolina Press, 2000).

[37] See Brandt, "Racism and Research," for a historical overview of the study.

[38] Martha Solomon Watson, "The Rhetoric of Dehumanization: An Analysis of Medical Reports of the Tuskegee Syphilis Project," in Reverby, ed., *Tuskegee's Truths*, pp. 251-265, quote on p. 260.

JULIE A. GREENBERG

INTERNATIONAL LEGAL DEVELOPMENTS PROTECTING THE AUTONOMY RIGHTS OF SEXUAL MINORITIES

Who Should Determine the Appropriate Treatment for an Intersex Infant?

1. INTRODUCTION

As the essays in this book illustrate, the medical treatment of intersex children is undergoing an intense examination. Doctors, psychologists, psychiatrists, sociologists, historians, ethicists, and intersex activists have all weighed in on the debate about the physical, psychological, sociological and ethical implications of early genital surgery. Before the last decade, the accepted medical protocol granted to physicians almost complete control concerning treatment decisions and the child's best interests. Physicians told parents little about their child's condition and many medical professionals advocated deceiving intersex patients about the exact nature of their conditions to protect them from psychological harm.[1]

During the last 10 years, this protocol has come under heavy attack. Although a number of experts have exposed flaws in the traditional approach, the debate about the appropriate treatment model is far from over. Comprehensive studies addressing this issue do not exist and because of ethical restraints limiting research in this area, the issue is unlikely to be resolved soon.[2]

Those involved in the debate now support three alternative protocols: (1) the model that has existed for the last 40 years, which emphasizes the need for early surgical and hormonal intervention to conform the child's body to societal norms and minimizes the information given to the child and parents to avoid psychological trauma; (2) a "middle ground" approach that emphasizes the need for disclosure of complete information to the parents and deference to the parental decision about whether surgical or hormonal treatment would be in the best interests of their child; and (3) a complete moratorium on all surgical and hormonal treatments that are not medically necessary so that the child, when she reaches the age of consent, can determine whether she wants to elect to undergo any surgical alteration.

Until comprehensive retrospective studies are conducted that clearly establish which approach best protects the interests of the intersex infant, positions are likely to become more polarized. Given the interests at stake and the intensity of the debate, legal institutions will likely be called upon to weigh in on the debate.

S.E. Sytsma (Ed.), Ethics and Intersex, 87–101.

Legislatures may be asked to enact statutes[3] and in the absence of legislative action, courts will be asked to intervene. Thus far, no country has enacted controlling legislation and Colombia is the only country where the highest court has rendered an opinion on this issue. Therefore, if courts are asked to resolve the legal, medical and ethical issues surrounding the treatment of intersex children, the outcome is far from clear.

This chapter explores how courts may resolve this issue if they are brought into the controversy. Part I provides a brief summary of the current debates about the treatment model that best protects the interests of intersex infants. Part II describes the doctrine of informed consent as courts have traditionally applied it in medical determinations on behalf of children and others who are not competent to make medical decisions on their own behalf. Part III describes how the Constitutional Court of Colombia, the only high court that has ruled on this issue, applied the law of informed consent in the context of surgical alteration of intersex infants. Part IV explores how courts in Europe, Australia and the United States are likely to resolve this issue if they are asked to intervene. Although no appellate courts in these jurisdictions have been confronted by this precise issue, recent decisions by the European Court of Human Rights, Australian courts, and the United States Supreme Court may shed light on the probable outcome. Part V concludes that the legal arena may not be the optimal forum in which to resolve this complex personal and ethical dilemma.

2. THE CURRENT DEBATE OVER THREE ALTERNATIVE MODELS

2.1 The Dominant Protocol

The dominant treatment protocol developed during the 1950s, due in large part to the influential work of John Money.[4] Money hypothesized that children are born without a fixed gender identity. He believed that children develop a gender identity that conforms to the gender role in which they are raised, as long as that gender role matches the appearance of their genitalia. Therefore, he encouraged physicians to surgically alter infants born with genitalia that do not conform to male or female norms. Money believed that if surgeons sculpted "normal-appearing" genitalia and administered appropriate hormones, and parents raised the child in the gender role that conformed to the surgically created genitalia, the child would develop an unambiguous gender identity, and severe psychological trauma would be avoided. Critical to this protocol is the requirement that intersex children be raised without any ambiguity about their gender. Therefore, physicians traditionally encouraged parents to hide the truth about the child's intersex condition. In addition, to avoid trauma to the parents, physicians often told parents less than the whole truth about the child's condition and guided parents toward the decision the physician believed was optimal.

Until the 1990s, physicians believed that they were uniquely qualified to determine the best interests of the parents and the child. By disclosing selective information to the parents and advocating support for only one treatment model, physicians controlled the ultimate outcome. As recently as 1995, major medical associations supported the selective disclosure of information to the parents and outright lying to the intersex patient about the nature of her condition.[5] Now, few would advocate in favor of hiding information from the parents or lying to the intersex patient. Changes in bioethical norms have shifted to a model favoring complete disclosure.

Although some recent comments indicate that many doctors are questioning the traditional protocol,[6] the most recent by the American Academy of Pediatrics (AAP) official publication supports this model.[7] Supporters of this treatment protocol believe that living with ambiguous or anomalous genitalia would lead to ostracism from peers, the potential weakening of the bond that parents are able to form with their child, and severe psychological trauma for the intersex child.

During the last decade, the traditional treatment model has been challenged by a number of intersex adults and researchers studying gender identity formation and the consequences of genital surgery. Intersex adults who were treated in accordance with the dominant model have asserted that the standard protocol often results in physical and psychological harm. They assert that genital surgery may result in a loss of reproductive capacity, a loss or diminishment of erotic response, genital pain or discomfort, infections, scarring, urinary incontinence and genitalia that are not cosmetically acceptable. In addition to physical complications, the dominant treatment protocol may exacerbate an intersex person's sense of shame by reinforcing cultural norms of sexual abnormality.[8] A number of researchers who are studying gender identity formation also believe that surgical alteration should not be undertaken on the assumption that infants are born with the ability to develop either a male or female gender identity. Some recent studies indicate that gender identity is not completely malleable and may be influenced or controlled by prenatal factors.[9]

Based upon these concerns, opponents of the dominant model have proposed two alternatives. One approach calls for a complete moratorium on all genital surgeries that are not medically necessary. The other model supports an approach that emphasizes the importance of providing complete information to the parents of the intersex child and deferring to parental decision making.

2.2 Complete Moratorium on all Surgeries that are not Medically Necessary

Some intersex activists and experts have called for a complete moratorium on all infant intersex surgeries, except for those that are truly medically necessary, until retrospective studies prove that the benefits of such surgeries clearly outweigh the potential risks. Supporters of a complete moratorium believe that the traditional model results in stigma and trauma. They believe that under the current approach, which emphasizes the "normalization" of the infant's genitalia, parents will experience guilt and shame over giving birth to an "abnormal" baby and the intersex child will experience a sense of rejection. Those who support a moratorium, question the traditional assumption that concealing or downplaying the existence of the intersex condition will help the family lead a "normal" life. In addition, they believe that relieving the parents' anxiety over the birth of their intersex child should not be accomplished by surgically altering the child to fit societal norms. Instead, they emphasize that parents should be educated, provided with complete information about their child's condition, and offered appropriate professional counseling and peer support. In addition, this group believes that children, when they reach the appropriate age, should be provided complete information and the option to decide for themselves whether they want to undergo surgery. Those calling for a moratorium believe that medical treatment of a child's intersex condition should be limited to treatment of conditions that pose an actual risk to the child's physical health.[10]

Those who support a complete moratorium recommend that: (1) experts assess the likely gender identity of intersex infants; (2) intersex children be raised in the recommended gender identity; (3) parents be educated and put in touch with people who can provide counseling and support; and (4) surgical intervention be delayed until the children reach an age when they can decide for themselves whether they want any surgical alteration.[11]

2.3   The "Middle Ground" Approach

Others have called for a "middle ground" approach.[12] Those who support a compromise position believe that the dominant model defers too much to the treating physicians, but a complete moratorium would not be in the best interests of all intersex children. This group believes that physicians should not be making life-altering decisions for their patients that may affect their ability to reproduce and achieve sexual satisfaction, and potentially lead to physical and emotional complications. This group rejects the call for a complete moratorium, however, because they are concerned that the untreated intersex child may suffer psychological trauma that is more detrimental than the potential risks of surgery. This group believes that parents who are fully educated about all the risks and benefits of the different protocols are in the best position to assess what is in their child's best interests.[13] Therefore, they believe that parents, and not physicians, should have the complete authority to determine the appropriate treatment for their children. In other words, this group supports the parents' right to decide, as along as the parental decision is based on a true informed consent. This approach is supported by the British Association of Paediatric Surgeons.[14]

3.   THE DOCTRINE OF INFORMED CONSENT

The informed consent doctrine preserves patients' rights to make medical decisions on their own behalf. The doctrine requires that patients be fully informed of all the material risks associated with the proposed medical treatment before their consent to a procedure is considered valid. The doctrine protects individuals' rights to bodily integrity and self-determination. In the case of incompetents or minors who are too young to understand and balance the risks and benefits of a particular medical choice, informed consent is required of a surrogate, typically the minors' parent(s).[15]

Parental decisions on behalf of their children are generally accorded great deference to protect family privacy and parental authority. Typically, courts are not involved in medical decisions involving children, so long as the parents and the physicians agree on the appropriate treatment. Court intervention in parental decisions is rare because legal institutions generally presume that parents will make decisions that will be in the best interests of their children.[16]

In some circumstances, however, when parents are seemingly unable to make a decision based solely upon the best interests of their child and the potential gravity of the consequences of the medical treatment are particularly severe, courts may carefully review parental consent to the treatment of their child. The classic case requiring close scrutiny is the involuntary sterilization of a minor or incompetent adult. Sterilization, without the patient's consent, involves a significant invasion into the patient's right to autonomy. In addition, parents may be motivated by their own concern about having to care for a grandchild should their incompetent child become pregnant or father a child. Therefore, courts will carefully scrutinize these decisions to ensure that the best interests of the child are being protected.[17]

Genital surgery on an intersex infant involves similar autonomy issues. These surgeries may result in involuntary sterilization, decreased capacity to achieve sexual satisfaction, and serious long-term medical complications. Therefore, these surgeries have the potential to permanently and dramatically infringe upon the intersexual's right to bodily integrity and self-determination. In addition, because parents may be making decisions at a time when they are suffering distress about giving birth to and raising an "abnormal" child, it is difficult for parents to objectively determine the treatment that would be in their child's long-term best interests. Therefore, if courts are asked to determine whether parents should have the ability to consent to surgical alteration of their intersex children, they will need to resolve complex ethical issues.

4.   INFORMED CONSENT FOR THE SURGICAL ALTERATION OF AN INTERSEX CHILD: THE COLOMBIA DECISION

Only one high court has directly ruled on whether the traditional protocol is legally acceptable.[18] Because of a Court decision in 1995, doctors in Colombia were concerned about potential liability for performing genital surgery on intersex infants. Therefore, in two cases in which the physicians recommended genital surgery to the parents, the physicians refused to proceed without a court order. The parents of the two children sought court authority for the procedures to occur.

The Constitutional Court of Colombia considered the evidence supporting the traditional model as well as evidence that critiqued this model and supported a moratorium on infant intersex surgeries. The Court concluded that the contrary opinions put the law at an impasse: to prohibit surgeries until the children reach the age of consent would be engaging in social experimentation, but to allow the surgeries to continue under the standard protocol would not ensure that the best interests of the children are protected.

To overcome this impasse, the court settled on a compromise approach. The Colombia court allowed parents to continue to consent to surgeries, but the court insisted that procedures be developed to guarantee that parents are consenting solely based upon their child's best interests and not their own self-interest. The court suggested that legal and medical institutions develop informed consent procedures that guarantee that the child's interests are the only concern. To ensure that the consent is truly informed, the court required that it be "qualified and persistent" and any procedures developed must meet the following requirements:

(1) The consent must be in writing.

(2) The information provided must be complete. The parents must be informed about the dangers of current treatments, the existence of other paradigms, and the possibility of delaying surgeries and giving adequate psychological support to the children.

(3) The authorization must be given on several occasions over a reasonable time period to make sure the parents have enough time to truly understand the situation.

The Colombia Court decided that surgical modification of intersex infants must be treated differently from other types of parental consent cases because the traditional model does not ensure that parents are in the best position to make a decision on behalf of their intersex children. The Court was concerned because parents typically lack information about intersexuality, intersexuality is viewed as a disease that must be "cured," and treating physicians convey a false sense of urgency to provide a quick cure. The Colombia court recognized that under these circumstances, parents could not easily distinguish their own fears and concerns from considerations of the "best interests" of their child.

The Colombia court decided that protecting the human rights of the infant required it to strike a balance between allowing parents full autonomy to consent to surgical alteration on behalf of their intersex infants and barring all intersex surgeries. Therefore, the court called upon legal and medical institutions to establish "qualified and persistent" informed consent procedures that protect the rights of the intersex child until comprehensive studies clearly establish the course of treatment that is in the child's best interests.[19]

5. INTERNATIONAL LEGAL DEVELOPMENTS

Colombia is the only jurisdiction in which the highest court has addressed the issue of parental authority to consent to surgery on behalf of an intersex child. Given the paucity of cases and legislation on point, it is impossible to predict with certainty how the courts of other nations would resolve this issue. Recent trends, however, indicate that international institutions are calling for greater protection of children's legal rights and greater respect for everyone's right to autonomy. In addition, legal institutions are generally enhancing the protections provided to other sexual minorities. None of these developments provides direct evidence of how courts in nations other than Colombia would rule if they were asked to resolve this issue. The international trend toward greater protection of the rights of children and sexual minorities and a more expansive interpretation of the right to privacy and autonomy, indicate, however, that other courts may adopt an approach similar to the approach adopted in Colombia.

International recognition of the need to enhance the legal protection provided to children is reflected in the *Convention on the Rights of the Child*, which was adopted by the General Assembly of the United Nations on November 20, 1989.[20] This convention recognizes that children, because of their vulnerability, need special care and protection and reaffirms a child's special need for legal safeguards. The dominant medical management protocol for intersex infants practiced in many nations today does not ensure the protection of an intersex infant's fundamental human rights as defined in the Convention. Current medical practices regarding intersex infants may violate Articles 2, 3, 12, and 16 of the Convention.

Article 2 requires that children should not be discriminated against on the basis of sex. Current medical practices may violate that obligation. The current protocol emphasizes the need for males to be able to engage in satisfactory sexual intercourse over their potential desire to procreate. An XY infant, who is born with a phallus that is considered to be too small for penetrative sex in adulthood, is assigned the female sex. The genitalia are altered to appear "female" and the testicles are removed, even though such removal results in the sterilization of an otherwise fertile male. For XX children, the need to procreate, rather than the ability to engage in satisfactory sexual intercourse, is emphasized. An XX infant, who is capable of reproducing, typically is assigned the female sex to preserve her reproductive capability, regardless of the appearance of her external genitalia. If her "phallus" is considered too large to meet the guidelines for a typical clitoris, it is surgically reduced, even if the reduction reduces or destroys her capacity for satisfactory sex. In other words, males are being defined by their ability to penetrate and females are being defined by their ability to procreate. This protocol treats XY and XX children differently based upon gender stereotypes about the proper roles from men and women and could be considered a violation of Article 2.

Article 3 requires that in all actions concerning children, the best interests of the child shall be a primary consideration. The traditional medical protocol emphasizes the need to "normalize" the child. One of the motivations for "normalizing" the child is to ease the psychological discomfort of the parents and enhance their ability to bond with their child. Surgical alteration of a child that may result in involuntary sterilization, diminished capacity for sexual satisfaction, and a gender assignment that may be contrary to the child's gender identity does not ensure that the best interests of the child are a primary consideration and thus the traditional protocol may violate Article 3.

Article 12 protects children's rights to have their opinion taken into account in any matter affecting them. The traditional protocol ensures that children do not have input into decisions that have a profound effect on their lives, including their ability to procreate and achieve sexual satisfaction, because these decisions are being made when the child is too young to participate in the decision making process.

Article 16 protects children from interference in their right to privacy. Procreative decisions are considered a fundamental privacy right under the United States Constitution and the laws of many other nations. A court could potentially find that surgeries that result in involuntary sterilization infringe on the child's fundamental right to privacy under Article 16.

The *Convention on the Rights of the Child* provides enhanced safeguards to protect the rights of children. If the medical treatment of intersex infants is eventually litigated, courts may refer to the terms of the Convention and determine that surgical alteration of intersex children, as practiced under the traditional model, improperly infringes on the rights of children.

In addition, other legal developments in Australia, Europe, and the United States, in cases involving other sexual minorities, including transsexuals and homosexuals, indicate that these jurisdictions may be more likely to provide enhanced protection to intersex children. Just as the rights of children are being recognized, sexual minorities, who historically have been subjected to discriminatory treatment, are now being accorded greater legal protection.

5.1 Australia

The courts in Australia have not been asked to determine whether parents have the ability to consent to genital surgery on behalf of their intersex infants. The Family Court of Australia has addressed, however, the rights of intersex persons in other related areas. The most recent decisions by the Family Court indicate that if it were asked to resolve the issue of infant genital surgery, it would likely place significant emphasis on the intersex infant's right to autonomy.

In 1979, *In Marriage of C. and D. (falsely called C.),*[21] Australia issued a decision that provided the least respect for the rights of intersex persons when it ruled that, an intersex person was neither a man nor a woman for purposes of determining his ability to marry. In this case, a wife sought an annulment of her marriage of 12 years claiming that her husband was not legally a man. The husband was a true intersexual with an XX chromosomal pattern and a combination of male and female biological aspects.[22] The husband had undergone a number of surgeries to modify his external sex organs and to remove his breasts so that his external appearance would be male. The court granted the wife's petition for annulment on the grounds of mistake because she believed she was marrying a male. Although the husband had male gonads and genitalia, he had the chromosomal configuration typical of a female. Therefore, the court concluded that he was neither a male nor a female.[23]

In 2003, in *Attorney General v. Kevin,*[24] the court rejected its decision in 1979 and greatly expanded the rights accorded to intersex and transsex persons. In determining that a female-to-male transsexual was a male for purposes of marriage, the court recognized that changes in social attitudes, advances in medical research, greater respect for the rights of children and international expansion of the right to privacy supported a finding that transsexuals are entitled to marry in their self-identified sex role.

In addition, Australian courts have been asked twice to determine the court's role in decisions by teens to undergo medical treatment that would physically alter their sex attributes to bring their bodies more into conformity with their gender identity. The judges in each case found that the teen's decision must be reviewed by a court, even if all the parties involved in the treatment decision are agree. The judges required court supervision because they found that there was a significant risk of making the wrong decision and the consequences of a wrong decision would be particularly grave.[25] The courts were concerned about the biological, social, and psychological consequences of the proposed intervention.

In its most recent decisions, the Family Court of Australia has followed the international trend of providing enhanced protection to sexual minorities and greater respect for the rights of children to privacy and autonomy. In addition, the court has indicated that it requires some type of judicial oversight of surgical or hormonal treatment that would alter a person's sex attributes because of the potentially grave consequences. Therefore, if Australian courts are asked to determine the appropriate treatment protocol for intersex infants, they are likely to follow the same approach as the Colombia court and require some type of oversight of the decision.

5.2 Europe

Although the European Court of Human Rights (ECHR) has not directly addressed the autonomy rights of intersexuals, it has resolved a number of disputes between member states and their transsexual[26] citizens seeking legal recognition as their self-identified sex. Recent ECHR decisions involving transsexuals illustrate the evolving expansion of the rights accorded to persons who fail to conform to sex and gender norms.

Transsexuals have made claims for decades that countries that refuse to grant transsexuals legal rights that comport with their self-identified sex violate Articles 8 and 12 of the *Convention for the Protection of Human Rights and Fundamental Freedoms (CPHRFF).*[27] Article 8 relates to privacy and Article 12 relates to the right to marry and found a family.

Before its decisions in *Goodwin v. United Kingdom*[28] and *I v. United Kingdom*[29] in 2002, the ECHR consistently held that denying transsexuals the right to be legally recognized as their self-identified sex did not violate the *CPHRFF*. In 1986, the Court, by a 12-3 margin, decided in favor of the state.[30] Although the Court continued to rule in favor of the state and against transsex claimants, over time, the number of justices ruling in favor of the state diminished. In 1990, the margin was reduced to 10-8,[31] and in 1998, in an 11-9 decision, a sharply worded dissent indicated that based upon societal and scientific developments, the court might soon reject its earlier decisions. In 2002, the ECHR unanimously rejected its earlier decisions and ruled that states that deny transsexuals the right to be recognized as their self-identified sex violate Articles 8 and 12 of the *CPHRFF*.[32] In 2004, the European Court of Justice made a similar ruling.[33] In 2004, Great Britain, which for decades has been one of the countries that provided sparse protection to transsexuals, joined other European countries and passed sweeping legislation to provide transsex persons expansive legal rights that recognize their self-identified sex.[34]

5.3   United States of America

Two recent developments in U.S. courts indicate that the U.S. may be moving towards providing greater legal protection to sexual minorities. First, the U.S. Supreme Court has expanded its conception of the right to liberty under the U.S. Constitution. In addition, recent decisions involving discrimination against gays, lesbians, and transsexuals indicate that the courts are now unwilling to allow discrimination based upon stereotypes of what constitutes a man or a woman.

The Supreme Court's decision in *Lawrence v. Texas,* in 2003, indicates that the court is willing to expand its conception of the right to liberty, which is protected by the Fifth and Fourteenth Amendments to the U.S. Constitution.[35] These amendments apply only to actions by the government, so the *Lawrence* decision would not apply directly to a parental decision to consent to surgical alteration of their intersex child. The reasoning and language in this decision indicate that the court supports the view that autonomy rights, especially regarding issues of sex must be protected. Because of ambiguous language in *Lawrence*, it is difficult to determine the exact implications of the decision. It is possible, however, that *Lawrence* portends a trend in the U.S. to acknowledge the importance of sexual self-determination.

In *Lawrence v. Texas*, the state of Texas adopted a statute that criminalized sodomy between two people of the same sex. The Supreme Court declared the statute to be unconstitutional because it unduly burdened an individual's right to liberty. According to the Court, a person's right to liberty is implicated because:

> These matters involving the most intimate and personal choices a person may make in a lifetime, choices central to personal dignity and autonomy, are central to the liberty protected by the Fourteenth Amendment. At the heart of liberty is the right to define one's own concept of existence, of meaning, of the universe, and of the mystery of human life.[36]

The state's right to criminalize same-sex sodomy is clearly distinguishable from the parental right to consent to genital surgery on behalf of their intersex child. But, by using expansive language to define the liberty interest and by overruling precedent that had narrowly defined the liberty interest, the Supreme Court indicated its willingness to provide greater protection to choices that are central to dignity and autonomy, including issues related to sexuality.

Another line of cases in the United States, involving statutes that prohibit discrimination because of "sex," have also greatly expanded the rights of sexual minorities to be free from discrimination based upon sex stereotyping.[37] Before the last decade, U.S. courts consistently ruled that "sex" discrimination statutes did not protect sexual minorities, such as homosexuals and transsexuals, from discriminatory actions.[38] Recently, courts are determining that discrimination based upon sex stereotyping about the proper roles for males and females constitutes unlawful "sex" discrimination.[39] None of these statutes specifically apply to intersex genital surgery, but the underlying rationale of these cases could be used by intersex persons if they are being surgically altered to conform their bodies to male and female stereotypes.

As previously discussed, the underlying basis for the dominant treatment protocol is in part based on inappropriate sex-role stereotypes because XY and XX infants are treated dissimilarly. For a male, the dominant concern is that the XY male have an "adequate" penis so that he can engage in intercourse. For an XX infant, the dominant concern is reproductive capability, rather than the capacity to engage in satisfactory sex. In other words, males have been defined by their ability to penetrate and females have been defined by their ability to procreate. This penetration/procreation gender stereotype is further reinforced by the medical community's emphasis on the need for a female to have an acceptable looking clitoris over her need for sexual satisfaction. Creation of a sensitive clitoris and a vagina that properly lubricates during sex is not the primary concern during female genital modification surgery. A successful surgical modification of a female is not defined as one that will likely result in her ability to achieve sexual pleasure; instead, it is defined as one that results in the creation of a proper sized clitoris (that may not be as sensitive as the unaltered clitoris) and a vagina that will allow penetration by a male's penis. Thus, the dominant model is based upon sex stereotypes.

Nothing in current U.S. legislation or case law specifically prohibits the continued use of the traditional treatment protocol. Recent cases regarding homosexuals and transsexuals, however, have indicated that U.S. jurists believe that sexual minorities should receive greater protection under the U.S. Constitution and some federal and state statutes. These cases could portend a trend to provide greater protection to intersex infants and could be used as persuasive authority to convince legislatures to adopt statutes or courts to rule in favor of providing greater protection to intersex children.

6. WHO SHOULD DECIDE?

The major difference between the alternative proposals turns on whether the ultimate decision makers should be physicians, parents, the intersex child, when she reaches the age of consent, or the courts. Until comprehensive studies are conducted that clearly indicate whether early genital surgery typically results in the potential for greater benefit or harm to the child, the decision cannot be left to physicians or delayed until the child reaches an age where she has the capacity to consent. Therefore, the remaining choices are granting the authority to parents to decide or requiring some type of review of parental decisions. Some experts believe that parents are uniquely qualified to make this decision, while others believe that it will be impossible or difficult for parents to divorce their self-interest from the child's best interests. Therefore, until studies more clearly indicate the model that is most beneficial for the intersex child, some type of oversight of parental decisions is desirable. The question remains, however, whether it is in the best interests of the child to have the courts provide this review or whether the oversight should be undertaken by an institution other than a court.

When faced with this issue, the Colombian court wisely decided that new decision models must be created to protect the rights of the children. It did not, however, mandate judicial oversight of these matters. Instead, the court encouraged legal and medical institutions to develop informed consent procedures that would result in a consent that is "qualified and persistent." The court set minimal requirements for a qualified and persistent consent and required that: (1) the consent be in writing; (2) the parents receive full information about all the uncertainties involved in the alternative treatment protocols; and (3) the parental authorization must be given on several occasions over a reasonable time period.[40]

Judges are not experts in this area and some may not have heard of intersexuality, much less have a thorough understanding of the complex physical and psychological consequences that may accompany the different treatment models. Although some recent court decisions indicate a trend towards greater respect for people's right to control their gender identity and sexuality, a number of other decisions illustrate that courts may choose to ignore experts and rely on their own prejudices in sensitive areas involving sexuality and gender.[41] For example, some courts presented with scientific evidence about the nature of transsexuality have chosen to ignore the scientific evidence in favor of sources such as Webster's dictionary.[42]

The case that best illustrates the problems that may arise if this issue is litigated in the courts is a 1993 decision from the family court of Australia. *In re A* involved an intersex child with Congenital Adrenal Hyperplasia (CAH), who had been raised as a girl.[43] At puberty, A began to virilize and he self-identified as a boy. When A was 14 ½ years old, he sought surgical treatment to bring his physical appearance in line with his gender identity. No one opposed the procedure. A's desire was supported by his parents and the medical treatment team, which included a surgeon, an endocrinologist, a psychiatrist and a psychologist. Because the procedure would result in the sterilization of A, court approval was sought.

The court determined that although A had a general understanding of the problems involved with the proposed surgery, the court was not convinced that he was sufficiently mature to fully appreciate and objectively assess the various options. The court also decided that the parents did not have the power to consent on behalf of their child and the treatment decision required court supervision. The court decided that court authorization was necessary as a "procedural safeguard" because it was not clear which decision would be in the child's best interests and an incorrect decision would yield particularly grave results.

Although the court decided that granting A's request was the correct decision, the court seriously considered denying the petition. The court stated:

> It is clear on all the material that the various treating experts regard this…as being highly desirable in A's interests. I had nevertheless considered the possibility of rejecting the application on the basis that it is only another three and a half years until A attains 18 years and at that stage it would be open to him to make his own decision.[44]

The court ultimately relied on the psychologist's evidence that delaying the surgery for three years posed a significant risk that A would commit suicide or suffer severe and irreparable psychological trauma. This possibility caused the court to grant A's petition. It is unclear how many other judges would have substituted their own judgment for that of the affected parties. Given that the judge in *In re A* was "sorely tempted," this possibility cannot be ignored.

Because judges are unlikely to have the knowledge to decide these issues and these requests may force judges to confront their own stereotypes about sex and gender, allowing one judge to determine the appropriate treatment for an intersex child is not ideal. Therefore, a fourth treatment protocol may be the best alternative to follow until comprehensive studies clearly indicate whether early genital surgery results in the potential for greater harm or good for the child. Instead of allowing a doctor, the parents, or a judge to control the outcome, a fourth alternative is to require the formation of committees to advise parents on alternative treatment options. These committees should consist of experts from all the relevant disciplines, including endocrinologists, paediatricians, psychologists, and sociologists as well as intersex adults who have experienced the different treatment protocols and parents who have been faced with this decision. These committees can serve four critical needs:

- They can provide guidance to the parents;
- They can ensure that any parental consent is qualified and persistent;
- They can gather data on the outcomes of different treatment models; and
- They can provide continuing education to intersex persons, parents, and treating physicians.[45]

By working together, advocates of each treatment model will be able to accomplish at least some of their goals. Those who support the traditional model will be able to continue to treat those patients whose parents consent, but physicians will no longer have to be concerned that they may later be sued because they failed to provide enough information for the consent to be truly informed. Those calling for a moratorium will not be able to halt to all surgeries, but they will know that a number of surgeries that would have otherwise been performed will not occur and that those that are performed will provide enhanced safeguards for the child. Those who call for parental control of these decisions will be satisfied that the decision still rests with the parents. Finally, all will be reassured that the ultimate decision will not be rendered by judges who may or may not be knowledgeable about these issues and who may render a decision based upon their own prejudices or stereotypes.

Julie Greenberg, Professor of Law at Thomas Jefferson School of Law, San Diego, California, U.S.A.

NOTES

[1]   Alice D. Dreger, "Ambiguous Sex—or Ambiguous Medicine? Ethical Issues in the Treatment of
      Intersexuality, *Hastings Center Report* 28 (1998): 27; Suzanne J. Kessler, *Lessons from the
      Intersexed* (1998).
[2]   Sharon Sytsma, "Ethical Dilemmas in Retrospective Studies on Genital Surgery in the Treatment of
      Intersexual Infants," *Cambridge Quarterly of Healthcare Ethics* 13 (2004): 394.
[3]   South Africa has considered whether to legislate in this area. *South African Press Association*,
      "Legislation Mooted to Regulate Intersex Surgery," 2004 WL 99626478. The city of San Francisco
      has also held hearings on this issue. "Historic Intersex Human Rights Hearing in San Francisco,"
      www.intersexinitiative.org/news/000119.html
[4]   John Money, "Hermaphroditism: Recommendations Concerning Case Management," *Journal of
      Clinical Endocrinology and Metabolism* 4 (1956): 547-556; John Money, Joan Hampson, and John
      Hampson, "An Examination of Some Basic Sexual Concepts: The Evidence of Human
      Hermaphroditism," 97 *Bulletin of Johns Hopkins Hospital* 97 (1955): 301-319.
[5]   Alice D. Dreger, *Hermaphrodites and the Medical Invention of Sex* (1998).
[6]   Martin T. Stein, David E. Sandberg, Tom Mazur, Erica Eugster and Jorge J. Daaboul, "A Newborn
      Infant With a Disorder of Sexual Differentiation," *Pediatrics* 114 (2004): 1473.
[7]   American Academy of Pediatrics Policy Statement, "Evaluation of the Newborn with Developmental
      Anomalies of the External Genitalia," *Pediatrics* 106 (July 2000): 138.
[8]   Intersex Society of North America. http://www.isna.org/library/recommendations.html
[9]   William G. Reiner and John P. Gearhart, "Discordant Sexual Identity in Some Genetic Males with
      Cloacal Exstrophy Assigned to Female Sex at Birth," *New England Journal of Medicine* 350 (2004):
      333.
[10] Alyssa Connell Lareau, "Who Decides? Genital-Normalizing Surgery on Intersexed Infants,"
      Georgetown Law Journal 92 (2003): 129; Hazel Glenn Beh and Milton Diamond, "An Emerging
      Ethical and Medical Dilemma: Should Physicians Perform Sex Assignment on Infants with
      Ambiguous Genitalia?" *Michigan Journal of Gender and Law* 7 (2000): 1; Bruce E. Wilson and
      William G. Reiner, "Management of Intersex: A Shifting Paradigm," 9 *Clinical Ethics* 9 (1998): 360;
      Kenneth Kipnis and Milton Diamond, "Pediatric Ethics in the Surgical Assignment of Sex" *Journal
      of Clinical Ethics* 9 (1998): 398; Milton Diamond and Keith Sigmundson, "Management of
      Intersexuality: Guidelines for Dealing with Persons With Ambiguous Genitalia," *Archives Pediatric
      Adolescent Medicine* 151 (1997): 1046; Cheryl Chase, "Surgical Progress is not the Answer to
      Intersexuality," *Journal Clinical Ethics* 9 (1998): 385; http://www.isna.org/drupal/agenda
[11] http://www.isna.org/drupal/agenda
[12] Jorge Daaboul and Joel Frader, "Ethics and the Management of the Patient with Intersex: A Middle
      Way," *Journal of Pediatric Endocrinology and Metabolism* 14 (2001): 1575.
[13] S. F. Ahmed, S. Morrison, I. A. Hughes, "Intersex and Gender Assignment; the Third Way?" *Archives
      of Disease in Childhood* 89 (2004): 847.
[14] British Association of Pediatrics Statement, *Statement of the British Association of Pediatric Surgeons
      Working Party on the Surgical Management of Children Born with Ambiguous Genitalia.*
      http://www.baps.org.uk/documents/Intersex%20statement.htm (July 2001).
[15] American Academy of Pediatrics, Committee on Bioethics, "Informed Consent, Parental Permission,
      and Assent in Pediatric Practice, in Policy Reference Guide," *Pediatrics* 95 (1995): 314.
[16] *Parham v. J.R.*, 442 U.S. 584, 602 (1979).
[17] *In the Matter of Romero*, 790 P.2d 819 (Colo. 1990); *Estate of C.W.*, 640 A.2d 427 (Pa. Super. 1994).
[18] Sentencia No. SU-337/99; Sentencia No. T-551/99.
[19] *Ibid.*
[20] 1989 *Convention on the Rights of the Child.*
[21] (1979) 35 F.L.R. 340.
[22] *Ibid.* 342.
[23] *Ibid.* 345. The court stated: "I am satisfied on the evidence that the husband was neither man nor
      woman but was a combination of both, and a marriage in the true sense of the word...could not have

taken place and does not exist." *Ibid.* As a non-man/non-woman the implication of this court's holding is that he could not marry anyone at all.

24 *Attorney General v. Kevin*, Family Court of Australia (2003) 172 FLR 300.

25 *In Re A*, Family Court of Australia (1993) 16 FLR 715 (involving a request by an intersex teen who had been raised as a girl but whose body virilized at puberty who sought to further masculinize his body to bring it into conformity with his gender identity); *Re Alex*, Family Court of Australia (2004) 31 Fam LR 503 ¶ 176(involving a transsex teen who sought sex modification surgery).

26 A transsexual is someone whose known biological sex markers are all congruent at birth, but who has a gender self-identity that does not conform to these biological factors.

27 *European Convention for the Prevention of Human Rights and Fundamental Freedoms*, signed 4 Nov. 1950, entered into force 3 Sep. 1953.

28 *Goodwin v. United Kingdom*, European Court of Human Rights (2000) 35 E.H.R.R. 18.

29 *Case of I. v. the United Kingdom*, European Court of Human Rights (2002) 36 E.H.R.R. 53.

30 *Rees v. United Kingdom*, European Court of Human Rights (1987) 2 FLR 111.

31 *The Cossey Case*, European Court of Human Rights (1991) 2 FLR 492.

32 *Goodwin v. United Kingdom*, European Court of Human Rights (2002) 35   E.H.R.R. 18; *Case of I. v. the United Kingdom*, European Court of Human Rights (2002) 36 E.H.R.R. 53.

33 *K.B. v. National Health Service Pensions Agency and Secretary of State for Health*, European Court of Justice (2004) Eur. Ct of Justice 0.

34 *See* Gender Recognition Act, 2004, Eliz. II, c. 7 (Eng.).

35 *Lawrence v. Texas*, 539 U.S. 558 (2003).

36 *Lawrence v. Texas*, 539 U.S. 558, 574 (2003).

37 A number of federal statutes prohibit "sex" discrimination. See e.g., Title VII of the Civil Rights Act of 1964, 42 U.S.C. § 2000e-2(a)(1) (prohibiting employment discrimination); Title IX of the Higher Education Act, 20 U.S.C. § 1681 (prohibiting discrimination in education); The Equal Credit Opportunity Act, 15 U.S.C. § 1691 (prohibiting discrimination in by lending institutions).

38 See, e.g. *Wrightson v. Pizza Hut of Am., Inc.*, 99 F.3d 138, 143 (4th Cir. 1996); *Williamson v. A. G. Edwards & Sons, Inc.*, 876 F.2d 69, 70 (8th Cir. 1989); *DeSantis v. Pacific Tel.& Tel. Co.*, 608 F.2d 327, 329-332 (9th Cir. 1979); *Sommers v. Budget Marketing Inc.*, 667 F.2d 748 (8th Cir. 1982); *Holloway v. Arthur Andersen*, 566 F.2d 659 (9th Cir. 1977); *Dobre v. Amtrak*, 850 F. Supp. 284; *Doe v. U.S. Postal Serv.*, 1985 WL 9446 (D.D.C. 1985); *Terry v. E.E.O.C.*, 1980 WL 334 (E.D. Wis. Dec. 10, 1980); *Powell v. Read's Inc.*, 436 F. Supp. 369 (D. Md. 1977); *Voyles v. Davies Med. Ctr.*, 403 F. Supp. 456 (N.D. Ca. 1975), aff'd mem., 570 F.2d 354 (9th Cir. 1978); *Grossman v. Bernards Township Bd. of Educ.*, [1975] 11 E.P.D. (CCH) P10,686 (D. N.J. 1975), aff'd mem., 570 F.2d 319 (3rd Cir. 1985).

39 See, e.g., *Nichols v. Azteca Rest. Ent. Inc.*, 256 F.3d 864 (9 thCir. 2001); *Rene v. MGM Grand Hotel, Inc.*, 305 F.3d 1061 (9th Cir. 2002); *Schmedding v. Tnemec Co. Inc.*, 187 F.3d 862 (8th Cir. 1999); *Heller v. Columbia Edgewater Country Club*, 195 F. Supp. 1212 (D. OR 2002); *Samborski v. West Valley Nuclear Serv., Co.*, 2002 WL 1477610 (W.D.N.Y. June 25, 2002); *Centola v. Potter*, 188 F.Supp.2d 403 (D. MA 2002); *Ianetta v. Putnam Investments*, Inc., 142 F.Supp.2d 131 (D. MA 2001); *Jones v. Pacific Rail Serv.*, 2001 WL 127645 (N.D. IL 2001); *Smith v. City of Salem*, 2004 WL 1745840 (6th Cir. 2004); *Schwenk v. Hartford*, 204 F.3d 1182, 1201 (9th Cir. 2000); *Rosa v. Park West Bank & Trust Co.*, 214 F.3d 213 (1st Cir. 2000); *Johnson v. Fresh Mark, Inc.*, 2003 WL 23757558 (N.D. Ohio Jan. 30, 2003); *Doe v. United Consumer Financial Serv.*, 2001 WL 3350174 (N.D. Ohio Nov. 9, 2001).

40 Sentencia No. T-551/99.

41 See e.g., *In re Estate of Gardiner*, 42 P.3d 120, 124 (Kan. 2002); *Littleton v. Prange*, 9 S.W.3d 223, 226 (Tex. App. 1999); *Kantaras v. Kantaras*, 884 So. 2d 155 (Fla. Dist. Ct. App. 2004).

42 *Gardiner*, supra note 38.

43 Family Court of Australia (1993) 16 FLR 715.

44 *Ibid.*

45 These committees must be mindful of the problems that may develop when ethics committees are asked to render decisions about medical treatment. *See, e.g.,* Robin Fretwell Wilson, "Hospital Ethics Committees as the Forum of Last Resort: An Idea Whose Time Has Not Come," *North Carolina Law Review* 76 (1998): 353.

MILTON DIAMOND AND HAZEL GLENN BEH

THE RIGHT TO BE WRONG

Sex and Gender Decisions

1. INTRODUCTION

A series of events occurred within a very short period and prompted consideration of the ethical dimensions of how, when, and why individuals, institutions or governments decide to get involved in people's lives. In particular we began to question if they should get involved with allowing, or not allowing, people to make major decisions regarding their own bodies. This is an essay reflecting such thoughts. It involves consideration of two tenets of medical practice: *Relieve pain and suffering;* and *First, do no harm.*

In order of occurrence, the events started when we were considering a legal case involving a 13-year-old female.[1] Alex, as the judge sitting on the case called her, had successfully argued in an Australian court that, in accordance with her wishes, she could live as a male and obtain the necessary medical help to achieve this. This means Alex, from that time on, would be getting hormones to prevent typical female puberty and at the age of sixteen years will receive androgenic hormones to virilize bodily and facial features. At the age of eighteen Alex will be eligible to obtain a hysterectomy and ovariectomy to stop any menses and feminization, and eventually to have a phallus constructed if he so wishes. The appropriate legal and professional psychological and medical experts, consulted prior to the decision, have made these recommendations. Religious and other factions, however, immediately challenged the decision. They complained Alex was too young to make such a choice, that the procedures would lead to later regret, and most crucially, would end Alex's ability to have children.[2]

The second instance involved a legal suit brought against a gender clinic by someone who had surgically and socially transitioned from living as a male to living as a female. Alan Finch, at the age of twenty-one had applied to the clinic for help with a desire for sex reassignment surgery (SRS). Therapists at the clinic vetted Mr. Jones's situation and approved of the transition. Surgeons subsequently removed his penis and testicles and in their stead fashioned a vulva and vagina. After living as a woman for eight years Mr. Finch decided it had been a mistake and now feels he should never have been allowed to transition and he ought to live as a man.[3] Mr. Finch blames the psychiatrists who counselled him and is suing the clinic at which they worked. Although he admits to having lied to the therapists during his meetings

S.E. Sytsma (Ed.), Ethics and Intersex, 103–113.

with them, he claims they should have realized he was conflicted over his gender. The clinic is protesting the suit saying, on the one hand, that the therapists involved had followed established procedures, and in any case, this had all occurred prior to the expiration of the statute of limitations. According to records, indeed, the clinic professionals did adhere to professionally approved procedures.[4] The local government is presently conducting a clinical review of the complaint and relevant occurrences.[5] In the meanwhile, factions both supporting and ridiculing the original transition, the secondary one, and the claim against the clinic have come forward.[6]

The third case involved a tragedy. David Reimer, while still an infant had his gender changed. A botched circumcision to repair phimosis of his penis resulted in its destruction. His parents were advised that life as a male without a penis would be intolerable and that he should be raised as a girl. They were told that he would then develop satisfactorily as a female (Diamond and Sigmundson, 1997; Colapinto 2000). This did not happen. David consistently objected to his life as a girl and repeatedly asked to live as the boy he felt to be. His life became so miserable that, at the age of 14, without knowing of his history, he threatened suicide unless he could live as a male. While he subsequently grew to live and marry as a man at the age of 25, he continued to have flashbacks to his early troubled life so that he eventually committed suicide at the age of thirty-eight.[7]

The practice of sex reassignment in similar cases when a penis has been lost due to infant trauma or accident, or when it is considered unusually small, is still current. It also occurs in many cases of intersexuality without the child's consent.[8] The correctness of this practice is a subject of current professional and lay debate. Some physicians still hold to its justification; while others, particularly those individuals who feel they were ill-served by such treatment, object (Diamond, 2004). We say more of this below. David's story is better known as the case of John/Joan and received wide coverage from many media.[9]

The fourth case is more mundane and also more common. A married father of two wrote to one of us (MD) seeking advice. For this discussion we call him Phil Johnson. At his age of 42 Phil said that he was finally seriously thinking of transitioning to live as a woman. Although having thought for years about transitioning, he felt he had come to a junction in his life where he had to make a decision. However, he was conflicted. On the one hand, Mr. Johnson feared that by transitioning he would lose his wife and children, and on the other, he felt driven to follow a life long compulsion. Whether he stays with his family and sacrifices his gender desires or denies his family aspirations involves a decision with both positive and negative consequences. But Phil felt at a choice-point and a decision had to be made. Under certain jurisdictions those who transition, if married, are obligated to divorce. In other cases, those who transition cannot later marry someone of the sex from which they changed. Not only does Phil's conundrum involve legal repercussions, but also similar cases have become part of the "same-sex marriage" argument with positions strongly held by those for and against the legality of transsexual change and subsequent marriage.[10]

In the first two cases the gender shift was at the request of the individual involved and in the third it was imposed from without. The fourth case is yet to be resolved. The types of transitions involved are not unique. Over the last several decades such cases have become the fodder of tabloids, television chat shows, documentaries and more. The Internet has become home to scores of communities that offer space for questioning, ventilation, counseling, and discussion on all sides of the relevant issues. In all of the cases, and others like them, outside individuals and groups have felt called upon to voice their opinions as to the right or wrong of these actions and choices. Some even want governmental agencies to regulate such conduct.

Three of the foregoing four cases involved individuals usually called *transsexuals*. They were said to be suffering from a condition medically called Gender Identity Dysphoria (GID) or Gender Identity Disorder. In brief, gender identity disorder is defined as the strong and persistent disturbing belief for at least two years that one is actually a member of the opposite sex (Frances et al., 1995). In David Reimer's case, he too wanted to change his gender, but it was to regain something taken away from him. While not usually identified as such, it might be said that he had an imposed disturbance of gender identity.

A basic question arises for all of these cases. Who should or should not have a right to dictate, or even have a say, in how one lives and what a person may do with his or her own body?[11] Should the voices of individuals, religious groups, political factions, or even families have determining weight in other people's decisions of such personal bodily alteration?

Those who protest against the requests often feel they are acting in the best interests not only of the individuals concerned, but also of society in general. Considering cases such as Alex's, it is plausible that a minor might change his or her mindset with increasing age and maturity. There is also logic in believing that adults, like Alan Finch or Phil Johnson, who have lived a life in one gender might regret leaving it to live in another. And experience has shown that physicians and other trained professionals usually have knowledge that should be taken into account when making life-altering decisions. There is certainly reason to accept that one might grieve over loss of genitals, facility, or opportunity. Further, it is probable that the full repercussions of any particular action might not be known or ever be known. But is it really likely that the individual involved has not considered most of the relevant matters brought up by others? Is it truly logical to believe these criticisms and objections, as well as others that might be more salient to the person involved, have not been thought of and examined?

From the point of view of the individuals concerned, there surely are important factors to consider. In Alex's case, aside from the public clamor, there is scientific evidence to complicate matters. Minors who desire sex/gender change frequently change their minds as they get to adulthood. It is also true that a majority of those considering a gender reassignment as minors, when adult manifest as persons demonstrating homosexuality without the gender dysphoria (Green, 1987; Zucker, 2004). Thus, for the adolescent, even allowing reversible treatment and permitting the adolescent to present in the opposite sex has future consequences if it solidifies a gender presentation that might have otherwise been later abandoned.

Alan Finch's situation is unusual since most transsexuals following surgery express satisfaction and delight at the outcome (Smith, et al., 2005). Only a minority experiences regret. This case is further clouded by not knowing what induced Mr.

Finch to originally desire a sex change so deeply that he would lie to the therapists regarding his life situation and motivation.

In Phil Johnson's case there are obvious family aspects of any decision that will affect others as well. Phil presents with pro and con issues of his own that must be resolved. His situation is not rare.

The original treatment for David Reimer was predicated on several points of faulty logic. The first was a belief that individuals are psychosexually neutral at birth and will adapt to any gender in which they are reared. The second was that any individual without a penis should be raised as a girl. From the start of his imposed transition, David objected to his treatment. The continued imposition of his management against his desires might even be considered child abuse. Nevertheless, the thinking that led to David's management is still used in dealing with many cases of intersexuality where ambiguous genitalia or a micropenis is present, or when genitalia are missing, as in cloacal exstrophy (Reiner, 2004).

In addition to any personal reason that might be involved, a justification offered by those that refer to the need for society's involvement in these personal decisions arises from the fear that certain actions provide a negative role model for others, or might serve as a precedent and challenge to a basic tenet held dear. They think this is reason enough to impose legal regulations on what individuals can and cannot do. Many social, governmental, and religious institutions, for example, are threatened if people make unique and atypical gender choices even if as minor as dressing in the clothes of the opposite sex. Other factions are disturbed if they or those they represent are not involved in decision making. For instance, psychotherapists or physicians might object if those among their number are not consulted regarding any gender transition. However, the role modelling has effect only on those persons who are themselves considering options regarding a possible transition. In that regard, we see it as any other educational source. We also do not believe that such actions are attractive enough to the average "onlooker" that they will be taken as behaviors to be emulated.

Some among the criticizing public base their objections on religious grounds. They quote biblical verse claiming the body is a holy temple[12] or they contend that man is made in God's image.[13] Some also think that procreation is a religious obligation and that a voluntary surrendering of reproductive ability is sinful. For many reasons individuals of different religious persuasions think the body should not be altered.

Regardless of the source of criticism, the heart of the issue is, should final decisions on instances such as the ones presented be left to government, agencies, factions, physicians, psychologists, priests, counsellors, or any other than the person particularly involved? We think not.

Certainly we think that parents or family can have a say and openly express their opinions. Yes, we think any and all groups might be consulted if that is the wish of the individual. Yes, we think interested groups should be free to offer advice and suggestions for alternate solutions to the situations faced by those like Alex, Alan, David, or Phil. And we think it is prudent to postpone the enactment of any of the actions associated with similar cases until a suitable interval of time has passed between the decision and desired action. We also think it proper that organizations such as the Harry Benjamin International Gender Dysphoria Association (HBIGDA) establish guidelines for the transition process for transsexuals, and respective medical associations have standards for specific medical procedures.[14]

To the extent that physicians or other professionals can predict that an individual or a population is at risk for later regret, they have an ethical obligation to identify that risk and counsel the patient appropriately. For example, studies of women undergoing tubal sterilization reveal that approximately 14% will have some degree of regret in later years. The age at which sterilization occurs strongly correlates with the likelihood and degree of later regret: young women are significantly more likely to regret the decision (Schmidt et al., 2000). Yet no one would suggest that medical or other professionals should deny all younger women the choice to be sterilized because they are more vulnerable to later regret. Instead, this finding warrants extra emphasis on pre-surgery counseling for younger individuals.

We believe the ultimate decision to proceed or not should be left to the competent and mentally mature individual involved regardless of whether doing so is in keeping with the desires or advice of the public, any specified institution, or involved professionals. In terms of making decisions regarding one's own body, we believe every individual has a right to be self-determining; every one has a right to even be wrong.

Our thinking in all these cases is that rational individuals ought have authority to make even life-altering choices when it involves their bodies, regardless of public acceptance or rejection. This holds as long as these persons are then ready to live by any consequences and not hold others liable for that determination. As enunciated by philosophers such as John Stuart Mill we consider these actions as a basic tenet of individual freedom.

Mill, in his essay entitled *On Liberty* expressed it thus:

> "The sole end for which mankind is warranted, individually or collectively in interfering with the liberty of action of any of their number, is self-protection. That the only purpose for which power can be rightfully exercised over any member of a civilized community, against his will is to prevent harm to others. *His own good, either physical or moral, is not a sufficient warrant. He cannot rightfully be compelled to do or forbear because it will be better for him to do so, because it will make him happier, because, in the opinions of others, to do so would be wise, or even right.*" (Emphasis ours.) [15]

Our discussion now turns to an opposite extreme regarding bodily integrity—a discussion of intersexed persons and how they are often treated. Intersexed individuals are persons with apparent anatomical admixtures of male and female biological characteristics. Such persons are not rare. Estimates of their frequency in the population vary. A conservative approximation is that an intersexed child occurs in about one per two thousand people and is recognized at birth by genitals considered ambiguously male or female (Blackless et al., 2000).[16] Since the 1950's and 1960s early surgical intervention for such individuals often was imposed. Predicated on the misguided belief that such genitals provoked a medical emergency, intersexed infants were subjected to surgery to "normalize" their genital appearance. These surgeries were frequently done without the parents being notified of the reasoning for the operations.

In most cases the surgery involved sex-reassigning the infant from male to female since fabrication of female appearing genitals was easier than structuring male genitals. Such surgeries were also imposed when a male infant's penis had been severely mutilated by trauma (as in David Reimer's situation) or was considered significantly small (Beh and Diamond, 2000). These procedures were often instigated without informed consent of the parents in the belief that withholding information about the ambiguities and sex reassignment would foster a more satisfactory upbringing for the child. It was thought that if the parents didn't know, they would not prejudice the infant's upbringing. These practices, while less frequent, still occur.

When parents were informed of the prospect of surgery and sex reassignment they were often told that the "normal" looking genitalia would dictate the child's gender development, and that any innate gender propensity would be changed by upbringing. Despite a lack of confirming evidence, medical literature from the 1970s to the late 1990s had promoted this treatment. Supporting evidence is still scant and there is a great deal of evidence against the belief (Diamond, 1999). Much depends upon the particular intersex condition being considered.

A significant number of intersexed persons were raised in their sex-reassigned gender and then, on their own, either switched to their opposite or instead elected to see themselves, not as male or female, but as intersexed.[17] Many of the intersexed infants that had surgery, even if staying within their assigned gender, have come to criticize such treatment. Many of the original surgeries had to be redone and many surgeries reduced the erotic sensitivity of the genitals.[18] Why, these intersexed individuals ask, couldn't they be allowed to live as they were born? Many question what right the surgeons had, with or without permission of their parents, to decide to subject them to surgery? Groups of intersexed individuals, such as those of the Intersex Society of North America (ISNA), A Kindred Spirit, and Bodies Like Ours have formed and voiced objection to such treatments.

Arguments supporting reconstruction of the genitals are based on the beliefs that humans are psychosexually neutral at birth and that they fare better in life if their gender and genitals match. Reconstruction of the genitals and sex reassignment is, therefore, justified. Little evidence has been offered to substantiate that claim, however. In contrast, neurological and biological studies support the premise that humans are, in keeping with their mammalian heritage, primarily predisposed and biased to interact with environmental, familial, and social forces in either a male or female mode.[19] Further, there is no evidence from medical or other records that intersexed individuals with ambiguous genitalia faired poorly if no surgery was imposed.

Physicians further justify their surgeries on the premises that growing up with ambiguous genitalia would lead to uncertainty on the part of the child as to its gender, and that the ambiguous genitalia would elicit unflattering and derogatorily shaming comments from others. There is only untested theory bolstering the belief about gender development, and only anecdote about the occurrence and effect of unflattering and shaming comments.

There are major ethical problems with "normalizing" ambiguous genitalia without informed consent of the individual involved. The most significant is that doing so ignores the possibility that the child, when an adult, might have a different concept of what is "normal" and what is desirable. And collusion in the surgery by well-meaning parents does not rectify the situation. Indeed, it might make it worse if the mature child comes to wonder why he or she could not be loved as they were born. There are many cases where those who had such surgery as infants later rue the procedures and the thinking that went with it. In cases of infant intersexuality, we think the most ethical stance is to hold open the infant's surgical future when any proposed change is not medically, but only cosmetically, at issue. At a later date, the child can then elect or decline any appropriate surgery (Beh and Diamond, 2000).

We thus present two sides of an issue: where those who wish to change their bodies meet with social criticism and where those who involuntarily had their bodies modified criticize the social forces that led to their unwelcome surgery. In both types of situations, the critics claim they are looking out for the best interests of the individuals involved, the public good, or both. When a decision is in keeping with social norms, the populace and most professional groups generally approve and consent is tacit. When an individual's choice is unpopular, however, it causes consternation and unease. Evidence for this is not difficult to come by. Cosmetic or psychiatric surgery obtained by minors is not uncommon in the United States in instances other than transsexual considerations. According to the American Society of Plastic Surgeons the number of cosmetic surgeries performed on people under the age of 18 exceeded 74,000 in 2003, a 14 percent increase from 2000. In 2003 some 3,700 breast-augmentation surgeries were performed on teenage girls and almost as many teenage boys had their breasts reduced.[20] All that was generally needed to obtain these operations was the financial ability to pay and the consent of parents or guardians. For those that wanted to go contrary to the usual in terms of gender, however, roadblocks of all sorts existed. Males and females, thus, are denied surgery if it is associated with a desire to change their sex, but not if it is to enhance gender stereotypes. And surgery toward "normalization" is promulgated when genitalia are believed to be unusual and differ from the norm.

We accept that those who chose might be making a mistake they will later regret. Yes, there might be repercussions difficult to remedy. But mistakes happen even when actions are made following the best of intentions. Regrets are not only for taking the road less travelled, but for taking the highway as well. And there are honest differences of opinion as to those persons who make the right decision and those who make wrong. Who is to say?

In discussion of this matter we can even call upon a concept of freedom in its broadest sense and immortalized in our country's central documents. The constitution starts off with our ancestor's desire to "secure the Blessings of Liberty to ourselves and our Posterity" and the Declaration of Independence declares: "We hold these truths to be self-evident: that all men are created equal; that they are endowed by their Creator with certain unalienable rights; that among these are life, liberty, and the pursuit of happiness."

If liberty is to mean anything it must offer freedom from external restraint or compulsion. A person's liberty must be seen as a condition of legal non-restraint of natural powers.[21] And as liberty is an inalienable right it cannot be surrendered or transferred.[22]

We thus think it is unethical to make bodily modification of adult or mature minors difficult or illegal when it is desired, and we think it equally unethical to impose, encourage, and promote it in infants when it has not been proven justified and when many on whom it has been imposed criticize the practice even to the point of claiming that it is harmful. People have a right to modify their bodies when they so choose and not have it modified without their expressed informed consent.

A parallel issue needs be considered in this discussion since the individual is not a completely independent agent. The transsexual who wants surgery, or the intersexed individual who doesn't, must interact with different professionals, usually psychotherapists and physicians.

While we presume informed patients with decisional capacity have the right to make medical treatment choices that may bother or offend the larger society, we must also acknowledge the professional's right and obligation to act within his or her conscience in cooperating with those choices. Professional obligations can serve as a legitimate limitation on patient autonomy. Nevertheless, we feel that patient autonomy should be paramount even, or perhaps especially, when exercising choice, which may result in later regret. Yet, patients do not and cannot make medical treatment decisions alone, because medical treatment, by its nature requires the participation of others who are obliged to follow their own conscience and are bound by rules of professional conduct. Thus, informed consent from competent patients may not alone suffice. Professional medical ethics, and the ethical codes of other helping professionals, preclude providing treatments for which there is no indication and those that offer no possible benefit.[23] Patients are not entitled to treatments "simply because they demand them" and physicians or others "are not ethically obligated to deliver care that, in their best professional judgment, will not have a reasonable chance of benefiting their patients."[24]

Admittedly, in some cases it might be difficult for transsexuals who desire counseling, hormones, or surgery, to everywhere find professionals willing and able to provide these services. However, there is no shortage of qualified specialists who are willing to serve. How to keep the intersexed individual from imposed surgery, however, is more problematic. Having a knowledgeable and understanding pediatrician is a place to start.

In summary, we think it is appropriate to call upon long held professional guidelines for those in the helping professions. In the first set of instances we offer *"Relieve pain and suffering."* The psychic pain and suffering of those diagnosed as transsexuals is well documented. The advice for the second set of instances, where individuals have not themselves requested surgery, is to refrain: *"First, do no harm."* The obligation for these decisions ultimately remains with the individual, and yes, every person has a right to be wrong.

Support for this work has come from the Eugene Garfield Foundation, Philadelphia, Pennsylvania.

EDMUND G. HOWE

ADVANCES IN TREATING (OR NOT TREATING) INTERSEXED PERSONS

Understanding Resistance to Change

1. INTRODUCTION

The core ethical question regarding the needs of persons born with intersexed conditions is whether they should have surgery during infancy. This question has been controversial for some time. The most critical concern is how these infants can best gain an intact gender identity. Many have thought that these infants' gender identity will be most affected by the infants' sexual anatomy and the manner in which they are raised. Thus, early surgery has been advised (Porter, 1998). Others have argued that these persons' gender identity may be more influenced, at least in some cases, by genes or hormones (Imperato-McGinley, 1979). Indeed, some people believe that genes may play a greater role than previously imagined (Fleming, 2005).

Parents and care providers presently face many difficulties in deciding what to do for these infants. One problem is that little is known about the experiences of intersexed persons—whether they have had surgery or not (Glassberg, 1999). Thus, both those for and against early surgery currently can argue that if more persons who have remained silent came forward, their case would be stronger.

This problem was exemplified by an exchange that took place at a national ethics conference a few years ago. A person spoke against early surgery and asserted that persons should decide about surgery only after they are older and can make the decision on their own. One of the discussants said in response: "But there may be an overwhelming majority of intersexed persons who have had surgery during infancy and are happy with the results. Unlike those who are unhappy at having had this surgery and express this openly, these persons, though happier, may have chosen not to speak out. Thus, if this is true and surgery is now not carried out on infants, this may do intersexed persons as a whole much more harm than good."

S.E. Sytsma (Ed.), Ethics and Intersex, 115–137.
© 2006 *Springer. Printed in the Netherlands.*

This problem of deciding what to do now is also difficult because intersexed persons who have had this surgery during infancy report being unhappy with their surgical results. These persons report that they have less sensation in their genital organs than they would have wanted, or none at all. Yet, surgical techniques may have improved, and if so, it might now be possible to affect surgical results not possible previously (Farkas, 2001). Of course, the results for intersexed infants who have this surgery now will not be known for years.

In light of this uncertainty, how should care providers presently advise parents, and what should these parents decide? In this chapter, I shall address these questions in three sections. In the first section, I shall address the difficulty sometimes experienced in trying to gather intersexed persons and care providers together to discuss these questions. To discern the best practices possible, discussion between particularly both these groups would, of course, be optimal (Creighton, 2004, Cull, 2002, Cull, 2005).

In the second section, I shall discuss the three different ethical questions bearing on this core question involving early surgery. The first is whether this surgery should be done because it best helps these persons establish an intact gender identity. The second is whether this surgery should not be done because it impairs these persons' capacity for sexual fulfilment to too great an extent. The third is whether legal changes should be made to recognize a third sex, to at least some extent.

In the third section, I shall address what, in light of the above discussions, parents and care providers now should do; as I have already made clear, there are highly different views of this question now. Thus, as opposed to presupposing that I have the right answer, I shall ask what, if anything, I can add to the discussion of this core question—and the three others mentioned above—that has not been said fully before. I should add that my experience with intersexed persons and their problems is not substantial. Yet, since even those who have had this experience (whether as care providers or as patients) are divided, experience does not provide answers for these questions. Thus, the few thoughts I shall raise here may contribute to both present and future "solutions."

In the last part of the third section, I shall finally discuss some recent genetic research that suggests that in the future, the problem of whether or not to operate may become less difficult. According to this research, we may be able to better predict the gender identity that infants born with intersexed conditions will later assume. Doing so could enable us to avoid surgery on infants that endows them, anatomically, with the wrong gender.

However, as I shall discuss, even these recent developments would not necessarily solve this core problem of whether to give many of these infants early surgery. That is, there would still be some infants who would experience the tragic result of being endowed with the wrong anatomical gender. Thus, the ethical question will remain whether to accept this harm to these few infants, though their identity at the time of early surgery would not be known, or to not do this surgery on any infants for whom this particularly tragic outcome is a risk. In this third and last section, I shall focus particularly on this question.

2. DIFFICULTIES IN GATHERING INTERSEXED PERSONS AND CARE PROVIDERS TOGETHER TO DISCUSS THESE QUESTIONS

Several years ago, I became interested in the above questions (Howe, 1998). I then thought it most important to raise them for others to consider. Thus, I gave some talks on this subject, and shared the controversies as I understood them. I reported data and personal experiences intersexed persons had shared with me, which indicated that at least some intersexed persons were unhappy with the results of early surgery. In addition, I acknowledged in these talks that this might be the response of only a minority of these persons, but that regardless, their saying this should at the very least suggest that the pros and cons of this early surgery be openly re-considered.

I was surprised at the response I often got. Care providers frequently voiced hostility, whether or not they had been involved directly or indirectly with those who had done this early surgery. I should perhaps have expected this hostility, because even in the earliest debates, persons have responded with passion to these questions. The study I alluded to above, for example, suggesting the influence of hormones on one group of intersexed persons, was written in the *New England Journal of Medicine* in 1979 (Imperato-McGinley, 1979). In this study, children raised as girls, upon reaching puberty, mostly became boys. The authors of this study argued that this change was based on the children's surges of testosterone. Another author, however, stated in rebuttal: "...after 11 or 12 years of age, the boys may seek entertainment at bars and cockfights, whereas the girls continue to be restricted physically and socially. The question then is: Under these circumstances, why wouldn't [such a child] choose to be a boy?" (Bleier, 1984, at 840).

With care providers responding as strongly as they did, I sought answers. Why were care providers responding this strongly? I believe there are several possible answers. All care providers and intersexed persons who recognize these answers may be able to engage in more productive dialogues with each other.

I have already mentioned one reason for the hostile responses of care providers. Scientifically, we don't know at this time whether the majority of intersexed persons who have had early surgery do or don't feel that they have benefited (Creighton, et al., 2001). Indeed, many have spoken out strongly against this surgery, as I have said. Yet many more, of course, haven't spoken and perhaps never will. Whether happy or unhappy, they may prefer to keep "their condition" private, and reveal it only to their partners and care providers. They may, for example, not want their children to know.

A second reason for the strong responses is that it is unclear that those who are unhappy are unhappy due to having had early surgery. They may be unhappy due to other factors, but have no way of knowing if this is the case; there is no control group. Conversely, for those who are happier, the psychological principle called "cognitive dissonance" could apply. This principle holds that when a person holds conflicting views, s/he may rationalize away one of them—often unknowingly—if it causes him or her more pain. Doing so allows the individual to have less cognitive dissonance and therefore be less distressed (Matz, 2005). Thus, those who had this surgery and had or even still have pain as a result may have rationalized away this pain without knowing it, allowing them to feel happier. Nonetheless, these persons may unconsciously feel much like those who are unhappy after this surgery, since the former also lack a control group. They, too, don't know how they would feel if their experience had been the opposite of what it was. These persons, without surgery, may have been even happier.

Finally, some patients who report positive responses may feel otherwise but be untruthful to investigators because of interpersonal reasons. The patient, for example, may give a positive response because that is what s/he thinks the investigator wants to hear. Untruthful reports are particularly likely if the investigators seemed to the patient to have been associated in any way with those who previously have treated the patient. Intersexed persons in this situation may want to please their former care providers, of course, for many reasons. Patients may, for example, believe rightly that their care providers tried to do the best they could with the knowledge they had at the time, and patients may most appreciate the efforts of their caregivers.

Care providers considering whether to change their treatment of intersexed infants in light of the above considerations may, understandably, not by swayed by the present arguments against early surgery. Rather, they may feel unwilling to change what they have been doing, since the above feedback may not truly represent the response of most intersexed persons who have had early surgery. People who are not care providers may exhibit a similar reluctance. For instance, on several occasions I have presented these same concerns to large groups of lawyers. Despite these lawyers being most open to taking new legal initiatives, they felt reluctant to initiate strong changes in the law in light of this same uncertainty. These lawyers were most open, not surprisingly, to trying to make legal changes that would help insure that parents trying to decide whether to consent to early surgery for these infants are fully informed. (Enhancing persons' autonomy by increasing the information they have is, of course, a frequent legal endeavor. It was lawyers, in large part, for example, who "pushed for" new legal standards of informed consent decades ago. These new standards favored patients' interests over those of physicians.)

It is possible that the information most of these parents receive could be increased. They could be given better access, for example, to meeting intersexed persons who feel that they have had both good and bad responses to early surgery. However, it is unclear how much these parents or their infants would benefit from the parents receiving such information. I shall discuss the problems these parents now face, even with more complete information, in the third section of this chapter.

Finally, care providers who have performed this early surgery may find it hard, again for wholly understandable reasons, to discuss these questions. That is, when patients have had this surgery and are unhappy, this may mean that their surgeons harmed them. Most care providers, of course, devote their lives to helping their patients and pride themselves on this, as they should. To acknowledge, then, that as opposed to having helped these intersexed persons, they may have harmed them, must be exceedingly painful.

3. THREE IMPORTANT ETHICAL QUESTIONS

3.1   A. Is Early Surgery Necessary To Give Intersexed Persons An Intact Gender Identity?

The main reason for doing early surgery in the past has been to enable infants to be better able to identify themselves as members of one sex (Porter, 1998). It was assumed, more or less, that children's identity would follow from the genital anatomy they had acquired as a result of surgery, and then, from how they were raised. Over time, however, it became apparent that some persons, during adolescence or beforehand, developed a gender identity opposite the one with which they had been endowed. A most tragic example of such an instance is that of David Reimer, who lost his penis due to a "botched circumcision," underwent surgery, "became" and was raised as a girl, but subsequently experienced himself as a boy. He eventually got married, but not long ago, he took his life (Navarro, 2004).

The category of intersexed infants includes many different subtypes (Sultan, 2002). The gender identity infants acquire may not depend only on their sexual anatomy and how they are raised, but also (or instead) on their hormones and genes. Assessing what gender identity an infant will assume is thus, in some cases, both unknowable and complex.

When infants' diagnoses and prognoses can be determined, it is generally believed (it would seem) that ample time should be allowed prior to performing early surgery to acquire this information. Significant gains in making these determinations recently have been made (Biswas, 2004). Particularly when these determinations can't be made, several uncertainties remain. Schober has summarized these recently (Schober, 2004). Chief among these uncertainties are the following:

First, the best time for surgery is unclear. The tissue for surgery is of a "better quality" for some infants during their first two years of infancy and puberty, due to spurts of estrogen at both these times (Schober, 2004, p.698). With early surgery, there may be less psychological trauma but a greater likelihood of a need for "revision surgery." There is, however, no evidence that early surgery will result in a better outcome. Adolescents can, of course, indicate what they want. Yet, during adolescence, surgery will evoke anxiety. Surgery may be more difficult at a later time since the distance that the "vaginal sinus must be mobilized' is greater (Schober, 2004, p.698).

Second, the extent to which sexual responsiveness will be impaired by surgery is uncertain. Preserving areas in the genital region that are highly sexually sensitive due to greater nerve density may be more possible due to advances in surgery at this time. Still, data shows that after clitoroplasty, persons may experience not only decreased tactile sensation, but also "highly abnormal hot, cold and vibratory sensation" (Schober, 2004, p.700). Thus, the extent to which new surgical techniques can change loss of sensation is open to question. Ethically, preserving intersexed persons' maximal sexual responsiveness is important. As one author says in this regard, for instance, "…[W]e conclude that there are instances when…a decision to change the sex of rearing, serious though this may be, is less serious than leaving the child in a circumstance where normal sexual life can't be hoped for" (Dewhurst, 1984).

Which of these two ends, optimal gender identity or maximal sexual responsiveness, should prevail if they are in conflict? Schober says, "The inherent goal of this type of surgery is to provide the patient with positive psychosocial and psychosexual adjustments throughout life...this goal has remained unchanged..." (Schober, 2004, p. 698). These patients' acquiring an intact gender identity may be what should matter most, but even if this is true, the difficult ethical problem I indicated earlier will remain: Early surgery may result in some persons irreversibly becoming anatomically the "wrong sex." At what point, if any, is the percentage of persons to which this will happen so small that the outcome of acquiring the wrong sex, though foreseeable, should be accepted? Is it, for example, 5%, 1%, or none at all? This question is additionally ethically problematic, of course, because the acceptable percentage isn't known.

According to one estimate, the percentage of persons who have had surgery and feel that they have had a bad outcome is 8% (Dennis, 2004). A figure such as this, even if accurate and helpful in some respects, must be further broken down. In addition to the percentage that is unhappy due to their gender identity and the percentage that is unhappy due to decreased sexual responsiveness, there are additional sub-categories that should be determined. It might matter, for example, if the "bad outcome" group is more men or more women or more persons who are heterosexual or gay. Each of these particular considerations may make a difference for many reasons. One such reason is that persons in our culture have different attitudes toward men and women, as well as toward persons who are heterosexual and homosexual. I shall discuss these attitudes in greater detail subsequently.

Regardless of these distinctions, the overriding ethical consideration is the one I have already mentioned: Should overriding moral weight be given to protecting those worst off? If this were done, priority might be given to protecting persons from having genital surgery that could result in their anatomy being different from their eventual gender identity, even if this protection could only be given to one person. Of course, those not having early surgery also could be greatly harmed psychologically: they might not be able to form an intact gender identity, due in part to their continuing to have ambiguous genitalia until a later age. They may, in addition, face ridicule from other children or undergo other negative effects—once again, due to their having ambiguous sexual organs during their formative years (Minto, 2001).

What, if anything, can be added? I would suggest that there are two interventions that possibly could profoundly benefit these children even if they don't have surgery—interventions that haven't yet been adequately examined. The first intervention is early and persistent counseling of intersexed persons from virtually the time that they are born. The second is counseling for their parents during this same time. These interventions may, for example, markedly enhance these children's self-esteem, whether or not the children have an intact sexual identity. It may be also that their self-esteem is actually more important than their sexual identity. That is, these children may be able to feel good about themselves, even if during their early childhood they don't know what identity they will become, or choose to have, at a later time. Then, with good self-esteem, they may fare well, despite not having had early surgery, and despite their not having acquired an intact gender identity until later on than during their infancy.

3.1.1 Counseling Intersexed Persons From Infancy Through Early Adulthood

Some have recommended that intersexed individuals should have counseling as early on as possible and that this counseling should continue well into their adult lives (Slipjer, 2003). Others have related how important it is that in regard to their condition, intersexed children be adequately, incrementally informed (Dayton, 2004).   Both notions are well accepted, and both counseling and information can be titrated. Each can be given in bits and pieces, according to what children can understand, absorb, and use to be able to emotionally grow.

Most likely, there is expertise here regarding how best to counsel these children that has still to be fully developed. This expertise may involve both special skills and knowledge, much as, perhaps, such special skills and knowledge once needed to be developed to maximally help persons who were gay and trying to decide when, and indeed whether, to "come out."

When thinking of the skill required, I am reminded of an example I've cited before—an example that epitomizes for me the skill and sensitivity such a counselor can and should ideally have (Howe 1998, p. 341, citing Goodall, 1991). This counselor was informing a girl that she had androgen insensitivity syndrome (AIS). The counselor told her that all embryos are, in fact, initially girls, and thus, the building blocks that enabled her to grow merely had XY on them as a label. Then she showed her a film of a mother with AIS happily raising her two adopted children.

Another aspect of this counseling that may particularly need to be developed is that of finding the best means to help these persons deal with ongoing trauma. When, for example, persons have some chronic disabilities such as quadriplegia, these disabilities may remind them several times each day of the painful traumatic event which caused the disability. These persons' needs are different in some ways from those of other persons who had similar trauma but then got completely well. The former have no escape from these painful cues. Further, some intersexed persons may have new trauma every time they meet with others, whether these others are persons whom they know personally, or whether they are strangers. Both groups may respond in ways that cause the intersexed persons additional stress. Persons with intersexed conditions may be more prone to ongoing trauma, for example, if they do not undergo early surgery. They may be teased by other children. An example is a 6-year-old girl who had clitoromegaly. She wouldn't attend swimming classes at school so that other children wouldn't notice her spontaneous erections (Minto, 2001).

One approach to avoiding this trauma is, of course, early surgery. Yet, it is possible also that with counseling, children could learn to be able to handle these stresses without long-term negative effects. If these children differ in appearance only in their genital areas, this trauma may be in most part avoidable. If their condition affects their facial appearance, on the other hand, they may feel traumatized in their daily interactions every day.

Our understanding of the best therapy for trauma in recent years has radically changed. It used to be presumed, for example, that after disasters, the best therapy was immediate debriefing (Raphael, 2004). Now it is believed that debriefing may do more harm than good. Debriefing, it is now believed, may re-expose victims of past trauma to repeated traumatizing cues, even though this repeated trauma is only in their imagination; imaginary traumatization may have the same effect as their being re-traumatized many times. Thus, there is presently a need to determine for all persons undergoing trauma, and for intersexed persons, what kind of counseling is best.

What we know now better than we have before, however, is the extent to which psychotherapy can actually alter the structure of the brain (Paquette, 2003). This provides better theoretical ground for optimism regarding what we could accomplish by counseling intersexed persons as they grow up. Counseling by therapists with optimal skills as early on as possible, and then throughout the intersexed persons' early lives, could much increase the intersexed persons' ultimate happiness.

For many intersexed persons, if not most, psychotherapy may not be necessary. Intersexed persons may be as or more happy than most others (Morland, 2001, citing Bern, 1975). Still, this therapy might be most important for intersexed persons who otherwise wouldn't follow "this course" of happiness (Cull, 2005). In particular, psychotherapy might help all such persons to have optimal self-esteem. If their self-esteem is strong, as I have suggested, it may be less important that they feel secure in regard to their gender identity. This security, in turn, may make the argument for early surgery accordingly less compelling or may even suggest that, aside from "medical indications," early surgery shouldn't be done.

3.1.2 Counseling Intersexed Infants' Parents

Parents, of course, will be with these children most of the time. How parents respond to these children may affect the children much more than even counseling. Parents may respond by often feeling stress, as when they change these infants' diapers or tell other persons that their children are intersexed. If so, this stress may adversely affect their children profoundly. Parents may need help, too, to avoid this stress. If they can manage to avoid or even reduce it, doing so may benefit their children immensely, which would in turn reduce the arguments in favor of and/or the need for early surgery.

Enhancing children's self-esteem by loving them unconditionally is, of course, something all parents should do. I convey this message to parents using as an example what they must strive to do if their children play Little League Baseball. Many young children in their first years of play go to bat, stand at the plate, and never swing at the pitched ball. They hope that they will "walk" in this way and, thus, get on base. It is the parents' task to feel as proud of their children if the latter never swing the bat, as they would if their children were the best hitters on the team. Parents of intersexed infants face the same task and this is a task which, in either case, therapists can help them accomplish.

Applying this general concept to parents of intersexed children, more specifically, therapists could help such parents handle such stresses as those I have mentioned above. Therapists can also help parents change cultural attitudes that may be destructive. For example, therapists can help parents to be more accepting of gay persons. Research suggests that this therapy is needed. In one study, for example, parents of intersexed children were asked whether they would prefer for their children to have an intact gender identity or to have full sexual sensations. The author concluded on the basis of their responses that the vast majority of these parents linked a successful outcome for their children with the children becoming heterosexuals. Parents felt this, he believed, because they had an intolerance for "nontraditional gender function" (Dayner, 2004). This prejudice could, of course, be harmful to intersexed persons who are gay. Again, however, therapists can affect this.

Intersexed persons, some believe, may be more likely than non-intersexed persons to be attracted to persons of the same sex (Morgan, 2005). If true, this could occur as a result of many different factors. Some have speculated that intersexed persons may have stronger homosexual preferences on the average than others, because, for example, they retain a greater degree of identification with the "part of themselves" that is the same as others of the same sex—a part that the intersexed persons have lost when they "were made into" the opposite gender (Slipjer, 2003).

John Money, a clinician who has influenced much of the early thinking in this area, raises some additional possibilities in regard to why homosexual tendencies could occur (Money, 1998). He has suggested that persons may retain mental images or memories of parts of their genitals they have lost, much like persons who feel pain or other sensations in a limb they have lost, a phenomenon referred to as having sensations in a "phantom limb" (Money, 1998, p. 116). If, for example, an intersexed person with an extremely small penis has surgery, loses some of his penis, and is "made into a girl," this child might, according to Money, retain an image in her brain as if she still had a penis. This image could play a role in the gender of the sexual partner this child later chooses: this child, now a female, could choose women. Money has also suggested that such children may initially have, and then later retain, a mental image of their "idealized partner" (Money, 1998, p. 119). This too could contribute to these children's future choice of a sexual partner; though having had surgery, these children could later prefer partners of the same sex.

These possibilities are significant here because they illustrate additional reasons it may be especially important that intersexed persons' parents can accept homosexuality in their children. However, can therapists help these parents change their responses and attitudes this profoundly? The answer would seem to be unequivocally "yes." Parents, even without help, can change and become wholly accepting of children changing their gender identity. A "naturally occurring" example of such acceptance seemingly took place among the parents of the children raised as girls who, during puberty, became boys, as I previously mentioned. These parents accepted this change. Their attitudes "...involved amazement, confusion and, finally acceptance, rather than hostility..." (Imperator-McGinley, 1979, 1236).

If, of course, these children have multiple surgical operations, this too may adversely affect their self-esteem. Money states that in the "worst case scenarios," persons needing penile reconstruction may have to undergo surgery as much as 15 times (Money, at 118). Whether gender identity or self-esteem is ultimately most important, at least in this one context, may then be determined only if psychotherapy is given to some infants and their parents when these infants don't have early surgery, as I have suggested here. These infants and parents should not be used, of course, to try to answer this question (Lenning, 2004). If the parents make this decision on their own, however, psychotherapy can be offered because it unequivocally should be in both their and their infants' interests. Under these conditions and these alone, this research could be done.

3.2   Should The Negative Effects Of Surgery Preclude Early Surgery?

One effect of early surgery is psychological, as I just mentioned. The area on which there was surgery often becomes the focus of both patients' and others' attention. Children's focusing on their genitals early on—if and as they need recurrent, "revision" operations—may affect them the rest of their lives. As one person who has heard what many intersexed persons say in support group reports, this surgery may be a "constant reminder of difference" (Cull, 2005).

Again, however, there is no control group. Thus, even if early surgery affects children so that they later focus in a negative way and to a greater extent on their genitals than they otherwise would have, they might focus in this same way to the same or even a greater extent if they hadn't had the surgery. Early surgery, then, may or may not be more psychologically harmful—in the above way—than no early surgery.

Some believe that having early surgery differs also by implying to children having early surgery that something is "wrong" with them (Lenning, 2004). Whether or not this is true, the extent of this negative effect is and may remain open to debate. Still, even if having early surgery has this negative effect, it may again be that psychotherapy could play a substantial role in helping these children overcome this negative response.

Psychotherapy may be less helpful in cases involving the severing of nerves during surgery, a consequence that negatively affect intersexed persons' subsequent sexual responsiveness. Again, perhaps the most critical question is whether it is more important for intersexed persons to experience full sexual responsiveness, or whether it is more important for them to form an intact gender identity.

An intact gender identity may, as opposed to what I have suggested above, be necessary for persons to acquire healthy self-esteem. Persons may, indeed, be happier if they feel that they know which gender they are, and persons meeting them will also know better how to respond. The experience of persons who are transsexuals, and who have not been able to change their appearance from one gender to the other convincingly, can attest to the profound, ongoing stress persons may experience when their appearance causes others to feel uneasy. The uneasiness others feel in such situations often prevents them from knowing how to appropriately respond to the intersexed individual.

It is worth my commenting here on a possible aspect of others' responses, because this aspect bears on the overall importance of intersexed persons having an intact gender identity. I, like many others, may feel tempted to want to condemn others for responding in an uneasy and thus negative way. Yet, their responses may be to some extent involuntary. I recall in this regard a reaction I once had. I was introduced to a woman who had been a man. She had undergone surgery and taken female hormones. Nonetheless, before this surgery, she had already acquired a deep, masculine-sounding voice. When she spoke, I felt stressed. Her feminine appearance somehow clashed with the masculine sound of her voice and the clash immediately evoked anxiety. I imagine that is what it may be like for some people when they first learn that persons with whom they are talking are intersexed. The source of their uneasiness may be different, but the feeling may be involuntary all the same.

Identity, then, may indeed be more important than intersexed persons having the capacity for full sexual sensation. Yet, if the benefits of early surgery, particularly with psychotherapy, are equivocal, it may be that intersexed persons can acquire healthy self-esteem in the absence of having an intact early gender identity, as I have postulated above. If so, intersexed persons' capacity to enjoy maximal sexual pleasure throughout their lives may, correspondingly, be relatively greater. It may, perhaps, be of such importance that their loss of responsiveness should be the deciding factor in determining whether or not early surgery should be done.

One source of controversy in regard to this question is the actual effect of this surgery on sexual sensation. Emotions affect what persons "sexually feel." Thus, some have argued that when intersexed persons who have had genital surgery later find their sexual interactions unsatisfactory, this may be because they have underlying emotional concerns. They may, for example, have concerns about their appearance or be simply shy. Consequently, their decreased sexual responsiveness could be due to these reasons, rather than the surgery. Once again, they would not have a way of knowing the true cause.

Indeed, due to emotions, persons can even have a total loss of sensation (Gracely, 2003). Some persons experience this due to a mental illness called a conversion disorder. Others, not mentally ill, but having an extremely high capacity for hypnosis, can also experience loss of sensation. These people can use hypnosis even to undergo surgery, such as a Caesarian section, without having to have any general or local anesthesia.

In addition to decreasing the extent to which persons can feel sexual pleasure, psychological factors can also cause pain during sexual relations. Some intersexed persons who have had surgery report that they have pain during sexual intercourse. This pain, like their lack of pleasure, may conceivably be due (at least in part) to intersexed persons' emotions rather than their surgery.

Some have suggested that the above question, whether intersexed persons' decreased sensation is due to surgery or their emotions (and if the latter, to what extent) may be answered in part by considering as a ground for comparison the responses of transsexual persons who have had surgery. These persons may more often feel, it is claimed, that the effects of surgery have been positive. Even if this difference does exist, however, it is unclear what such a difference might mean. Surgery is, for instance, what transsexual persons deeply want. Thus, their happiness at being able to have this surgery could be a psychological factor resulting in their experiencing a better outcome. Cognitive dissonance, for example, may lead them to reduce or deny the importance of any loss of feeling that this surgery brings about. This same happiness may not be present, of course, among intersexed persons who have this surgery, especially if they have had it during their infancy as opposed to their having chosen to have it later.

Some have pointed out, analogously, that this same question of whether impaired sensation is caused by this surgery or intersexed persons' emotions (and if the latter, to what extent), may also be answered in part by finding out whether intersexed persons who have problems with sexual relations also have problems when they masturbate. If they experience a more satisfactory sexual response when they masturbate than when they have sex with a partner, for example, this might suggest that their lack of sensation is more due to psychological factors than to their surgery. What if, however, persons who are intersexed have diminished sexual responsiveness due (in part) to feelings such as inhibition or self-consciousness? Again, psychotherapy, as I have described it, could have a beneficial effect.

This discussion of how surgery affects intersexed persons' experience with partners raises, in turn, several additional considerations, such as whether surgery has a different effect on intersexed persons who are male or female, or heterosexual or gay. Having or not having surgery may affect intersexed persons' relationships with their partners differently, for example, depending on whether the intersexed person would have an enlarged clitoris or an exceptionally small penis without surgery, and also whether their partners would be heterosexual or gay. These considerations could, in some cases, be the deciding factors in deciding what patients, parents and/or care providers should do regarding surgery.

The arguments for and against this surgery may also differ, depending on intersexed persons' gender and whether they are heterosexual or gay. For example, if males have a small penis and do not have surgery, whether they are in a heterosexual or homosexual relationship, they can still (so they and their partners say) give full pleasure to their partners, as well as experience pleasure as fully or more fully than they could after surgery. Skeptics might claim that their partners aren't telling the truth, but are telling their intersexed partners what they most want to hear. While logically possible, this claim is implausible. There are innumerable couples who lack the capacity for "normal" sexual intercourse and report that they can fully give each other pleasure and many have, of course, also stayed together, apparently happy for years. The best example here is that of couples that include one person who has a profound physical disability.

Similar questions can be asked in regard to women who have and haven't had surgery to reduce the size of an enlarged clitoris. The most prominent questions are: what difference does an enlarged clitoris make, and does the woman's experience generally differ whether she is having sexual relations with a male or female? The answers may or may not differ depending on how greatly the clitoris is enlarged, and whether or not answers do differ in this way may be an important issue. A greatly enlarged clitoris may affect other children's responses to the intersexed individuals, a problem illustrated by the example of the 6-year-old girl who would not go in the swimming pool. In the past, the degree of enlargement has sometimes been a decisive factor in making the decision that this surgery should be done. If, of course, having an enlarged clitoris makes no difference in intersexed persons' later lives, or generally adds to the sexual pleasure they experience with others, it may be that clitoris size should no longer be construed as a problem for those with an enlarged clitoris in the same way it has in the past. As a result of this change in the way and/or extent to which an enlarged clitoris is viewed as a problem, the arguments for surgery might be altered accordingly. Presumably, the argument in favor of surgery would then be reduced and dealt with differently, as it has in the past. Some intersexed persons who have an enlarged clitoris and have not had surgery have reported that their partners (on the basis of what they have told them), as well as themselves, find the enlarged clitoris a source of exceptional pleasure. Again, their partners may be "just" saying this, but since (in these cases) their partners obviously can accept these intersexed persons and their anatomy as they are, and since the partners enjoy having sexual relations with them, this possibility seems implausible. Yet, for mutually satisfactory sexual relations to occur, as I have just suggested, intersexed persons' partners must be able to emotionally accept intersexed persons being as they are. If the partners of intersexed persons feel emotional discomfort with intersexed persons' genital anatomy, this would most likely impair these partners' capacity to fully enjoy their sexual relations with these intersexed persons. Likewise, if these partners felt discomfort, intersexed persons would most likely detect this. Intersexed persons detecting that their partners felt discomfort would most likely then impair their capacities to full enjoy sexual relations with these partners, as well. Indeed, some potential partners may have more difficulty than others in emotionally accepting intersexed persons having an exceptionally small penis or enlarged clitoris. This acceptance may differ, depending on what gender intersexed persons are and whether they prefer partners of the same or the opposite sex. Yet, there may be an advantage to some potential partners having this difficulty. When intersexed persons have not had surgery, their partners must be willing to accept this. If intersexed persons have not had this surgery, then they have, as it were, a kind of built-in "screening device" or means of screening out partners who, for one reason or another, can't emotionally accept them as they are. This possibility raises the question of whether partners who can accept intersexed persons' genitals as they are may have more to offer as lifelong partners than others who can't. If so, this screening may be desirable. If not, then, of course, it is not. Clearly, these partners must at least be able to overcome anxiety that would significantly interfere with their being able to fully enjoy sex. Even if partners who can accept intersexed persons' anatomy when they don't have surgery are deeper and this, therefore, works to intersexed persons' advantage as a screening device, intersexed persons have many other valid reasons to still have surgery, especially during their adolescence or as adults.

The extent to which partners would accept intersexed persons as partners if the intersexed persons have not had surgery also is unknown. The rate of acceptance may be much greater than parents and care providers have imagined. If this is the case, the argument in favor of not doing surgery may, of course, also, be correspondingly stronger.

3.3   Should Intersexed Persons Be Allowed By Society To Be A Third Sex?

I recall having a discussion with an intersexed person who believed that our society should accept a third sex. She believed that this acceptance should include establishing in public places three bathrooms: his, hers, and others'. I tried to persuade her that if she truly wanted to further the interests of intersexed persons, her advocating this third sex might not be the best approach, because she might lose credibility.

Whether or not I was right, her believing that society should change to this degree illustrates the conviction—shared by many intersexed persons—that society should allow them to be as they are. One intersexed person, for example, has expressed this attitude, saying, "...[G]iven the choice of 'male', 'female', [or] 'intersex', I would unhesitatingly select 'intersex'...." (Lenning, 2004, citing Mairi MacDonald at http://www.ukia.co.uk).

Some societies in this and previous times have accepted a third sex. In Australia, for example, persons now can choose not to indicate their gender on their passports. Since ancient times, other cultures have accepted that intersexed persons are separate from males or females. Perhaps the best-known example of this practice is Tieresias, who told the future to Oedipus. Tieresias was considered, as this example illustrates, to be able to see what others couldn't see.

Anthropologists have also described other cultures in which societies give intersexed persons special roles. These societies may, for example, give intersexed persons special status as healers. It is perhaps worth asking why these societies have tended to view intersexed persons as having exceptional insight, like Tieresias, or exceptional qualities which would equip them to be special healers. It is worth considering the possibility that it isn't solely coincidental that societies sometimes attribute to intersexed persons these exceptional qualities. Societies' doing this could reflect that indeed, these persons tend to have exceptional insight and/or capacities for caring and healing. Morland claims, in fact, on the basis of empirical data, that individuals who have "an androgynous gender identity" are "happier, more socially competent and more intelligent than those with a fixed, stereotypical gender" (Morland, 2001). His empirical basis for making this claim has, however, been questioned (Minto, 2001).

If Morland were right about his claims, why would intersexed people exhibit the qualities he mentions? Intersexed persons, like many others (such as those with serious disabilities) may have, of course, a markedly different experience from others. This experience may give them unique insights. They may, for example, be better able than most others to distinguish what is more important in living from what is not. They may, for example, be more able, on the average, to enjoy others more on the basis of admirable human qualities than on the basis of how they look.

Others have offered more far-reaching speculations as to why intersexed persons could have exceptional positive qualities. The writer Virginia Woolf claimed, for instance, that intersexed persons are more likely to have the strengths of each gender. She wrote in *A Room of One's Own*: "Coleridge perhaps meant this when he said that a great mind is androgynous. It is when this fusion takes place that the mind is fully fertilized and uses all its faculties" (Woolf, 1989, p. 98).

If Woolf is correct, there may be many reasons, both physical and psychological, for intersexed persons' exceptional positive qualities. If, for instance, intersexed persons happen to experience themselves first as members of one gender, and later of the other, they may acquire unique awarenesses as a result. This possibility is suggested, for example, by Herculine Barbin, who lived in the nineteenth century, first as a girl, and then as a boy. He wrote in his diary that as a result of his early experiences as a girl, he had an exceptionally great understanding of women. As a man he described the unique capacity to understand women that he felt he had acquired. He said regarding one woman, " I can read her heart like an open book" (Lorraine, 1996, p. 263).

Why might this possession of unique qualities matter? It may not. There is, after all, a danger that even though these speculative attributions are positive, they will further stereotype intersexed persons. I believe that the possession of unique qualities matters because such qualities—like ambiguous genitalia—may be another important aspect of the intersexed person's identity. The importance of the wish to be recognized as a third sex is important on two levels. One is legal. Even if this does not occur, it is also important of course, that societies accept these persons as they are. Societies' not accepting them should not, for example, be a reason for intersexed people to decide to have surgery. They should also not have to have surgery as infants to escape children's prejudice. Rather, parents should teach their children to be as accepting of intersexed children as they should be of children of other ethnic groups and races. If, of course, society became more accepting, this could tip the balance in favor of parents not choosing for their infants to have surgery at an early age.

Societies' prejudice against these individuals may, however, be less open to change than might be imagined, since there are unusual hidden factors at stake. Many persons feel insecure regarding both their gender identity and their capacity to "perform" sexually. The latter concern often involves their sexual organs. Men may feel threatened regarding their gender identity, for example, when others so much as even imply that these men have a feminine gesture, such as lifting their little finger when they drink from a glass. Women, correspondingly, may be offended if others imply that they are dressing in a masculine way. Men worry about the size of their penises and women worry about the size of their breasts.

Persons of both sexes may psychologically "project" their worries about their gender identity and sexual adequacy onto others, such as persons who are intersexed. As with their children, if and when they do this, this is as or more harmful to themselves.

The best hope that this prejudice may become less over time may be that as more intersexed persons meet with others (such as care providers) to discuss together what should be done, more members of society will get to know intersexed individuals, personally. Then, whether or not the intersexed individuals have exceptional qualities, persons in society could be expected to fear and stereotype them less. This would, of course, be a second benefit of intersexed persons and care providers meeting together more, in order to try to resolve these questions together.

4.   WHAT SHOULD PARENTS (AND CARE PROVIDERS) DO NOW?

The first legal change, if any, that this society makes will not be, I would guess, recognizing intersexed persons as a third sex. Rather, it would be giving parents greater access to full information prior to their having to decide whether to consent to their intersexed infants having early surgery. Even if parents are more fully informed, however, as I have suggested, it is still unclear what decision they should make.

Some therapists believe that when persons face difficult decisions, they ideally need three things: persons who have knowledge regarding their situation (e.g. care providers), persons who are at the same time going through what they are so that they aren't then alone, and persons who have gone through what they have and done well, or at least done acceptably and survived.

If parents have greater access to persons who are facing the question of early surgery for their infants at the same time as parents are themselves, parents will not be so alone. And if parents have greater access to intersexed persons who have had and have not had early surgery, such access may help parents as well. This last opportunity, may, however, possibly do greater harm. Depending on who they meet, this opportunity may make parents' decision more difficult or leave them feeling more pessimistic regarding the optimal results.

Still, however, even if parents had these three things, the question of how they should decide will remain. If at all possible, it would seem that parents and care providers should take the time necessary to try to discern these infants' diagnoses and prognoses prior to carrying out what is, of course, irreversible surgery (Ogilvy-Stuart, 2004). This would be most advisable for numerous reasons. In some cases, for example, the diagnosis might suggest strongly what the infant's later gender identity will be. In the case of infants born with 5a-reductase deficiency in which those raised as girls "became boys during puberty," for example, infants might be expected overwhelmingly to later identify themselves as males (Imperato-Mcginley, 1979, Reiner, 2004).

Other realities identified might also carry moral weight. One example here, for instance, is that of intersexed persons having the capacity to become pregnant (Tegenkamp, 1979). If pursuing the possibility of arriving at a diagnosis takes a longer time, parents may want to take this into consideration when they name their infant. They may also want to think carefully about how they wish to handle such concerns as birth announcements (Ogilvy-Struart, 2004). A name that is both "male and female" may, of course, be preferable. I shall say more later about one less obvious reason why giving such a name may be optimal.

Some would argue, of course, that unless intersexed infants have a diagnosis that makes surgery necessary for medical reasons, parents should defer surgery until these children can decide for themselves. If parents do this, they could raise these children as if they were the gender that care providers would assume they would be when performing early surgery. The other option, absent early surgery, is for these parents to raise these children as persons with a third, indeterminate gender and let them later decide what, if either, gender they want to be. If, having done this, after some years and/or during adolescence, it seems for some reason best for the child to have surgery, this can then be done. As I have mentioned, in some cases this surgery may be more successful during adolescence, due to a surge of estrogen at that time (Schober, 2004).

If and when these children decide they want surgery (which would obviously involve changing their gender), they and their parents must decide whether to stay with the same friends or to move and, as it were, "start anew." It may or may not be preferable if the child is to become the opposite gender to be able to have a new start. If a new start occurs, however, and the child's name is one that both genders use, at least this aspect of the child's identity can stay the same.

The primary importance of deferring surgery during infancy until a later time, such as the child's adolescence, is not necessarily that doing so would better respect these children's autonomy, as some persons, such as Schober, have asserted (Schober, 2004). This value is nevertheless important, since deferring surgery until adolescence would, of course, then allow these children to choose. An alternative value which may warrant even greater moral weight here, however, is that at a later time the child may know better what his or her gender identity is or will most likely be.

Practically, there is a profound difference between the two alternatives mentioned above. The difference is this: if respecting the child's autonomy is the value given greatest priority, it might be necessary to wait until the child is a certain age to decide whether or not to have surgery. This age might be, at the very least, the age at which the child legally can be a "mature minor." This determination that a child is a mature minor usually is made now not on the basis on the child's chronological age, but rather, on the basis of the child's emotional maturity. Still, this judgment usually is not made unless the child is 14 or older. A child might show an unequivocal preference to be a boy or girl, however, long before this, as at age 10 or 11. If so, it might make more sense to allow them to have surgery then.

If these children want to have surgery at any later age, there is, of course, also the possibility that before having surgery that would irreversibly change their anatomy, they could live as the opposite gender or their "gender-to-be" on a "trial basis." This would be somewhat equivalent to what transsexual persons do prior to undergoing surgery. Intersexed children then could better discern whether this surgery would result in a gender change that they really want.

Although this "trial basis" approach might be preferable to not living as the opposite gender prior to undergoing surgery and changing one's gender identity, it also could prove misleading. If, for example, these children moved at the same time as adopting this trial of a different gender identity, they might be unhappy due to the move, but mistakenly think that their unhappiness is due to their change in gender. This move might involve, for example, these children losing their friends. They could then mistakenly think that their unhappiness from this loss of friends is instead due to losing their previous gender. This difference might become clearer over time. Taking into account all their options, which include not making this gender change at this age, not moving, and not adopting a gender change on a trial basis, their taking this risk may, however, be the best that they could do.

The age at which these children should change identities, if it appears that this is what they should do, should also be determined by such factors as the effects of hormones at this time in their lives. The ideal time might in some cases be adolescence, when changes such as girls' breast development and the deepening of boys' voices occurs. The other option is, of course, early surgery. I have spelled out the options other than early surgery in great detail, while hardly discussing early surgery at all, because early surgery has been most common in the past.

How, then, should parents and these children's care providers decide whether or not to perform early surgery? Ethically, in many contexts in which other factors are considered equal, it is assumed that if possible, irreversible actions should be avoided. In this instance, however, this condition of other things being equal can never be met. Both early surgery and no early surgery will result in irreversible changes.

What moral weight, then, if any, should this consideration of irreversibility have in this context? Some children, and perhaps the great majority of them, may gain from early surgery. These children would be irreversibly harmed by not having it. They may, for example, have psychological problems with forming a sexual identity and have problems being teased by other children, as I have discussed. Both of these problems—and others—may or may not be reducible by counseling. Still, a small minority will be greatly harmed by having early surgery if they later identify themselves as members of the opposite gender. Whose interests, then, should prevail: the greater group or this much smaller number?

There is an ethical principle of justice according to need that gives greatest priority to meeting the needs of persons worst off. This principle may support or require protecting the needs of even just a few persons if they are vulnerable to experiencing much greater harm than others. In the case of intersexed infants who undergo surgery, this principle applies. Those intersexed infants who undergo surgery and later change their gender identity are much worse off than other intersexed persons, though at the time their surgery is done, their identity isn't and couldn't be known. The approach of not doing early surgery to protect these few might be warranted under this principle, then, even though not doing early surgery would prevent many more intersexed persons from having possibly great benefits from early surgery.

The philosopher John Rawls introduced an imaginary exercise that may be most applicable here (Rawls, 1971). Rawls asks what reasonable persons would decide if they were under a "veil of ignorance" such that they didn't know what state they were in. They might be rich or poor, healthy or ill, and might be deaf and blind and have no arms or legs. Most persons, Rawls maintains, would opt for a policy that would protect them if they were worst off so that even in this event they would still be able to enjoy their life.

If this imaginary veil of ignorance were applied to this question regarding early surgery, and if Rawls is right, reasonable persons would opt here to protect those worst off. This would mean that they would not risk having early surgery and then possibly ending up among those few who had been "made into" the "wrong" and, indeed, opposite gender. They would rather take their chances on not having early surgery, and hope that with psychotherapy for them and their parents, they could then still do well.

If this moral value of justice according to need is given the greatest ethical priority, this might mean, however, not only withholding early surgery except in cases in which it was clear what gender these infants would become. It might also be ethically obligatory to try to offset the potential negative effects on all the other children resulting from their not having early surgery. This offsetting could be done, as I have suggested, by offering all these children and their parents opportunities for counseling, as I have discussed above.

Could this allocation of resources be justified? I would argue that it could, particularly for two reasons. The first reason is based on the same moral principle that underlies the withholding of early surgery in the first place, namely, the principle of justice according to need. Intersexed children who have surgery and then develop a gender identity opposite to that of their anatomy are the intersexed persons worst off. Yet, if intersexed children who don't have early surgery can't acquire an intact gender identity as a result of not having had early surgery, they, though "less worse off," are among the worst off, as well. They too, then, might have a greater claim than most others on societies' limited resources on this same basis.

The second reason is based on the principle of fairness, or more specifically, a kind of compensatory justice. That is, intersexed children who do not have early surgery may be worst off without this surgery largely because of society's prejudice that persons must be one gender or the other to be "ok." Society in this sense, then, may greatly contribute to these intersexed children's initial and later difficulties. Thus, society may have a greater moral obligation to these persons than to others to try to compensate them for the harm it has caused. Society may have a moral obligation to try to help offset this negative effect.

It may be that in the future it will become more feasible to predict the gender identity intersexed children will develop. The frequency with which infants now develop gender identities opposite to those that their care providers have predicted may be rare. The number may become even less. Research suggests, for example, that perhaps to a greater extent than many have expected, intersexed person's gender identity may be genetically caused (Dennis, 2004). If so, as more of the genes that affect gender identity are identified, care providers' capacities to accurately predict which gender intersexed infants will assume will increase.

Three kinds of evidence suggest that genes may play a greater role than previously thought. The first kind comes from a rare bird called a zebra finch that genetically is a male on one side of its body but is a female on the other. If hormones totally determined this bird's gender, this couldn't be the case. The second kind comes from a researcher who switched the forebrains in Japanese quail embryos before their gonads began to develop. If only hormones directed these birds' gender development, this change shouldn't have affected these birds' subsequent sexual behavior. In males, however, it profoundly did. The third kind is findings suggesting that transsexualism runs to a greater extent in families. It is possible, perhaps, that this tendency has other causes, but still, a genetic influence may be one of them. Dennis summarizes the possible implication of all the above developments as follows: "in mammals, male and female brains start traveling down different developmental paths from the outset, before hormones have entered the picture" (Dennis, 2004, p. 391).

What, however, if this is the case? What if the degree to which intersexed children will develop a gender identity as male or female can be better predicted? Would this increase the argument for doing early surgery? It might not. The ethical argument I have posed above in regard to protecting those intersexed persons worst off will remain. Even under these new conditions, some infants who have had early surgery still will end up having anatomically been made into the "wrong" gender. The ethical question this still poses is whether, at any point, the need to protect these persons should no longer be overriding. The answer may be, based on the principle of justice according to need, never.

5. CONCLUSION

The core ethical question now posed in regard to intersexed persons is whether they should have early surgery. Up until recently this question has not been discussed to the degree it ideally should. Even now there are difficulties getting together intersexed persons and care providers at the same table.

Intersexed persons who have had surgery and aren't happy with their results may not take fully enough into account the lack of information these care providers had and still have. Care providers who have done and do this surgery on these children still have sound reasons for believing that surgery may be these infants' best course. Care providers may find it emotionally difficult, understandably, even to consider the possibility that decisions they have made, and are still making, are wrong. As Money has said, summarizing this situation for both parents and care providers, "[This is a situation in which] you're damned if you do and damned if you don't" (Money, 1998, p.114). This question remains, of course, particularly agonizing for parents faced with this decision. As one parent expressed, "Will she hate us for letting her have the surgery? Or will she thank us for having it done when she was young enough not to know?" (Navarro, 2004).

I have discussed three key questions related to whether care providers should do early surgery. These are whether early surgery is essential to enable these children to acquire an intact gender identity, the degree to which this surgery impairs intersexual persons' sexual responsiveness at any age, and whether legally intersexed persons who want to should be able to be a third sex.

The extent to which early surgery is necessary to enable intersexed children to acquire an intact gender identity is uncertain. It is also unclear whether to give greater importance to their acquiring an intact gender identity or to their acquiring healthy self-esteem. It may be that they can obtain optimal self-esteem whether or not they have an intact gender identity. It may be also that this is particularly likely if both they and their parents have ongoing counseling from the time that these children are infants.

It is unclear how both early and later surgery will affect these persons' sexual responsiveness. This lack of clarity is due in part to the fact that persons' sexual experiences may depend on the feelings they have in interpersonal contexts. It is likely that if intersexed persons do not have surgery, they will be able to experience sexual pleasure to a greater extent. This may be possible, however, only if they have partners who can accept them and their sexual organs as they are. The extent to which potential partners can and will accept intersexed persons as they are—without having surgery—may be much greater than parents and care providers imagine, but is, in any case, largely unknown.

Intersexed persons, like all persons, should be able to take full pride in being just as they are. Creating this reality even to a small extent may require our society to allow intersexed persons to be able to identify themselves legally as a third sex, as is done in Australia. What may be even more important, however, is that members of this society come to accept intersexed persons as "ok" as they are, whether intersexed persons have surgery or not.

Parents and care providers will continue to face agonizing decisions regarding early surgery. Ethically, there are now arguments for and against early surgery that may be made and there is no way that these can be unequivocally resolved. I have highlighted in this discussion some implications of giving greatest moral weight to the principle of justice according to persons' needs. I have suggested that giving greatest priority to this moral principle, as I suspect Rawls would, would result in two conclusions: First, early surgery shouldn't be done. Second, when these infants don't have early surgery, psychotherapy should be offered to them and their parents as early on as possible, and until these infants reach adulthood.

I have suggested that society should fund this counseling for two reasons: First, intersexed children who do not have early surgery may be among those within society that would be worst off, particularly without this therapy for them and their parents, even though they would not be as badly off as infants who had early surgery and then changed their gender. Second, society may have a special moral obligation to these children because it has a culturally based prejudice that persons must be one or the other gender to be "ok." This belief may contribute to intersexed persons being harmed most substantially. This belief that these children aren't "ok" without having surgery may, for example, become for these children a self-fulfilling prophecy. To the extent that it can, society may have a moral obligation to try to help offset negative effects it has caused.

Edmund Howe, Professor, Department of Psychiatry, Uniformed Services University of the Health Sciences, Bethesda, Maryland, U.S.A.

REFERENCES

Ahmed, S.F., S. Morrison, and I.A. Hughes. "Intersex and Gender Assignment; the Third Way?" *Archives of Disease in Childhood* 89: 9 (Sept. 2004): 847-50.

Baratz, Arlene B. "Sex Determination, Differentiation, and Identity: To: The Editor." *The New England Journal of Medicine* 350: 21 (May 2004): 2206-07.

Berenbaum, Sheri A., and David E. Sandberg. "Sex Determination, Differentiation, and Identity." *The New England Journal of Medicine* 350: 21 (May 2004): 2204-06.

Bern, S.L. "Sex Role Adaptability: One Consequence of Psychological Androgyny." *Journal of Personality and Social Psychology* 31 (1975): 634-43.

Biswas, Krishna, et al. "Imaging in Intersex Disorders." *Journal of Pediatric Endocrinology and Metabolism* 17: 6 (2004): 841-5.

Bleier, Ruth. "Why Does a Pseudohermaphrodite Want to be a Man?" *The New England Journal of Medicine* 301: 15 (Oct. 1984): 839-40.

Creighton Sarah M., et al. "Meeting Between Experts: Evaluation of the First UK Forumfor Lay and Professional Experts in Intersex." *Patient Education and Counseling* 54 (2004): 153-7.

Creighton, Sarah M. and Catherine L. Minto, "Managing Intersex." *British Medical Journal* 323 (Dec. 2001): 1264-65.

Creighton, Sarah M., Catherine L. Minto, and Stuart J. Steele. "Objective Cosmetic and Anatomical Outcomes at Adolescence of Feminizing Surgery for Ambiguous Genitalia Done in Childhood." *Lancet* 358 (Jul 14-2001): 124-25.

Cull, Melissa L. "Commentary: A Support Group's Perspective." *British Medical Journal* 330 (2005): 341.

_____. "Treatment of Intersex Needs Open Discussion." *British Journal of Medicine* 324: (April 13-2002): 919.

Dayner, Jenifer E., Peter A. Lee, and Christopher P. Houk. "Medical Treatment of Intersex: Parental Perspectives." *The Journal of Urology* 172: 4 (Part 2 of 2, Oct. 2004): 1762-65.

Dennis, Carina. "The Most Important Sexual Organ." *Nature* 427: 29 (Jan. 2004): 390-92.

Dewhurst, John, and R.R. Gordon. "Fertility Following Change of Sex: A Follow-Up." *The Lancet* (December 22/29-1984): 1461-62.

Dreger, A.D. *Hermaphrodites and the Medical Intervention of Sex* (Cambridge, Mass: Harvard University Press, 1998).

Farkas, A, B. Chertin, and I. Hadas-Halpren. "1-Stage Feminizing Genitoplasty: 8 years of Experience with 49 Cases." *The Journal of Urology* 165: 6 (June 2001): 2341-46.

Fleming A. and E. Villain. "The Endless Quest for Sex Determination Genes." *Clinical Genetics* 67: 1 (2004): 15-25.

Goodall, J. "Helping a Child to Understand Her Own Testicular Feminization." *Lancet* 337: 8732 (5 January 1991): 33-55.

Gracely, R.H. "Is Seeing Believing? Functional Imaging of Hysterical Anesthesia." *Neurology* 60: 9 (May-2003): 1410-1.

Howe, E.G. "Intersexuality: What Should Care Providers Do Now?" *The Journal of Clinical Ethics* 9 (Winter 1998): 337-344.

Imperato-McGinley, Julianne, et al, "Androgens and the Evolution of Male-Gender Identity among Male Pseudohermaphrodites with 5a-Reductase Deficiency." *The New England Journal of Medicine* 300: 22 (May 1979): 1233-37.

Lenning, Alkeline Van. "The Body as Crowbar." *Feminist Theory* 5: 1 (2004): 25-47.

Lorraine, T. "Ambiguous Bodies/Believable Selves: The Case of Herculine Barbin." In *Interaction and Identity* (New Brunswick, N.J: Transaction Publishers, 1996):259-271.

Matz, D.C. and W. Wood. "Cognitive Dissonance in Groups: The Consequences of Disagreement." *Journal of Personality and Social Psychology* 88: 1 (2005): 22-37.

Mairi MacDonald, Mairi. http://www.ukia.co.uk .

Minto, Catherine, et al. "Management of Intersex: A Reply." *Lancet* 358: 9298 (Dec. 2001 [internet]).

_____. "The Effect of Clitoral on Sexual Outcome in Individuals who have Intersex Conditions with Ambiguous Genitalia: a Cross-Sectional Study." *Lancet* 361 (April 2003): 1252-57.

Money, John. "Case Consultation: Ablatio Penis." *Medical Law* 1 (1998): 113-23.

_____. "Re: Editorial: Gender Assignment and the Pediatric Urologist." *The Journal of Urology* 163:3 (2000): 926-27.

Morgan John F., et al. "Long Term Psychological Outcome For Women With Congenital Adrenal Hyperplasia: Cross Sectional Survey." *British Medical Journal* 330 (2005): 340-1.

Morland, Iain, "Management of Intersex," *Lancet* 358: 9298 (Dec. 15-2001): 1-2. [internet]

Meyer-Bahlburg, H., et al. "Attitudes of Adult 46, XY Intersex Persons to Clinical Management Policies." *The Journal of Urology* 171:4 (April 2004): 1615-19.

Navarro, Mireya. "When Gender isn't a Given." *The New York Times* (Late edition-final) Column1: Page 1: section 9 (Sept. 19-2004): [internet]

Ogilvy-Stuart A.L. and C.E. Brain. "Early Assessment of Ambiguous Genitalia." *Archives of Disease in Childhood* 89 (2004): 401-7.

Ozcakar, Levent, et al. "Compartment Syndrome after Substitution Vaginoplasty: An Onerous Medical Complication." *Plastic and Reconstructive Surgery* 112: 7 (Dec. 2003): 1947-75.

Paquette, V., et al. "'Change the Mind and You Change the Brain:' Effects of Cognitive Behavioral Therapy on the Neural Correlates of Spider Phobia." *Neuroimage* 18: 2 (2003): 401-9.

Porter, Roy. "Body of Evidence," Review of *Hermaphrodites and the Medical Invention of Sex* by Alice Dreger (Cambridge, Mass.: Harvard University Press, 1998) in *Nature* 393 (28 May 1998): 323-324.

Raphael, B., and S. Wooding. "Debriefing: Its Evolution and Current Status." *Psychiatric Clinics of North America* 27: 3 (2004): 407-23.

Rawls, John. *A Theory of Justice.* (Cambridge, Mass.: Harvard University Press, 1971).

Reiner, William G. and Bradley P. Kropp. "A 7-year Experience of Genetic Males with Severe Phallic Inadequacy Assigned Female." *The Journal of Urology* 172: 6 (Pt 1) (2004): 2395-8.

Schober, Justine M. "Sexual Behaviors, Sexual Orientation and Gender Identity in Adult Intersexuals: A Pilot Study." *The Journal of Urology* 165: 6 (Part 2) (June-2001): 2350-53.

_____. "Feminizing Genitoplasty: A Synopsis of Issues Relating to Genital Surgery in Intersex Individuals." *Journal of Pediatric Endocrinology and Metabolism* 17 (2004): 697-703.

Slipjer, Froukje, M. "Clitoral Surgery and Sexual Outcome in Intersex Conditions." *The Lancet* 361 (April 12-2003): 1236-37.

Sultan, Charles, et al. "Ambiguous Genitalia in the Newborn." *Seminars in Reproductive Medicine* 20: 3 (2002): 181-8.

Tegenkamp, T. R., et al. "Pregnancy without Benefit of Reconstructive Surgery in a Bisexually Active True Hermaphrodite." *American Journal of Obstetrics and Gynecology* 129 (Oct 1-1979): 427-8.

Wisniewski, Amy B., et al. "Complete Androgen Insensitivity Syndrome: Long-Term Medical, Surgical, and Psychosexual Outcome." *The Journal of Clinical Endocrinology and Metabolism* 85: 8 (2000): 2664-69.

Woolf, Virginia. *A Room of One's Own.* (New York: Harcourt, Inc., 1989).

Zucker, Kenneth J. "Re: Sexual Behaviors, Sexual Orientation and Gender Identity in Adult Intersexuals: A Pilot Study." *The Journal of Urology* 168: 4 (Part 1) (Oct-2002): 1507-08.

TIMOTHY F. MURPHY

EXPERIMENTS IN GENDER:

Ethics at the Boundaries of Clinical Practice and Research

1. INTRODUCTION

In 1967, the Reimer family in Winnipeg took their twin sons to a physician for a commonplace surgery. The twin boys, Brian and Bruce, suffered from a constriction of the penis foreskin, and the family physician recommended circumcision as a resolution to this problem. During Bruce's circumcision, the physician mishandled the electrocautery blade and destroyed the boy's penis. His parents were distraught, to say the least, and Brian's circumcision never took place. The Reimers had great difficulty imagining what it would be like for their son to grow up without a penis. Through television, they learned about John Money and his views that boys could be transformed into girls through early-age interventions. The family contacted the Johns Hopkins psychologist, and he offered further details of his view that gender identity is open to change. Rather than have the boy face the psychic and social damage of having no penis, he recommended the child be raised as female.[1] Persuaded, the Reimers came to the decision that because of the injury Bruce would be better off as a girl, and so began one of medicine's most fateful experiments in gender.

With consent from the parents, Money helped make the arrangements to have the child's testes removed and a vaginal cleft formed when the child was about 23-months-old. Money directed the parents to treat the child henceforth as female in all matters. Accordingly, the parents renounced the child's birth sex, and 'Bruce' became 'Brenda,' long hair and frilly dresses included. As Brenda approached puberty, the parents gave the child estrogen, and breast development occurred. If all went according to plan, later surgery to create a vaginal canal would finalize the interventions necessary to transform the child from male to female.

This bold intervention occurred in the context of a debate in the psychological sciences about the malleability of gender. On one side, some parties believed that psychological development and socialization played the dominant roles in the emergence of one's felt sense of being male or female, and Money was a leading expositor of this view. On the other side, some researchers believed that biology played an irreducible role in the emergence of gender identity.[2] Yet even these

S.E. Sytsma (Ed.), Ethics and Intersex, 139–151.

skeptics could not blink away the reports that Money started publishing in 1972, reports that a child born male could enter fully into a female identity.[3]

It is, of course, one thing to report that a male child – a little more than two years old–can be coaxed into female-typical behavior and it is another thing to know that the child goes on through puberty, adolescence, and adulthood with an unequivocal female identity. As years passed, the skeptics wondered about the absence of follow-up studies confirming exactly this transformation for the Reimer child, but Money and his colleagues published no such long-term reports. A persistent psychologist, Milton Diamond, finally located 'Brenda Reimer' for an interview with the now-adult twin in 1995, and published an article about his findings in 1997.[4] Diamond learned that, far from being a success, the gender intervention had failed and had failed early on. What's more, the attempt to re-assign the child's gender had imposed an enormous psychological cost on the child and the family. The parents roiled in doubt about the propriety of their choice for years, and the child felt ostracized to the point of attempted suicide. In 1980, on the advice of a family physician, 'Brenda's' father disclosed to his child the story of the circumcision accident and subsequent gender transformation. The 13-year-old immediately reclaimed a male identity and chose David as his name. Even though he had known that the experiment in gender transformation had failed, John Money remained professionally silent and continued to cite his original studies about the Reimer child as evidence that early-age interventions could shape a child's gender identity and behavior.

2. THE ETHICS OF CLINICAL INNOVATION

Many people were ultimately involved in the gender re-assignment of David Reimer: his parents, his psychologist, the clinical team that agreed to carry out the castration, physicians who saw the child for medical care and who prescribed hormones, as well as family members and educators who treated the child as female. Even so, no independent and disinterested review body evaluated the risks and benefits of re-assigning the child's gender. Indeed, the intervention took place before key developments that now guide contemporary thinking about clinical innovation and research. In 1979, the National Commission for the Protection of Human Subjects in Biomedical and Behavioral Research issued the *Belmont Report*, which made a number of recommendations regarding ethics standards in clinical innovation and research.[5] In the 1970s, the U.S. government put regulations in place that require prior review and approval of research as a way of protecting the rights and welfare of human subjects.[6]

Looking back at case like that of David Reimer opens the door to all kinds of 'what if' questions. What if the Reimer family had never found out about John Money's gender theories? What if a physician had–early on–counseled the Reimer family to love their son in spite of his injury and to protect him from the cruelties that might be his lot? What if a well-meaning relative had refused to go along with the re-assignment and spilled the beans to the child about the surgery? These questions cannot be answered in any definitive way, of course, and can be distracting precisely to the extent they can be multiplied indefinitely. By the same token, it can make sense to pursue counterfactual questions if they are instructive about how standards have come into place or how standards hold up when tested by cases from history.

It is exactly this kind of testing by history that I want to pursue here with regard to contemporary oversight standards: what if some kind of independent evaluation – of the kind that is required today for biomedical research–had been required for the gender re-assignment of Brenda Reimer in the late 1960s? Would that kind of review have stood in the way of the intervention or altered its course in any meaningful way? And is any part of this case useful for a consideration of the standards we use today?

The *Belmont Report* described a threshold at which, the Commissioners thought, medical interventions should receive oversight and approval before going forward. This threshold is, as such matters usually are, open to interpretation. Depending on how one interprets the threshold, one could make the case–when talking about the Reimer case using these standards–that the gender re-assignment did not need prior review and approval or that, even if it did, the review process could have let the transformation go forward. What is perfectly clear, however, is that review by a disinterested committee would have given the proposed gender re-assignment considerable more scrutiny than it got and, very likely, increased significantly the disclosures made to the Reimer parents in the name of informed consent.

Considered as a retrospective thought-experiment, the case of John/Joan case–as David Reimer's case is sometimes known[7] –shows how contemporary standards could have improved the conduct of this experiment even as they leave a free hand for clinical innovation. The case also shows the ways in which contemporary ethics standards governing clinical innovation are a matter of continuing debate.

3. THE ETHICS OF CLINICAL INNOVATION

With a few exceptions, research scandals have proved the impetus for defining and implementing ethical standards for research with humans. For example, in the early 1970s, a Public Health Service study of "untreated syphilis in the male Negro" (this study is far better known as the 'Tuskegee syphilis study') elicited strong federal interest, to the point that a National Commission for the Protection of Human Subjects in Biomedical and Behavioral research was convened.[8] Using specific definitions of research and human subjects, the Commission marked off a domain of investigation that requires prior review and approval, and these recommendations found their way into federal regulations.[9] Henceforth, local Institutional Review Boards (IRBs) would be charged with the task of protecting the rights and welfare of human research subjects.

The National Commission's *Belmont Report* introduced a key distinction between clinical innovation and research into its analysis.[10] In general, the Commission wanted a system of prior review and approval in order to detect and deter objectionable research, a system that would work against needless risk and degrees of risk incommensurate with possible gains in knowledge or therapy. By the same token, the Commission was aware of the importance of leaving a free hand for clinicians in regard to the sometimes novel approaches necessary in treatment decisions. Not even the most ambitious practice guidelines and treatment recommendations can capture the complexities of clinical treatment. Accordingly, the *Belmont Report* defined *research* as the activity designed to test hypotheses, permitting conclusions to be drawn that develop or contribute to generalizable knowledge. By contrast, the Report defined medical or behavioral *practice* as the diagnosis, treatment, or therapy accorded to particular individuals. Variations in clinical practice, the Commissioners concluded, do not constitute research, according to this standard, so long as the focus of the innovation is on the clinical care of an individual, as against making a general contribution to knowledge. The Report goes on to say specifically: "The fact that a procedure is 'experimental' in the sense of new, untested, or different, does not automatically place it in the category of research."

In terms of evaluating Money's gender intervention with Bruce Reimer, the applicable standard–was the effort to change the child's gender a form of clinical treatment or research?–would depend on what the people behind the intervention had in mind. Money and his colleagues might have contended that they simply wanted to offer novel care on behalf of the individual child and that they were not looking to answer the question about gender interventions in any definitive way. In this sense, the gender intervention would simply be meeting the clinical needs of an individual child, on terms provided for in the *Belmont Report*. Even the radical novelty of the intervention would not have necessarily invoked the requirement of prior review and approval, or so Money and his colleagues might have argued. This is not to say that those involved in the gender transformation would have to be unaware of the implications of his treatment in order to invoke a clinical exemption to the standard of prior review and approval. Money certainly understood that a successful gender re-assignment would have significance in terms of understanding psychosexual development. It is merely to say that it might have been possible for someone in Money's shoes to argue that the primary goal of the gender re-assignment was avoiding the trauma he foresaw in the boy's life if he grew up without a penis (whether or not this expectation was necessarily or even remotely correct). So understood, the *Belmont Report* would not seem to require that the intervention that John Money charted for Bruce Reimer receive prior review and approval if it were–which it was not–being conducted according to the terms laid out by the National Commission.

While the Commissioners were sensitive to the importance of clinical innovation, they were also mindful of the need for evaluating innovations that would radiate from one practitioner to wider professional use. In some medical disciplines (surgery, for example), a series of case reports can be as persuasive as any other evidence in defining therapeutic success and motivating other practitioners to adopt novel techniques. Yet both as a matter of ethics and science, it is important that healthcare not get ahead of the limitations that case reports sometimes conceal. For this reason, the Commission recommended that radically new procedures should "be made the object of formal research at an early stage, in order to determine whether they are safe and effective." In other words, clinicians are free to innovate in clinical care, but they also have an ethical obligation to look at the results of their innovations in a systematic way.

Clinicians need a range of freedom in which to respond to the individual needs of their patients. It is unwise to require prior review and approval for all diagnostic and therapeutic choices that depart from approved uses, written guidelines, or received wisdom and, so, the *Belmont Report* protects this clinical freedom in its ethical advisories. But this clinical freedom doesn't mean that clinical practitioners should behave in ways that fail to protect the rights and welfare of their patients and clients. The words of the *Belmont Report* are as apt in this regard now as when they first appeared in 1976: novel clinical innovation should undergo formal evaluation as soon as possible.

How quickly should this happen? In fact, the *Belmont Report* makes no specific recommendations on timing for this kind of formal evaluation. In general, the Report as a whole stayed away from questions of research priorities and the speed at which they ought to go forward. One way to answer this question about conducting formal research at an "early stage" is to say that research ought to begin in a way that is proportionate to the risks and benefits of the intervention. In other words, risky interventions should be studied as quickly as possible, especially if other clinicians are likely to try the intervention with their own patients.

For his own purposes, John Money did attempt to follow Brenda Reimer's progress, but his relationship with the child was strained, to put it mildly; the child first showed resistance to seeing Money at age 7. And no wonder: in his office the psychologist confronted the child with uncomfortable issues and asked the twin children to engage in sexual rehearsal play, something he thought essential to the emergence of sexual identity.[11] Eventually, Brenda simply refused to have anything to do with Money, and that was the end of Money's attempts to follow the child's development. This meant that the case reports of success would go uncorrected until Milton Diamond's reports appeared many years later.[12]

4.   WHAT IF THERE HAD BEEN AN IRB?

To continue this thought experiment further, suppose John Money had taken the proposal to reassign the gender of Bruce Reimer before an IRB. Suppose further that Money planned to conduct a series of gender assignments like the one he planned for Bruce Reimer, taking in 5 – 10 children over a period of time, and studying them at various intervals afterward. In other words, what if Money had planned his gender interventions as research with human subjects as defined by contemporary federal definitions? Several factors would bear on an IRB's decision, but the case can be made that uncertainty in several key areas could justify going ahead with this kind of study or at least not closing the door to it necessarily.

Bruce Reimer was not the only male child to have been assigned as female at a very young age. Other clinicians have done the same thing with other children, and to the extent that the outcomes of this intervention remain obscure, there is at least an argument that they should be able to continue doing so under some circumstances, so long as they are persuaded that the benefits outweigh the risks. In making its proposal, the research team of the time might have pointed to unsettled questions in the professional literature about the extent to which gender might be influenced by socialization. To be sure, they might also have pointed to possible damages to a child because of the loss of a penis. The researchers would have the burden of proof to show that the proposed intervention carries benefits commensurate with its risks, but a researcher might have then–and might even today–persuade an IRB that children with anatomical injuries or intersex conditions are good candidates for this kind of intervention given the psychological damage they face in the future. They could have argued, too, that gender re-assignment carried fewer risks than facing life with an intersex condition or genital anomaly.

This is not to say, again and insistently, that there would be no debate about these issues, because there were researchers arguing against Money's position, who maintained that gender identity is not open to postnatal influence.[13] And there are scholarly commentators and gender activists who have argued against uncautious gender assignments on the grounds that they are unnecessary and harmful.[14] But it is to say that it is possible to make a case for a proposal along these lines that could, in principle, pass muster with an IRB. This is all the more possible because IRBs are not a centralized decision-making body. They are local committees, staffed mostly by volunteers who will have a broad range of views about the interpretation of standards governing research. Not all IRBs must come to the same decisions for their work to be morally defensible.

To be sure, an IRB worth its salt would ask lots of hard questions about any such proposed research. Among other things, federal regulations charge IRBs to ensure that research does not unnecessarily expose subjects to risk, that risks are reasonable in relation to any anticipated benefits, that the selection of subjects is equitable, that informed consent is secured, that research is monitored for safety, and that privacy and confidentiality are maintained.[15] An IRB reviewing a protocol involving the sex re-assignment of young children would be entitled, therefore, to ask exactly how the intervention worked in favor of the child's well being. An IRB doing its work well would have surely asked whether the Reimer family had been advised about the far-reaching implications of the intervention, not only for the child but for themselves and other members of their family who would be affected in altering their beliefs about the child's gender. They might have asked whether these children, who lost their penises as infants to accidents, were the best candidates for this research, as against children with ambiguous or intersexed genitalia and atypical chromosome endowments. It would have certainly taken pains to ensure that the researcher apprised families of other treatment modalities that were available, and what advantages and disadvantages these had compared with the proposal favored by the researcher. What options are there for parents wanting to help protect male children who lose their penises for reasons of developmental anomaly or accident? A diligent IRB would surely have asked, too, about what the parents could expect if the intervention failed in the sense that the child continued to identify as male, no matter how many social cues – name, expectations, dress–pointed him toward femininity.

An effective IRB would also have wanted to know how the study would be monitored over the years to ensure that problems were picked up at the earliest possible time–and to the extent they were significant–used to modify the planned intervention. What threshold did the researchers recognize as failure, and how would they respond to such a failure in a way that would protect the well-being of the children? They might have asked, too, how emerging data would be integrated into decisions about entering other subjects into the study. In other words, how would the researchers know a failure when they saw one and how would that failure influence care and enrolment decisions further down the research track? Lastly, a diligent IRB would also want to ensure that appropriate standards of privacy and confidentiality were in place.

In short, a diligent IRB would have asked for assurance about a number of issues related to the child's well being, the informed choice of the parents, and the oversight of the research. None of these issues by itself poses an insuperable obstacle to a study that wants to look at whether interventions after birth offer a means of shaping a child's gender identity. This point can be underlined by noting that the failure in the Reimer case did not disturb equipoise, even as it raised very serious questions about the specific interventions carried out under Money's auspices. Equipoise refers to indeterminacy within a community of practitioners about whether or not one particular drug, device, or treatment is better than another. It is this indeterminacy that is the moral justification for asking subjects to face the risks of unstudied or understudied interventions.[16] Given what indeterminacies there are about the emergence of gender identity, a research protocol along these lines could be expected to make an interesting and perhaps important contribution to knowledge. The question at issue is whether it is better–all medical, psychological, and social issues considered – to assign infant males who have lost their penises as female. That the intervention with Bruce Reimer failed is not definitive evidence that disturbs equipoise, or to put it another way, is not evidence that gender re-assignment is inferior to any other course of action taken with regard to the psychological well-being of boys in similar circumstances. It may be that the intervention with Bruce Reimer came too late at 2 years of age or that that there was insufficient environmental support for the child's gender re-assignment. Indeed, another case in the literature suggests that a child's gender can be successfully reassigned.[17] The danger of case reports is, of course, that they offer anecdotal evidence, rather than evidence that can be taken into account by clinicians as a whole and incorporated credibly into their work.

When viewed retrospectively through the lens of contemporary research standards, the John/Joan case shows that early gender re-assignment might be compatible with protections of the rights and welfare of research subjects, and an IRB would be within its rights to accord a diligent researcher the right to pursue exactly this question, assuming there are good theoretical reasons to expect success, assuming that the right subjects are used, the right methods are used, that meaningful results to meaningful questions can be obtained, and so on. What the case also shows is the high thresholds that should be met before any such experimentation goes forward. Too much is at stake and there are too many unanswered questions to assume that it is somehow automatically better for a child to be raised as a female without ovaries or uterus rather than as a male without a penis.

5. CONCLUSIONS

John Money was a pioneer in psychosexual development, and he has made many durable contributions to the psychological sciences. For example, it was Money himself who introduced the term 'gender identity' to designate one's felt sense of being male or female.[18] This language made it easier to see essential distinctions between anatomy and psychological identity. Money also did important work in providing a framework for distinguishing males and females according to behavioral thresholds at which they typically respond to stimuli.[19] Even his willingness to undertake studies in psychosexual development cut against an academic grain that did not give its full attention to these matters at the time.

Unfortunately, the Bruce Reimer case was not John Money's only scrape with professional ethics. In the late 1980s, Money co-authored a case study of one of his patients, only to have the man recognize himself in the book, *Vandalized Lovemaps.*[20] The man objected not only to this public exposure but also to the label of pedophile that Money applied to him.[21] He was sure that anyone who knew him would see past the pseudonym Money had deployed. The National Institutes of Health agreed with the complainant and found that misconduct had occurred. It is, however, his scientific silence on the failure of Bruce Reimer's gender reassignment that really stains Money's legacy.

In 2003, in response to criticism of his role in Bruce Reimer's gender re-assignment, Money put matters this way: "I have never done a circumcision, which operation I classify as a mutilation. I do not experiment on baby boys by amputating their genitals in order to raise them as females. I am not a surgeon. I do not do reconstructive surgery. I do not do sex reassignment surgery. I do not prescribe hormones. I do not exploit patients for financial or academic gain. I have no tyrannical power over Johns Hopkins or any of its physicians. I am a pediatric medical psychologist, and my job is to help people in crisis, as much as is possible."[22]

As a psychologist, it is true that Money would not perform circumcisions, castration, prescribe hormones, or do any other work that–as a matter of professional licensing standards–falls to physicians. But it remains true nevertheless, that Money was the chief architect of Bruce Reimer's gender re-assignment, and his after-the-fact denials of responsibility are simply not credible. It is an unanswered question, of course, whether those who were involved with carrying out the castration, prescribing hormones, and so on acted in ways that they felt were in the best interests of the little boy whom they were constructing as female. But in any case, John Money was not the only party to this experiment.

It is not only the children who face gender re-assignment that might be helped by an oversight committee. In a sense, these committees work to protect researchers, too, by protecting them from poor choices or from initiating ill-considered therapies. Seeking prior review and approval for this kind of innovation from an independent body, would have had the value–at least–of formalizing the rationale for the intervention, putting it in print. By seeing the proposal in the context of a formal justification, the intervention could be debated by all the clinicians involved more clearly and moved forward, hopefully, on its merits rather than simply by force of personality and the enthusiasm of personal beliefs. That is not a negligible benefit for clinical innovators themselves

Certainly, the Reimer case is easy enough to find fault with in retrospect, but the value of applying federal regulations retroactively–as a thought experiment–is not primarily about condemning past clinical choices. For that, in any case, we would need a fuller theory of what it means to practice objectionable clinical care in a time that did not have the standards of review that are currently in place. No, the value of considering past clinical care in light of contemporary standards is also in the way it allows us to assess standards in terms of their current adequacy.

It turns out that the question of gender interventions with children is still an open question, which means that even now, with a system of review required for research involving human subjects, we must still ask how that system applies, if at all. The *Belmont Report* carves out a domain of clinical innovation that does not require prior review and approval. Even at this stage of our knowledge, could a clinician make the case that he or she could go ahead and try a gender re-assignment in the name of taking care of an individual patient? There are ways to argue yes and no in answer to this question.

The clinician might argue that each element of the intervention is taken 'off the shelf,' that there is nothing new in what he or she would do in the name of the gender reassignment. The clinician might also argue that because of being in private practice and well outside academics that he or she has no interest in making a contribution to generalizable knowledge, but that he or she only wants to take care of an individual patient. Of course, to look at things from the other side, the clinician might well know that that the outcome would–by its very nature–be consequential for the debate about the scientific and ethical value of early-age gender interventions. In this sense, the clinician might see that it would be virtually impossible to carry out this intervention and not make a contribution to knowledge, no matter what the outcome: a simple case report would be of interest in lots of professional journals. It turns out that there is no clear and bright line between what does and what does not make a contribution to generalizable knowledge.

Putting gender re-assignments before an IRB would probably do more good (for the parents and children involved) than harm (to the clinician in terms of loss of time and opportunity). The IRB would at least be able to debate the question of risks and benefits and make the outcome of that debate known to the clinician. What are–in their totality–the knowable psychological and physical risks of full-scale gender re-assignment, and why are these ultimately less significant than the putative benefits? At the very least, an IRB should make clear that parents making choices about children with ambiguous or damaged genitalia should have the opportunity to weigh other approaches (e.g., counseling and perhaps some reconstructive surgery later) to their child's anatomical non-conformity, other choices that might equally well serve the child's interests.

A promising middle way might also be mentioned here: when they want to go forward with innovations that they think do not trigger the need for IRB review, some clinicians are turning to 'innovative therapy committees.' These committees are usually institutional or professional committees to which clinicians turn for peer guidance about the advisability of novel treatments and therapies. These committees will only be as good, of course, as the intellectual scrutiny they focus on various proposals. While a full accounting of these kinds of committees is still yet to be made, at first blush, it seems that these committees could offer constructive peer-to-peer counsel about the advisability of novel techniques, in circumstances that do not call for IRB prior review and approval. It should be kept in mind, of course, that if clinicians are truly interested in making contributions to generalizable knowledge, they probably should be dealing with IRBs and not innovative therapy committees. At the very least, if innovative therapy committees focus on clinical treatment that does not, properly speaking, trigger IRB review, they could very well help protect patients from innovations that are ill-considered or not yet ripe for implementation. Such an approach might well serve candidates for early gender re-assignment.

A review of the Reimer case does not, of course, foretell the future of early-age gender reassignment. A re-visitation of the standards that trigger the need for prior review and approval will not do that either. It may be that changes in social context will foretell the future of gender re-assignment better than anything else. For example, the failure of David Reimer's gender re-assignment seems to have pushed some psychologists, surgeons, and pediatricians away from the idea that males born without a penis are at a disadvantage so profound that their psychological integrity and well-being can only be rescued by gender reassignment. Advances in the reconstruction of injured genitalia are also doing their part to undermine the desirability of gender re-assignment. Gender activists have complained about early-age surgeries, and psychologists and medical clinicians have given them a hearing. These developments have forced a conversation that extends far beyond the issue of protecting children in the research setting. All things considered, social accommodation of genitally atypical children may well be a better approach to their well-being than surgical and hormonal interventions. At the very least, people charged with oversight of frontier medicine should do well to keep these changes in mind, no matter whether they are clinicians, members of innovative therapy committees, or members of IRBs.

6. EPILOGUE

While the second edition of the *Encyclopedia of Bioethics* was being planned, I approached the editor about including an entry on 'gender identity disorder.' He declined, saying that the editors wanted to avoid a focus on particular diseases or disorders. That was an entirely reasonable editorial approach so I went back to him with a proposal for a broader entry on 'gender and gender identity disorder,' offering an entry that would try to open up discussion about the intersection of gender and theories of health and disease more generally. Square in the middle of that discussion sits the question of gender plasticity and the ethics of gender interventions with children (among other things). This revised proposal proved more agreeable to the editor, and the entry eventually appeared in the 1994 edition of the *Encyclopedia*. I'm genuinely sorry it did. I look back on this entry with more regret than any other piece of writing I have ever done. This is not simply the regret of looking back at work done in haste or hubris. My regret is tied to the way my conclusions depend on scientific reports that have proved unfounded. When the *Encyclopedia* appeared, David Reimer had thrown off his female identity some 15 years earlier. In writing my entry, I had relied on scientific reports known by their author at the time to be incorrect but who had taken no steps to retract them.

My 1994 entry says, for example, that prevailing developmental theories suggest that a child's gender – the gender of any child, not merely children with ambiguous genitalia or intersexed traits – is moldable through early application of medical and psychological methods.[23] I cited Money's 1972 case report as evidence of the plastic nature of human gender identity. In 1994, twenty-two years out, Money's attempt to assign a female gender to Bruce Reimer had more than failed, and yet academics, clinicians, and researchers like myself still had no word from the researcher that the experiment had proved a spectacular failure.

Diamond and Sigmundson's 1997 article changed all that. In the most recent edition of the *Encyclopedia of Bioethics*, which appeared in 2004, my discussion now points out that gender assignment in children has not been well studied and that "Physicians should propose gender interventions to parents [of children with ambiguous genitalia or atypical genetic traits] only after a rigorous evaluation of the risks and benefits. Among other things, practitioners should advise parents that some individuals live happily with atypical genitalia or intersex conditions and that gender assignment can be carried out later on if that is desired by the child. Parents need support as they think through decisions about gender interventions with their children, and this support should include nonpathological images of intersex children."[24]

Even though the *Encylopedia* now better reflects the state of knowledge about early gender assignment, I still wonder how many people turned to Money's work (and all the derivative work that depended on it, including my own 1995 work) and came away thinking that gender identity is easily manipulated, so long as one intervened very early in life and never wavered from treating a child as female or as male, depending on the desire outcome. How many people turned to these texts and walked away with the sense that transforming boys into girls and girls into boys was possible even if it was slightly complicated? How many ill-formed experiments in gender went forward as a result of the reports that the gender identity of children was open to postnatal intervention? What was my complicity, if any, in the spread of this misinformation?

I've had lots of opportunities to think about these questions, even during vacations far from the wintry Northern Hemisphere. In December 2002, I whiled away a few sunny hours on a beach in Sydney. One man who strolled along the beach was exercising his option to go without clothes (it was that kind of beach). He was in his late 30s and had testicles but no penis. Whether he lost his penis to accident, to disease, or to developmental disorder, he seemed entirely at ease as he splashed in and out of the water. From what I could tell, his lack of a penis didn't seem to make much difference to people around him either. It was perhaps unusual that he had no penis, but his appearance was intelligible. A moment's reflection makes it clear that anyone can lose any body part to injury or disorder, and that includes testicles, penises, breasts, nipples, and all the anatomical markers we use to mark and signify gender. Whatever problems this man might have had in the past by reason of his lost penis, he had no qualms about shedding his clothes in order to enjoy Australia's magnificent beaches. Judging from appearances, I suspect this man would not easily believe that his sex, gender identity, or gender role should be cast into doubt simply because he had no penis. It was not lost on me that–in his late thirties–this beachgoer was approximately the same age as David Reimer. What I could not known at that time was that David Reimer's life was already approaching its end.

In the early part of 2004, David Reimer committed suicide at age 38.[25] Speaking to the press, his mother "said she was still angry with the Baltimore doctor who persuaded her and her husband, Ron, to give female hormones to their son and raise him as a daughter." Because this 'doctor' went unnamed, I complained to the public editor of the *New York Times*, in which paper I saw the report of the suicide. This doctor, I protested, was no local practitioner toiling in obscurity far downstream from the headwaters of medical knowledge. This doctor was psychologist John Money, a leading theorist of human psychosexual development and a prolific contributor to the scientific literature. The public editor replied by saying that the *Times* had picked up the article from a wire service and that someone apparently unfamiliar with the details of the case had written the article. Had the *Times* written the article, the editor said, more information might have been disclosed. I hope that's right. As a matter of full disclosure in regard to a landmark case in human psychology, I hope that John Moneys' obituary–when it comes–will include his landmark experiment with a young Canadian boy, David Reimer by name.

Timothy Murphy, Professor, Department of Medical Education, College of Medicine, University of Illinois at Chicago, Illinois, U.S.A.

---

[1]   John Colapinto, *As Nature Made Him: The Boy Who was Raised as a Girl* (New York: Harper Collins, 2000).

[2]   Some commentators believe that biology has been wrongfully relegated to the sidelines as a determinant of virtually any human behavior or trait. For a critique of the 'tabula rasa' theory, see Steven Pinker, *The Blank Slate: The Modern Denial of Human Nature* (New York: Penguin, 2003).

[3]   John Money, and Anke A. Ehrhardt, *Man and Woman, Boy and Girl: The Differentiation and Dimorphism of Gender identity from Conception to Maturity* (Baltimore: Johns Hopkins University Press, 1972).

[4]   Milton Diamond, and H. Keith Sigmundson, "Sex Reassignment at Birth: A Longterm Review and Clinical Implications," *Archives of Pediatric and Adolescent Medicine* 151.3 (1997): 298-304.

[5]   http://www.hhs.gov/ohrp/humansubjects/guidance/belmont.htm

[6]   Robert J. Levine, *Ethics and Clinical Regulation of Research*, 2nd ed. (New Haven: Yale University Press, 1988) xi-xiii.

[7]   John Colapinto, "The True Story of John / Joan," *Rolling Stone* Dec. 11. 1997: 54-97.

[8]   James Jones, *Bad Blood: The Tuskegee Syphilis Experiments* (New York: Free Press, 1981).

[9]   45 *Code of Federal Regulations* 46.

[10]   http://www.hhs.gov/ohrp/humansubjects/guidance/belmont.htm

[11]   Colapinto, *As Nature Made Him* 97.

[12]   To identify and protect a domain of clinical innovation does not mean, of course, that the public is altogether without redress should clinicians go too far. Malpractice law would be applicable if a clinician departed from professional standards in a way that directly caused damages.

[13]   Colapinto, *As Nature Made Him* 45-46.

---

[14] Cheryl Chase, "Rethinking Treatment for Ambiguous Genitalia," *Pediatric Nursing* 25.4 (1999): 451.

[15] 45 *Code of Federal Regulations* 46.111.

[16] Timothy F. Murphy, *Case Studies in Biomedical Research Ethics* (Cambridge: The MIT Press, 2004) 18, 47.

[17] Colapinto, *As Nature Made Him* 223ff.

[18] John Money, *Gay, Straight, and In-Between: The Sexology of Erotic Orientation* (New York: Oxford University Press, 1988).

[19] Money, *Gay, Straight, and In-Between.*

[20] John Money, Margaret Lamacz, *Vandalized Lovemaps* (Buffalo: Prometheus, 1989).

[21] Colapinto, *As Nature Made Him* 240-244.

[22] John Money, *A First-Person Account of Psychoendocrinology* (New York: Plenum, 2003) 75.

[23] Timothy F. Murphy, "Gender and Gender Identity Disorders," *Encyclopedia of Bioethics,* Warren T. Reich, ed., vol. 2 (New York: Macmillan, 1994) 901-907.

[24] Timothy F. Murphy, "Gender Identity," *Encylopedia of Bioethics*, Stephen G. Post, ed., vol. 2, (New York: Macmillan/Gale, 2004) 943-948; 944.

[25] "David Reimer, 38, Subject of the 'John/Joan' Case, Dies," *New York Times,* May 12, 2004: A21.

WILLIAM G. REINER

PRENATAL GENDER IMPRINTING AND MEDICAL DECISION-MAKING

Genetic Male Neonates with Severely Inadequate Penises

1. INTRODUCTION AND BACKGROUND

Scientific ideas tend to emanate from observations, accumulated information, or intuition (immediate cognition). Utilizing the scientific method, hypotheses are generated, experiments are designed, data are collected, and information is gleaned from the interpretation of the data, invoking various constructs that more or less successfully appear to model the data themselves. Thus, elicited phenomenology generates the core of a new or greater idea which is explored, albeit piecemeal, until the various models–or, really, the multiplicity of data collected–are reformulated as theory from which new questions may arise that are interwoven with new conclusions. Conclusions, therefore, are supported not by the models but by an overall interpretation and understanding of the data collected, commonly by multiple researchers in multiple laboratory settings.

Sexual differentiation in animal species is just such a scientific idea. Observations and phenomenology have led to discoveries that in turn have led to theories or new ideas cloaked in hopeful optimism as well as in nagging doubts relative to our sense of understanding. What we know is that sexual differentiation in the human involves at the least a prenatal cascade of events and processes that are influenced by dozens of genes and gene products, hormones and receptor molecules, and are as well directed or modified by other aspects of structural embryogenesis (Vilain, 2002; Xu, Burgoyne et al., 2002; Grumbach, 2003; Reiner and Gearhart, 2004). Critical within these processes is the place of the brain and of the mind both in terms of developmental potential, prior to any but the most basic of genetic influences, as well as of the transformations that occur and the implications of those transformations, during the cascade of differentiation processes themselves. While it can be difficult in humans to successfully analyze these processes specifically, accumulated observations over time of people with errors of sexual differentiation– and the phenomenology of how we have socially dealt with such errors–may be very helpful to an overall understanding of the sexual differentiation of the mind and brain and how mind and brain may be one and how that "one" is unique, and male or female, and at the same time a part of the greater human experience.

S.E. Sytsma (Ed.), Ethics and Intersex, 153–163.

Errors of sexual differentiation comprise clinical entities that typically include specific disorders of primary embryogenesis (often including genital development specifically) as well as a variety of often unrelated intersex conditions (Vilain, 2002; Xu, Burgoyne et al,. 2002; Grumbach, 2003; Hines, 2003; Houk, Dayner et al., 2004; Reiner and Gearhart, 2004). Intersex itself is a generic term that for the most part includes problems of inadequate prenatal androgen effects in genetic males–and therefore inadequately virilized external genitalia–or inappropriate prenatal androgen exposure in genetic females–and inappropriately virilized external genitalia (Vilain, 2002; Berenbaum and Bailey, 2003; Grumbach, 2003; Hines, 2003; Reiner and Gearhart, 2004; Reiner and Kropp, 2004). At least, this is how clinicians have tended to understand intersex over the last half of the 20th Century. Disorders of sexual differentiation are generally rare. When present in genetic male newborns (specifically) they are commonly expressed, at least outwardly, by the absence of a penis, or more typically, the presence of a severely inadequate penis. Thus, there may be an underdeveloped single erectile body (corpus cavernosum) with a poorly formed glans penis, or two small corpora cavernosa, or a minimally formed phallic structure not much larger than a clitoris that curves markedly on erection, and so forth–typically with an absence of the corpus spongiosum (the spongy body that bears the male urethra). Clinically and practically speaking, these clinical entities do not include those of simple or even complex hypospadias, conditions usually involving a penis that curves on erection, with the urethral meatus not reaching the tip of the penis, but in the face of histologically normal testes. Rather, these conditions involve a severely inadequate penis that almost assuredly will not be adequate for sexual performance after puberty, even if surgically reconstructed, and often one or both testes are not normal either.

Major disorders of sexual differentiation in genetic males, then, can be caused by specific genetic defects, inadequate exposure to prenatal androgens, androgens that cannot act because their specific receptor molecules are absent or abnormal, or general or specific structural developmental disorders of genital embryogenesis itself (Vilain, 2002; Berenbaum and Bailey, 2003; Grumbach, 2003; Hines, 2003; Reiner and Gearhart, 2004; Reiner and Kropp, 2004). The most severe form of this latter disorder is a complex birth defect known as cloacal exstrophy, a condition with which the author has a large clinical and research experience. Cloacal exstrophy includes very severe developmental errors of early embryogenesis of the entire pelvis – that is, it is a full field-defect of pelvic development (Husmann, 1999; Mathews, Perlman et al., 1999; Reiner and Gearhart, 2004; Reiner and Kropp, 2004). Thus, newborns with this condition typically present with an omphalocele, a shortened small bowel, marked foreshortening of the hindgut with an actual admixture of hindgut and bladder tissues (and thus the term "cloaca"), and with this gut-bladder admixture open to the outside ("exstrophy") as though surgically incised in the midline and the cut edges sewn to the skin. Lower extremity and spinal cord anomalies can be present as well. These children commonly have absence of the internal and external genitalia–but not of the gonads. Genetic males with cloacal exstrophy, thus, present with an absent or nearly absent penis, but in the face of otherwise normal testes, androgens, and androgen effects (Mathews, Perlman et al., 1999; Reiner and Gearhart, 2004; Reiner and Kropp, 2004).

2. CLINICAL REALITIES OF ERRORS OF SEXUAL DIFFERENTIATION
IN THE GENETIC MALE

The etiologies of such diverse disorders of sexual differentiation imply molecular, cellular, tissue, organ, or systems involvement. The sexual differentiation error itself involves no life-threatening clinical issues, although other physiological errors may sometimes require emergent or urgent clinical intervention (Grumbach, 2003). The central *genital* issues facing the clinician who encounters such a newborn genetic male, and thus the critical data surrounding any medical decision-making, have focused on the sexual performance implications of the absent or severely inadequate penis, as perceived at birth (Tank and Lindenauer, 1970; Howell, Caldamone et al., 1983; Husmann, McLorie et al., 1989; Skoog and Belman, 1989; Lund and Hendren, 1993; Mathews, Jeffs et al., 1998; Glassberg, 1999; Husmann, 1999). Thus, if the clinical impression was one of genital ambiguity, if clinicians were unsure, in other words, of the future sexual identity of the child, genital issues became paramount. After all, surgeons could not construct a functioning penis but during the 50's and 60's they had developed innovative techniques for successful construction of a vagina and a vulva.

Disorders of psychosexual development and especially of the development of sexual identity (gender identity) have been inferred, or assumed, in these children. That is, it has been assumed that these major genital anomalies induce such an obstacle to psychosexual development that the genetic males will not be able to function socially as adult males. Psychosexual development would not be simply problematic but most likely severely abnormal. Indeed, conjuring images of severe psychosexual developmental trauma, the literature has sometimes suggested that suicide would be a high risk if these neonates were to be sex-assigned and reared male from birth (Husmann, McLorie, et al. 1989; Husmann, 1999).

During the 1950s an idea was formulated that gradually evolved into a clinical paradigm. This idea encompassed the notion that sexual identity is plastic in humans, at least in the newborn and early childhood periods (Money, 1972). The development of such identity, it was argued, depended upon sociological forces that determine a child's sense of self in sexual terms; thus, if the child were reared as a given sex and if the child's genitals were of that sex, then the child would experience psychosexual development typical of that sex. Matter, at least as formulated in terms of development, could determine Mind; the brain was but an object for behavioral engineering. Fundamental to this argument was the notion of human identity, and specifically sexual identity, as a *tabula rasa*, a blank slate, in the newborn (Money, 1972). How this conception wound its way out of the trends and trajectories of 20th-century socio-psychological dualism and its relationship to post-Enlightenment historicism are well beyond the scope of this manuscript. It is important to recognize, however, that this idea, or model, construed identity as a social construct that is at once plastic and malleable at birth but also permanent and constant at some later (though unclear) period.

The hallmark John/Joan case, as it first surfaced in reports and conferences during the 1960s, provided the foundation for clinical action, for application of the idea (Money, 1975). The details of this case and of its implications for clinical practice are well-known publicly (Colapinto, 2000), but in summary "John" was an identical twin who lost his penis to a traumatic infant circumcision, was converted to "Joan" surgically and socially and emerged later as a little girl and then an adolescent young lady. The simplicity of the conception and the implications of the successful outcome in this child dominated the clinical literature about sexual identity and intersex (and other errors of sexual differentiation) for decades. Clinicians were pleased, parents were happy, developmentalists were impressed, because this hallmark case proved the veracity of the model of neonatal sexual identity-plasticity, stimulating early formulations for clinical interventions that evolved into a workable clinical paradigm (Skoog and Belman 1989; Lund and Hendren, 1993; Glassberg, 1999). The model, as a clinical construct, was looked upon as a clinical blessing by pediatric endocrinologists and especially pediatric urologists, because it provided not only a path away from the clinical anxieties and helplessness surrounding the ambiguity of the genitalia (and thus of the sexual identity), but it also allowed the surgeon to utilize creative techniques to construct–not reconstruct, but construct–someone from a broken or incompletely formed child.

The clinical paradigm, of course, virtually always dictated sex-assignment of the genetic male to female rather than the other way around. Genital structures were feminized surgically at birth or in infancy: excess phallic and scrotal structural tissues were excised, and a clitoris, vulva, and labia were formed (the vagina generally was constructed a bit later); testes were surgically removed from genetic males. Yet there are rare cases with genetic females being born totally virilized. In such rare cases genetic female fetuses are exposed to so much prenatal male hormone, secondary to a genetic error in the adrenal gland (called congenital adrenal hyperplasia), that they are born looking like normal newborn boys, with a normal penis, foreskin, urethra, and scrotum. The scrotum is empty, of course, because they are genetic females and have internal ovaries but no testes. Even in cases of such complete virilization, the clinical teaching was to rear these (genetic female) children as female, perhaps engendering a bit of clinical confusion in some – after all, the genitalia in these rare children were completely normal male anatomically and physiologically. But the presence of normal ovaries and internal female structures implies potential fertility. In these children fertility overruled genitalia, and fertility was maintained at the expense of external genital anatomy. That the fertility of genetic males sex-assigned female was always lost–recall that sex-assignment to female from genetic male requires castration as well as feminizing genitoplasty–was dismissed, because fertility (at least at that time) was not possible without adult male sexual function anyway.

Outcome data tended to be singularly scarce or even absent. Of interest is that minimal outcome data–or data that conceivably could have been interpreted as bearing some importance to potential outcomes for this clinical paradigm–were published. First, animal studies did not seem to support this clinical paradigm for humans, in that psychosexual development and behaviors in animals were shown to be directly related to prenatal (or, in some species, early postnatal) androgen exposure – during the so-called Critical Period for imprinting (Phoenix, 1968; Goy 1972; Phoenix, 1973). Arguments for the social uniqueness and dominance of human culture superposed such animal data and were used to maintain the dominance of the paradigm in clinical practice, however. Second, Imperato-McGinley in 1979 reported a series of genetic males from 3 Dominican villages with a very rare deficiency of the 5 alpha-reductase enzyme, the enzyme which converts testosterone to the far more potent dihydrotestosterone (DHT) (Imperato-McGinley, Peterson et al. 1979; Imperato-McGinley, Peterson et al., 1979). It is DHT that actually virilizes external and internal genitalia prenatally (that is, DHT is required for the development of male genitalia). Thus, a deficiency of this enzyme leads to absence of DHT and thus absence of genital virilization–newborns with this deficiency are genetic males looking female, or mostly female, at birth and who were, therefore, sex-assigned female at birth. Testes are undescended. However, at puberty the testes secrete such high quantities of the less potent testosterone that these children experience progressive genital virilization during early adolescence anyway. In Imperato-McGinley's study 17 of the 18 adolescents transitioned completely to male sexual identity (the eighteenth mostly withdrew socially). Additional data began to accrue that prenatal androgen exposure in genetic females could at times lead to markedly male-typical gender role and interests (Dittmann, Kappes et al., 1990; Berenbaum and Resnick, 1997; Berenbaum, 1999; Hines, 2003).

Then, in 1996, Reiner published a 7-year follow-up on a child with mixed gonadal dysgenesis (Reiner, 1996)–a genetic mosaic condition typically with a karyotype of 46 XY/45 X-, a single small testis on one side and a streak gonad (like a scar) on the other side that is accompanied by internal female ductal structures (on the streak side), and typically with a severely inadequate phallus. This child was believed to be female at birth and reared unequivocally female. At age 14 years, however, after lifelong male-typical behaviors and interests, this child declared male sexual identity, transitioned to male identity socially and legally, and was at his request (or demand) surgically reconstructed as male. He was sexually attracted to– and later sexually active with–females exclusively. Subsequently, in 1997, Diamond and Sigmundson published a long-term follow-up of the original John/Joan case; the outcome was, in fact, a dismal failure (Diamond and Sigmundson, 1997). "Joan" transitioned to male at age 14 years after a miserable childhood, lived the remainder of his life as male, married and adopted three children, but committed suicide in 2004 after a series of difficult depressive, family, and employment problems (Colapinto, 2004).

A small flurry of case reports followed, appearing almost to be vying for the validity or success of the clinical paradigm. Numbers typically were small, methods tended to be problematic or not mentioned, and interpretations therefore were equally problematic (Bradley, Oliver et al., 1998; Schober, Carmichael et al., 2002).

Subsequently, Reiner published the first of several articles detailing his outcome data about sexual identity, initially with genetic male children with cloacal exstrophy and then with genetic male intersex children as well (Reiner, 2004; Reiner and Gearhart, 2004; Reiner and Kropp, 2004). A summary of his clinical experience found that of 73 genetic male children and adults ≥ 5-years-old, 60 were reared female from birth; 13 were reared male (Reiner, in press 2005). Almost all those reared female had been castrated within the first month of life, and all by age 3 months. Thirty-two (53%) of these 60 children sex-assigned female at birth have transitioned to male–about one-third spontaneously and about two-thirds after being told by a parent that they were "born a boy" (or "born with a Y chromosome"). *Spontaneous* declarations of male identity, along with transitioning to male socially, occurred as young as 4-½ years-old and as old as 12 years, although a few parents did not allow the transition to occur (at least at home). Of those children *informed* of their birth status (between 5-years-old and 18-years-old) all but 2 declared themselves male and successfully transitioned to male identity socially; the 2 who did not declare themselves male (now 15-years-old and 17-years-old) have persistently refused to discuss their sexual identity at any time since being informed of their birth status. Those who transitioned to male have undergone bilateral mastectomies, for all who had been treated with estrogen; additionally, each has expressed a strong desire for construction of a penis (as have the 13 reared male).

Of those same 60 children sex-assigned female at birth, 26 of 60 declared themselves female (43%). None of them is aware of their birth status, although maintaining such secrecy may not be possible forever. Additionally, all of the adolescents transitioning to male recognized sexual orientation towards females, often before declaring male identity. Of adolescents continuing to live as female, only one has been willing to discuss sexual orientation–which is also towards females. Finally, all 73 of the children showed mild, moderate, or severe male-typical gender role behavior throughout their development.

3. CLINICAL IMPLICATIONS AND THE STANDARD OF CARE

Several lessons can be learned from this clinical narrative, and other implications may be recognized with time, as we continue to learn of the diversity of prenatal genetic and hormonal foundations of human sexual differentiation. First, the medical exhortation to "above all, do no harm" generally must supersede the well-meaning desire to improve people's lives. As a second lesson, the patients must be the ones to ultimately define success or improvement–that is, outcome. As a third lesson, interventions–that is, those attempts to improve people's lives–must be evidence-based. Evidence-based approaches, long being central to clinical medicine, should also help patients define expectations and clinical outcomes. Evidence itself emanates from studies utilizing the scientific method, with the research utilizing the processes and goals of this method.

And what of the scientific method? It is important to recognize that the clinical paradigm sex-assigning genetic males to female (or clinically sex-assigning any newborn when we do not know what the child will ultimately recognize as sexual identity) was based neither on science nor clinical experience. It was based on an idea. The idea can be reduced simplistically but importantly to two parts: 1) sexual identity is a *tabula rasa*, and 2) a boy growing up without a penis will be a psychosexual developmental disaster. An important corollary to this idea was that a genetic male could be made into a fully functioning female, fully functioning anatomically, physiologically (with pharmacologic assistance), and psychosexually. One might well infer two additional implications of the idea: 1) a girl must be made up of rather simple stuff, and 2) a boy or a man is only as capable of living as male as his penis is functional.

While these latter implications might evoke socially humorous discussions, the idea itself is frighteningly simplistic, especially considering the complexity of the very social forces that supposedly determine the development of sexual identity and gender roles–and the broad range of human experiences and social exposures that developing children encounter. Indeed, with a large population and a rather generous population growth (by about 4 million births per year in the United States alone), observed psychosexual developmental variance in the greater population as a whole provides little support for the idea of sexual identity-plasticity, at any age. As an example, transgendered children recognize or at least prefer or adhere to a sexual identity at odds with their sex-of-rearing and their (otherwise) normal external and internal genitalia, and their corresponding gonads, for that matter. In another example, many of a rather large population of children, adolescents, and adults with spina bifida (a rather common birth defect) have neurological deficits eliminating both genital function and genital sensation–somewhat akin to having no genitalia, or no penis in boys; yet outcome studies in males with spina bifida does not support either psychosexual developmental disaster or the inability to be or be considered as male (Woodhouse, 2005). Additionally, suicide as a problem in males without a penis cannot be supported in any way by a review of the literature (Reiner and Kropp, 2004)–although suicide in general is a socially significant problem.

A fourth lesson learned is that clinicians must maintain intellectual vigilance about medical decision-making. Clinical skepticism can be a safety measure for their patients. As discussed, the clinical paradigm in question–that a child would become the sex-of-rearing as assigned if the genitalia correlated to that sex–was drawn from a model in search of data (Petersen, 2001). This was an unfortunate and unrecognized breach of the scientific method. Rather than posing a hypothesis, designing experiments to obtain data, and exploring a series of models each of which might fit the data more or less well, social and behavioral scientists advocated a mere *idea*–and thus they failed the clinicians. Clinicians, seduced mostly through a sense of helplessness in caring for these children, unwittingly conducted what were in essence experiments, as though looking for data to fit the model. Critical analysis of the idea itself by clinicians should have exposed its lack of foundation.

A fifth lesson learned is that a Standard of Care, once accepted, can be very difficult to dislodge, new evidence notwithstanding. On the other hand, when outcome data does successfully refute a Standard of Care, the ultimate loss of the treatment algorithm can lead to decision-making paralysis for some clinicians, entrenchment (or a reification of the original idea) for others, and clinical confusion, at the least, for many. But clinical care must continue. Children with errors of sexual differentiation continue to be born. Sex must be assigned for social and legal reasons, at the least. Parents, or some parents, will seek some kind of intervention for their children as infants. Therefore, we must develop clinical guidelines that are disease-specific and evidence-based, and we must thoroughly educate parents about the evidence that does exist and what we do not know.

Sixth, we have learned that sexual identity can certainly be independent of sex-of-rearing as well as independent of the presence of genitalia. As a corollary that is important to clinical interventions, removal of genitals, gonads, or parts of genital structures precludes their future reconstruction. While surgical reconstruction as a male–or delaying surgical reconstructions–does not preclude later reconstruction as a female (or male), surgical reconstruction as a female typically involves permanent surgical excisions. Additionally, puberty can be (markedly) delayed if necessary. Therefore, prepubertal gonads, whether ovaries or testes, can be maintained in a nonfunctional state indefinitely–until a child or adolescent can tell us who and what they are. And gonadal excision, of course, requires that a person receive post-pubertal lifelong sex hormone administration while precluding any hope of fertility.

Finally, if sexual identity is independent of sex-of-rearing, and of genitalia, then the primary lesson learned is that we must be flexible with any child whose neonatal phenotype defies our ability to predict who they are. We must assess and reassess such children, cooperating fully with parents in an environment of open communication and readily available information. For example, we have long recognized that adopted children can grow and develop with the knowledge that they do not know who their biological parents are. We can now recognize that children can grow and develop without parents knowing exactly who their child is. This is nothing new, of course–many parents have long recognized that their children can be totally unpredictable in psychosexual development, or in any aspect of development. Parents and clinicians should be capable of learning with the children and from the children.

4. PRESENT AND FUTURE CLINICAL IMPERATIVES

How can we determine appropriate interventions for a child with major disorders of sexual differentiation? Or, how do we cope with parents or our own anxieties about not knowing who the newborn child is? We must focus on the same approaches that direct all clinical medicine. We must observe and describe the data; we must hypothesize and then collect additional data; we must perform clinical trials with appropriate informed consent; we must critically evaluate and interpret the data and apply our interpretations clinically. We must, as clinicians, parents, and members of society, adjust and adapt and continue to critically analyze in order to seek and to achieve what is the good for the patient.

We are not functioning in a vacuum, however. And a new Standard of Care will develop–or rather several standards, each with some disease-specific character. We must stress that we do understand much about some clinical situations (hypospadias, for example), a fair amount about other clinical pictures (cloacal exstrophy, for example), and a little about many other situations (mixed gonadal dysgenesis, for example). We have learned that when we talk about surgically constructing an organ that can function sexually, we must focus on, "Function for whom?" If we speak of ambiguous genitalia we must ask, "Ambiguous to whom?" Similarly, when we speak about potential fertility we must have some idea about whether the people involved will care about or want their fertility. When we speak about identity, we must recognize that only a given person can know who he–or she–is.

These simple points can actually offer some guidance. For example, we have a great deal of evidence (not discussed here) that hypospadias generally does not involve problems of sexual identity, although technically hypospadias could be considered an error of sexual differentiation. We also have a great deal of evidence that males do wish to be able to function sexually. Therefore, surgical reconstruction of the hypospadiac penis appears quite warranted. Similarly, genetic males with cloacal exstrophy have demonstrated that they cannot be made into females, even if they may continue to live as female after neonatal sex-assignment to female. Additionally, such sex-assignment offers the additional burdens of requiring lifelong sex hormone administration along with the loss of any potential fertility. Therefore, genetic males with cloacal exstrophy should be reared male. These realities are not to deny potential psychosexual–or other–developmental hurdles.

On the other hand, in genetic male children with intermediate prenatal androgen effects (mixed gonadal dysgenesis, for example) sexual identity may be unpredictable. Many will recognize themselves as male if reared female, but some will likely recognize themselves as females. Indeed, it is conceivable that some may recognize themselves as female even if reared male, especially if prenatal male genetic and/or androgen effects are minimal. Therefore, if not virilized or if very minimally virilized, such children probably should be assigned female. Clinical caution should oversee any clinical interventions, however, especially for any surgical excision. Parents and patients must be allowed ample time to learn about the diagnosis and its implications and to explore their options. They must have free access to all available information as well as open communication as possible to willing other patients or parents of such patients. Informed consent–or at least informed assent–must be obtained from patients themselves whenever possible.

5. SUMMARY

Genetic male newborns with a severely inadequate penis but who have experienced some degree of prenatal androgen influence will often–but likely not always–recognize male sexual identity, independent of neonatal sex-assignment and sex-of-rearing and independent of the appearance or even of the presence of their genitalia. Gender role behaviors will typically also reflect such prenatal influences. Neurobiological ramifications of prenatal male genetic and hormonal influences must not be ignored or dismissed. Medical and especially surgical interventions must be designed around these clinical realities.

We as clinicians must provide evidence for any interventions. Parents and patients, or parents alone if the patients are preverbal, must be allowed to make an informed decision. If adequate evidence is not available, we must carefully educate the parents and other clinicians with all of the evidence that is available, proceed cautiously, and provide minimal and conservative interventions until the prenatal genetic, hormonal, and cellular imprinting is fully understood. Many interventions very well may have to await the child's ability to verbalize what is for them intuitive. Therefore, we will need to develop not one new clinical algorithm but several flexible algorithms that reflect what we know of clinical correlations between disease-specific generalities as well as individual nuances and specific realities--that is, correlations between the child's specific disease and the unique identity that only he–or she–can know.

William Reiner, Associate Professor, Department of Urology, and Adjunct Associate Professor, Department of Psychiatry, University of Oklahoma Health Sciences Center, Oklahoma City, Oklahoma, U.S.A.

REFERENCES

Berenbaum, S. A. "Effects of Early Androgens on Sex-typed Activities and Interests in Adolescents with Congenital Adrenal Hyperplasia." *Hormones and Behavior* 35.1 (1999): 102-10.
Berenbaum, S. A., and J. M. Bailey. "Effects on Gender Identity of Prenatal Androgens and Genital Appearance: Evidence from Girls with Congenital Adrenal Hyperplasia." *J Clin Endocrinol Metab* 88.3 (2003): 1102-6.
Berenbaum, S. A., and S. M. Resnick. "Early Androgen Effects on Aggression in Children and Adults with Congenital Adrenal Hyperplasia." *Psychoneuroendocrinology* 22.7 (1997): 505-15.
Bradley, S. J., G. D. Oliver, B. Avinoam, A. B. Chernick, and K. J. Zucker. "Experiment of Nurture: Ablatio Penis at 2 Months, Sex Reassignment at 7 Months, and a Psychosexual Follow-up in Young Adulthood." *Pediatrics* 102.1 (1998): e9.
Colapinto, J. *As Nature Made Him–The Boy Who Was Raised as a Girl.* New York: HarperCollins, 2000.
Colapinto, J. What Were the Real Reasons Behind David Reimer's Suicide? *Slate*, (2004).
Diamond, M., and H. K. Sigmundson, "Sex Reassignment at Birth. Long-term Review and Clinical Implications." *Arch Pediatr Adolesc* Med 151.3 (1997): 298-304.
Dittmann, R. W., M. H. Kappes, M. E. Kappes, D. Borger, H. F. Meyer-Bahlburg, H. Stegner, R. H. Willig, and H. Wallis. "Congenital Adrenal Hyperplasia. II: Gender-Related Behavior and Attitudes in Female Salt-wasting and Simple-virilizing Patients." *Psychoneuroendocrinology* 15.5-6 (1990): 421-34.
Glassberg, K. "Gender Assignment and the Pediatric Urologist." *J Urol* 161 (1999): 308-10.
Goy, R. W., and C. H. Phoenix. "The Effects of Testosterone Propionate Administered Before Birth on the Development of Behavior in Genetic Female Rhesus Monkeys." *UCLA Forum Med Sci* 15 (1972): 193-201.
Grumbach, M. M., I. A. Hughes, and F. A. Conte. "Disorders of Sex Differentiation" *Williams Textbook of Endocrinology.* R. H. Williams, P. R. Larsen, S. Melmed, K. S. Polonsky. Philadelphia: W B Saunders, 2003, 842-1002.
Hines, M. "Sex Steroids and Human Behavior: Prenatal Androgen Exposure and Sex-typical Play Behavior in Children." *Ann N Y Acad Sci* 1007 (2003): 272-82.
Houk, C. P., J. Dayner, and P. A. Lee. "Genital Ambiguity with a Y Chromosome: Does Gender Assignment Matter?" *J Pediatr Endocrinol Metab* 17.6 (2004): 825-39.
Howell, C., A. A. Caldamone, H. Snyder, M. Ziegler, and J. Duckett. "Optimal Management of Cloacal Exstrophy." *J Pediatr Surg* 18.4 (1983): 365-9.
Husmann, D. A., G. A. McLorie, and B. M. Churchill. "Phallic Reconstruction in Cloacal Exstrophy." *J Urol* 142.2 Pt 2 (1989): 563-4.
Husmann, D. A., and D. A. Vandersteen. "Anatomy of Cloacal Exstrophy, The Surgical Implications." *The Exstrophy-Epispadias Complex, Research Concepts and Clinical Applications.* J. P. Gearhart, Mathews, R. New York: Kluwer Academic/Plenum, 1999, 199-206.

Imperato-McGinley, J., R. E. Peterson, T. Gautier, and E. Sturla. "Androgens and the Evolution of Male-Gender Identity Among Male Pseudohermaphrodites with 5 Alpha-reductase Deficiency." *N Engl J Med* 300.22 (1979): 1233-7.

Imperato-McGinley, J., R. E. Peterson, T. Gautier, and E. Sturla. "Male Pseudohermaphroditism Secondary to 5 Alpha-reductase Deficiency--a Model for the Role of Androgens in Both the Development of the Male Phenotype and the Evolution of a Male Gender Identity." *J Steroid Biochem* 11.1B (1979): 637-45.

Lund, D. P., and W. H. Hendren. "Cloacal Exstrophy: Experience with 20 Cases." *JPediatr Surg* 10 (1993): 1360-8; discussion 1368-9.

Mathews, R., R. D. Jeffs, W. G. Reiner, S. G. Docimo, and J. P. Gearhart. "Cloacal Exstrophy–Improving the Quality of Life: the Johns Hopkins Experience." *J Urol* 160.6 Pt 2 (1998): 2452-6.

Mathews, R. I., E. Perlman, D. W. Marsh, and J. P. Gearhart. "Gonadal Morphology in Cloacal Exstrophy: Implications in Gender Assignment." *BJU International* 84.1 (1999): 99-100.

Money, J. "Ablatio Penis: Normal Male Infant Sex-reassigned as a Girl." *Arch Sex Behav* 4 (1975): 65-71.

Money, J., and A. Ehrhardt. *Man and Woman, Boy and Girl: The Differentiation and Dimorphism of Gender from Conception to Maturity.* Baltimore: Johns Hopkins University Press, 1972, 1-4, 118-123, 152-154, 176-179.

Petersen, E. "The Tangible Scientific Model as Quasi-experiment: Applying the 'Mediating Model' Concept to Johns-Hopkins Style Clinical Sexology of Gender Identity Formation": a Philosophy Seminar Lecture. La Jolla: University of California San Diego Philosophy Seminar, 2001.

Phoenix, C. H., R. W. Goy, and J. A. Resko. "Psychosexual Differentiation as a Function of Androgenic Stimulation." *Perspectives in Reproduction and Sexual Behavior.* D. M. Bloomington: Indiana University Press, 1968: 33-49.

Phoenix C.H., A. K. Slob, and R. W. Goy. "Effects of Castration and Replacement Therapy on Sexual Behavior of Adult Male Rhesuses." *J Comp Physiol Psychol* 84 (1973): 472-81.

Reiner, W. G. "Case Study: Sex Reassignment in a Teenage Girl." *J Am Acad Child Adolesc Psychiatry* 35.6 (1996): 799-803.

Reiner, W. G. "Psychosexual Development in Genetic Males Assigned Female: the Cloacal Exstrophy Experience." *Child Adolesc Psychiatr Clin N Am* 13.3 (2004): 657-74.

Reiner, W. G. "Gender Identity and Sex-of-rearing in Children with Disorders of Sexual Differentiation." *Journal of Pediatric Endocrinology and Metabolism* (In press, 2005).

Reiner, W. G., and J. P. Gearhart. "Discordant Sexual Identity in Some Genetic Males with Cloacal Exstrophy Assigned to Female Sex at Birth." *N Engl J Med* 350.4 (2004): 333-41.

Reiner, W. G. and B. P. Kropp. "A 7-year Experience of Genetic Males with Severe Phallic Inadequacy Assigned Female." *J Urol* 172.6 Pt 1 (2004): 2395-8.

Schober, J. M., P. A. Carmichael, M. Hines, and P. G. Ransley. "The Ultimate Challenge of Cloacal Exstrophy." *J Urol* 167.1 (2002): 300-4.

Skoog, S. J., and A. B. Belman. "Aphallia: its Classification and Management." *J Urol* 141.3 (1989): 589-92.

Tank, E. S., and S. M. Lindenauer. "Principles of Management of Exstrophy of the Cloaca." *Am J Surg* 119.1 (1970): 95-8.

Vilain, E. "Anomalies of Human Sexual Development: Clinical Aspects and Genetic Analysis." *Novartis Found Symp* 244 (2002): 43-53.

Woodhouse, C. R. J. "Myelomeningocele in Young Adults." *BJU International* 95 (2005): 223-230.

Xu, J., P. S. Burgoyne, and A. P. Arnold. "Sex Differences in Sex Chromosome Gene Expression in Mouse Brain." *Hum Mol Genet* 11.12 (2002): 1409-19.

KENNETH J. ZUCKER

GENDER IDENTITY AND INTERSEXUALITY

1. CLARIFYING THE PROBLEM

Gender identity is often conceptualized in a dichotomous manner: a person's basic sense of self as either male or female. Of course, it is not necessary, theoretically or empirically, to restrict the conceptualization in this way. One can imagine "third" (or even more) gender identities. Indeed, in recent years, some adults have characterized their subjective gender identity as "intersexed" (Schober, 2001). However, the vast majority of humans appear to differentiate rather strongly either a male or a female gender identity.

The origins and determinants of gender identity differentiation have long elicited rather pointed controversy and debate. The tendency to dichotomize the reason as either fully biological (the essentialist perspective) or psychosocial (the constructionist or socialization perspective) is well illuminated by the following two quotes: On the one hand, Swaab et al. (1992) asserted that gender identity is very difficult to change, "probably because...[it is] fixed in the brain" (p. 52). On the other hand, Thorne (1993) asserted that:

> While many still see gender as the expression of natural differences, the women's movement of the 1970s and 1980s launched a powerful alternative perspective: notions of femininity and masculinity, the gender divisions one sees on school playgrounds--the idea of gender itself--*all* are social constructions. Parents dress infant girls in pink and boys in blue, give them gender-differentiated names and toys, and expect them to act differently....peer groups...also perpetuate gender-typed play and interaction. In short, if boys and girls are different, they are not born, but *made* that way. (p. 2, italics in original)

But because the rearing of an infant as a boy or a girl is usually perfectly confounded with biological sex, researchers have long made the point that it is actually difficult to disentangle the relative contribution of biological and psychosocial influences. For some researchers, it was this methodological and interpretive dilemma that led to the study of children with physical

S.E. Sytsma (Ed.), Ethics and Intersex, 165–181.

intersex conditions in the hope of providing at least a partial resolution to this problem.

Regarding psychosexual differentiation in general and gender identity differentiation in particular, the study of children with physical intersex conditions has been characterized as an "experiment of nature." In fact, it might be more accurate to say that the study of such children represents a "quasi-experiment of nature and nurture." The "experiment" is not a formal one, as in random assignment procedures, but really an approximate experiment in which there are variations in both sexual biology and in rearing conditions, of which the researcher has only partial control.

2. WHICH SEX? WHICH GENDER?

For a long time now, the medical community has played an important role in making decisions about the "appropriate" sex and gender assignment of newborns with physical intersex conditions. As reviewed by Meyer-Bahlburg (1998, 1999, 2004), the standard guideline for such decisions has, for many years, been the so-called *optimal gender policy* of psychosocial and medical management, originally developed by Money, a medical psychologist, and colleagues in pediatric endocrinology at the Johns Hopkins Medical School in Baltimore, Maryland. This policy aimed to result in the best possible prognosis with regard to six variables: (1) reproductive potential (if attainable at all); (2) good sexual function; (3) minimal medical procedures; (4) an overall gender-appropriate appearance (e.g., the external genital configuration matching the assigned gender); (5) psychosocial well-being; and (6) a stable gender identity.

3. THE SEX-OF-REARING HYPOTHESIS

In the mid-1950s, Money and colleagues reported data on the psychosexual development of children born with physical intersex conditions. One aspect of the database concerned the gender identity differentiation of these youngsters. Based on a study of 105 youngsters with various types of physical intersex conditions, Money et al. (1957) concluded that "the sex of assignment and rearing is consistently and conspicuously a more reliable prognosticator of a hermaphrodite's [gender identity] than is the chromosomal sex, the gonadal sex, the hormonal sex, the accessory internal reproductive morphology, or the ambiguous morphology of the external genitalia" (p. 333). The importance of the gender-related psychosocial rearing environment had one important caveat, namely the advisability of an early decision about sex assignment. Money et al. (1957) recommended that when there was uncertainty about the appropriate sex of assignment, the final decision should certainly be made no later than 18-24 months, and argued that "uncompromising adherence to the decision is desirable" (p. 334).

It is now 50 years since Money and his colleagues first wrote about youngsters with physical intersex conditions (Money et al., 1955). Over these past five decades, a tremendous amount of knowledge has been acquired about the biological mechanisms that underlie normative physical sex differentiation and the various biological processes that cause atypical physical sex differentiation, i.e., the processes that cause the various forms of physical intersex conditions that comprise the contemporary taxonomic and nosological landscape. As well, we have also learned a great deal about the biological and psychosocial mechanisms that underlie both normative and atypical psychosexual differentiation, the component parts of which include gender identity, gender role, and sexual orientation (Ruble and Martin, 1998; Martin et al., 2002).

From an historical point of view, it is important to recognize that, at the time of Money's early writings, the term *gender identity* had not even been coined or conceptualized by social scientists. Indeed, Money (1955) himself did not use the term gender identity, but rather *gender role*, which he defined as "all those things that a person says or does to disclose himself or herself as having the status of boy or man, girl or woman, respectively. It includes, but is not restricted to, sexuality in the sense of eroticism" (p. 254). It was only later, in the early 1960s, that the term gender identity was coined by Stoller (1964), a psychoanalyst, and it was later adopted by Kohlberg (1966), a cognitive-developmental psychologist. Of course, this is not to imply that prior to the 1950s or 1960s people did not "have" a gender identity. Gender identity is such a basic aspect of the self that, for many, it seems so "natural" as to not require either personal reflection or classification by social taxonomists. People born with physical intersex conditions "forced" medical authorities to think more about how gender identity developed and many physicians were placed in the position where it seemed like they had to "decide" on a person's gender which, in the ordinary situation, appeared to occur so naturally.

It took some time before the theoretical implications of Money's initial clinical observations and conclusions took hold, but by the mid-1960s to early 1970s, it was widely embraced by social learning theorists and feminists. Indeed, the idea that gender identity resulted primarily, if not entirely, by psychosocial factors ("sex of rearing") was embraced by the environmental determinists of that time period (see Diamond, 1982).

It should, however, be noted that although the social environment appeared to be a strong determinant of gender identity differentiation, it is likely that this influence worked in concert with at least some biological parameters. Consider, for example, gender identity differentiation in one of the most common physical intersex conditions: congenital adrenal hyperplasia (CAH). In chromosomal females with this condition, excess prenatal exposure to androgen results in masculinization of the external genitalia. When such youngsters are reared as girls, one can examine whether or not the rearing environment can override the effect of excessive exposure to prenatal androgen (in comparison to unaffected chromosomal females). But, it should be noted that the effects of psychosocial rearing likely work in concert with other parameters (e.g., post-natal steroid treatment that blocks the overproduction of androgen, feminizing genital surgery in infancy or toddlerhood, etc.). More radical tests of the rearing environment are less systematic (e.g., one does not really have for comparison, at least in contemporary samples of girls with CAH, one group that randomly receives early feminizing genital surgery with another group that grows up with markedly masculinized-looking external genitalia). Thus, one does not know if gender identity differentiation differs as a function of the appearance of the external genitalia.

In this chapter, I will review the fate of the *sex-of-rearing* hypothesis and consider various points of controversy that have ensued.

4. POINTS OF CONTROVERSY

The sex-of-rearing explanation for gender identity differentiation in people with physical intersex condition was subjected to criticism early on and review articles by Diamond (1965) and Zuger (1970) represent two major critiques from the early period. Drawing on a variety of data sources, including experimental studies of lower animals, Diamond, for example, challenged the notion that humans were psychosexually "neutral" at the time of birth, but rather had biological predispositions to behave in a masculine or feminine manner and, by implication, suggested that gender identity itself had an in-born bias to move in one direction or the other.

4.1 5-Alpha-Reductase 2-Deficiency

In my view, the first substantive and systematic challenge to the sex-of-rearing hypothesis arose from the psychosexual study of patients with a newly discovered intersex condition, now known as 5-alpha-reductase 2-deficiency (5-ARD-2). In genetic males, this intersex syndrome, among other things, invariably results in marked ambiguity of the external genitalia at birth. During fetal development, an impairment of steroid 5-reductase activity, catalyzed by one of two enzymes (Russell and Wilson, 1994), leads to an underproduction in plasma dihydrotestosterone, which causes the incomplete masculinization of the external genitalia; however, because testosterone production is unaffected, masculinization of the internal reproductive structures is normal. Moreover, at puberty, there is relatively normal physical masculinization--both primary and secondary sex characteristics develop along male lines (e.g., the phallus enlarges to become, in some instances, a functional penis; the testes descend, if they had not done so already; the voice deepens; and there is an increase in muscle mass).

In behavioral sexology, 5-ARD began to receive a great deal of attention about 30 years ago. At that time, Imperato-McGinley et al. (1974) described a cohort of affected individuals from the Dominican Republic, in which the prevalence of the condition was unusually high because of in-breeding, who showed a gradual change in gender identity from female to male, i.e., they "switched" from living as girls/women to boys/men. Imperato-McGinley et al. noted that newborns with 5-ARD were often assigned to the female sex and subsequently "raised as girls." At puberty, the girls' physical masculinization was so striking that they became known locally as "*guevedoces*"–penis at 12 (years of age). Imperato-McGinley et al. commented that after puberty "psychosexual orientation" was male in all of the 18 individuals who had been reared as females (i.e., they perceived themselves as male, adopted a masculine gender role, and were sexually attracted to females). Imperato-McGinley et al. concluded that:

> The male sex drive appears to be testosterone related and not dihydrotestosterone related...and the sex of rearing as females...appears to have a lesser role in the presence of two masculinizing events--testosterone exposure *in utero* and again at puberty with the development of a male phenotype. (p. 1215)

In a subsequent article, Imperato-McGinley et al. (1979) provided additional details about their subjects, including a description of the community's social life, the community's behavioral expectations for children, and the gender role tasks of the community's adults. They interviewed affected individuals and significant others (e.g., parents, siblings, neighbors) "to discern any sexual ambiguity in the rearing of subjects raised as girls and to determine in these subjects the validity of the change to a male...gender identity and male...gender role" (pp. 1233-1234). Of 18 subjects "nambiguously raised as girls...17 of 18 changed to a male... gender identity and 16 of 18 to a male...gender role [during or after puberty]"(p. 1233). They summarized their data as follows:

The 17 subjects who changed to a male...gender identity began to realize that they were
different from other girls in the village between seven and 12 years of age, when they
did not develop breasts, when their bodies began to change in a masculine direction and
when masses were noted in the inguinal canal or scrotum. These subjects showed self-
concern over their true gender. A male...gender identity gradually evolved over several
years as the subjects passed through stages of no longer feeling like girls, to feeling like
men and, finally, to the conscious awareness that they were indeed men. (p. 1234)

Since these initial reports, similar accounts of gender change from female to
male have been described in cohorts of subjects from Papua New Guinea,
Mexico, Brazil, and the Middle East, as well as in single case or small series
reports (for reviews, see Wilson et al., 1993; Zucker, 1999; Wilson, 2001;
Cohen-Kettenis, 2005).

In some quarters, the reaction to the initial reports by Imperato-
McGinley and colleagues was not to dispute the veracity of the gender
change, but the explanation for it (see Zucker and Bradley, 1995). The initial
commentaries contained a great deal of discourse about the nature of the
gender assignment at birth, particularly among post first-generation
probands. For these probands, the family and community had acquired some
knowledge about the natural history of the condition, including the physical
masculinization that occurred at puberty. Thus, for these probands, it was
argued that they were not assigned unambiguously to the female sex and
reared as girls, but that the culture created both "third sex" and "third
gender" categories that would guide postnatal socialization. Money (1976),
for example, commented on the psychological significance of the "folk
prognosis" of "*guevedoces*." Money argued that since the parents rapidly
became aware of the impending physical masculinization at puberty that
they:

could not confidently assign a newborn hermaphroditic baby as a girl. Even if the birth
certificate was assigned female, the parents would know they were rearing a *guevedoce*
who would not look feminine after childhood. Even in the first generation in which
hermaphrodites appeared in two families in the family tree...before they could be
defined as *guevedoces*, parents would rear their child as one of ambiguous sex, not
knowing what to expect at puberty (p. 872).

Subsequently, Herdt (1990; Herdt and Davidson, 1988) made similar
arguments with regard to the social environment of 5-ARD individuals from
Papua New Guinea.

The rebuttal to Money by Imperato-McGinley et al. (1976) was, quite
interestingly, equivocal. On the one hand, they argued that

Money obviously does not know how the parents raised these children. Our interviews
with some of the affected males and their parents indicate that in the first generation, the
affected subjects...were raised as girls and there was no ambiguity on the part of the
parents as to the sex of the child at birth or in early childhood. They believed they were
raising a little girl. (p. 872)

On the other hand, Imperato-McGinley et al. also observed that because the condition had become better recognized, the

> villagers now either raise the subjects as boys from birth, rear them as boys as soon as the problem is recognized in childhood or raise them ambiguously as girls. Now that the villagers are familiar with the condition, the affected children and adults are sometimes objects of ridicule and are referred to as *guevedoce, guevote* (penis at 12 years of age) or *machihembra* (first woman, then man). (p. 1235)

How are we to best interpret the phenomenon of gender change among individuals with 5-ARD? On the one hand, some have read the data as suggestive of a strong main effect (to use the language of the factorial design) of biological influences on gender identity differentiation. On the other hand, it has been argued that the evidence is more supportive of interaction effects: that is, genetic males with 5-ARD have, despite their ambiguous genitalia at birth, male-typical prenatal masculinization, including putative central nervous system (CNS) effects, that predispose to postnatal behavioral masculinity. The response in the social environment augments this biological predisposition, which is augmented even further by the spontaneous physical masculinization that occurs at puberty. Among 5-ARD individuals raised from infancy as boys, the social environment certainly appears to work in concert with the putative prenatal masculinizing CNS effects (for reviews, see Wilson, 2001; Cohen-Kettenis, 2005).

How best to resolve these competing explanations? Here, it would be extremely useful to have natural history data on individuals with 5-ARD who are treated differently, both medically and psychosocially, than in the cultural groups noted above. For example, in the United States and Europe, it is possible that at least some 5-ARD individuals would be raised as girls on the grounds that the external genitalia will not masculinize sufficiently to permit comfortable (heterosexual) sexual functioning. Thus, in accordance with the optimal gender policy, such individuals would be castrated in infancy, receive surgical feminization of the genitalia, and be placed on feminizing hormones at puberty.

Unfortunately, the psychosexual development of 5-ARD individuals treated in this manner has been described rather poorly. The relevant case reports are scattered widely throughout the biomedical literature and reference to gender identity differentiation, as noted by both Zucker (1999) and Cohen-Kettenis (2005), is often described rather briefly within the context of more detailed accounts of the syndrome itself. Nonetheless, Cohen-Kettenis' (2005) updated review shows that there is more variability in gender identity differentiation among such patients than was reported in the initial cohort by Imperato-McGinley and colleagues.

From an interpretive standpoint, one could argue that, for those patients who had differentiated a female gender identity, the social environment vis-a-vis gender identity (along with the corresponding surgical feminization of the genitalia, etc.) overrode the prenatal hormonal masculinization and its putative CNS effects. But even this argument may not be strong enough because a number of case reports indicated that a female gender identity differentiated in the *absence* of any hormonal or surgical intervention prior to early adolescence or young adulthood (see Zucker, 1999). Thus, even under the circumstance of a masculinizing body habitus at puberty, if not earlier, these patients retained a female gender identity, a finding reminiscent of the female gender identity among late-treated women with CAH (Ehrhardt et al., 1968).

In summary, the data on gender identity differentiation among patients with 5-ARD are strikingly complex. On the one hand, the phenomenon of gender change first reported on by Imperato-McGinley et al. (1974) has been verified in several additional cohorts of patients, thus constituting an important replication of the original observation (Wilson et al., 1993). On the other hand, differentiation of a female gender identity also occurs in a minority of patients, even in cultures in which there is strong external pressure for the patient to change from living as a female to a male (Cohen-Kettenis, 2005). To some extent, this latter finding appears to challenge the now prevailing perspective in the literature on the psychosexual natural history of patients with 5-ARD, i.e., that gender change is inevitable subsequent to the masculinizing events that occur around the time of puberty.

To account for this variability in gender identity outcome, what are the best candidate explanations? One possibility is that variation in gender identity differentiation is related to the degree of prenatal hormonal masculinization of the CNS and, perhaps, to the degree of postnatal physical masculinization at the time of puberty and beyond. My reading of the literature suggests that this is an unlikely or satisfactory explanation. A second possibility is that the variation is accounted for by the classical sex-of-rearing hypothesis originally advanced by Money et al. (1957): For those patients who are unequivocally reared as females, a female gender identity ensues; for those reared ambiguously (along with the corresponding pubertal physical masculinization), a gender change ensues; for those reared as males from infancy onwards, a male gender identity ensues. Unfortunately, as I have argued elsewhere (Zucker and Bradley, 1995), this interpretation has been hampered by the absence of good prospective data and the reliance on post-hoc interpretations of the eventual outcome. As I also argued elsewhere (Zucker and Bradley, 1995), what is urgently needed is a psychometrically sound method of assessing the sex of rearing construct, in which observers can agree whether or not the affected individual is being raised unequivocally as a girl or as a boy or, alternatively, somewhere in between these two traditional modes of gender rearing.

4.2 Contemporary Empirical Studies and Reviews

For the various reasons noted above, I would argue that the gender identity data on 5-ARD have been equivocal in evaluating the sex-of-rearing hypothesis. Over the past few years, with the increased sophistication in the taxonomy of physical intersex conditions, it has become easier to evaluate gender identity differentiation on a syndrome by syndrome basis. New data sets include reviews on (1) chromosomal females with CAH, (2) chromosomal males with either complete or partial androgen insensitivity syndrome (CAIS or PAIS), (3) chromosomal males born with a micropenis, (4) XY or mosaic patients born with either mixed or partial gonadal dysgenesis (GD), and (5) chromosomal males born with either penile agenesis or cloacal exstrophy (CE), all of which allow for a more detailed appraisal of the sex-of-rearing hypothesis.

Here, I will summarize the general conclusions drawn from these reviews. Regarding chromosomal females with CAH, chromosomal males with either complete or partial AIS, and chromosomal males born with a micropenis, the sex-of-rearing hypothesis has received reasonable support: gender identity appears to differentiate largely in accordance with the gender assignment at birth (Dessens et al., 2005; Mazur, 2005). Nonetheless, it is important to consider some caveats in reaching this conclusion. Regarding chromosomal females with CAH, for example, the percentage who develop gender dysphoria is higher than the known base rates of gender dysphoria in unaffected adult females. As noted by Meyer-Bahlburg et al. (1996), the explanation for the increased rate of gender dysphoria is likely multifactorial. Regarding chromosomal males born with a micropenis, the number of patients who have been raised as girls (and for whom there are published outcome data) is strikingly small, so one has to be quite cautious in appraising the data (Mazur, 2005).

Mixed or partial gonadal dysgenesis is a physical intersex condition for which systematic data on psychosexual differentiation have been relatively lacking (Meyer-Bahlburg, 2005a). As an androgen resistance syndrome, it bears a number of similarities to 5-ARD, 17-beta-hydroxysteroid dehydrogenase-3 deficiency, and the micropenis syndromes of uncertain etiology. In recent years, several case reports have been published in which the patient initiated a gender change from female to male (Reiner, 1996; Birnbacher et al., 1999; Phornphutkul et al., 2000). The authors of all three case reports have interpreted the gender change as representing a challenge to the sex-of-rearing hypothesis.

As I have argued elsewhere (Zucker, 2002), however, one of the current methodological problems in the literature is a variant of what has been termed the "file drawer" problem in experimental research (Rosenthal, 1979). For a long time, it has been noted that journals are inclined to publish the results of "successful" experiments. Unsuccessful experiments are relegated to the file drawer. Because published findings may overestimate the success of a particular line of research, quantitative procedures were developed for computing the tolerance for filed and future null results. Regarding psychosexual differentiation among patients with physical intersex conditions, however, the file drawer problem is the exact opposite, namely, that cases of "unsuccessful" rearing are more likely to be published than successful cases, at least nowadays, because it is the unsuccessful cases that are deemed newsworthy. Thus, it is likely that clinicians and others would be less inclined to try and publish a case report in which gender identity differentiation remained consistent with the gender assignment at birth. As I will argue in detail below, it can also be argued that a gender change can be interpreted from various vantage points, including those that do not necessarily invalidate the importance of sex-of-rearing.

To my knowledge, there is only one systematic follow-up study of patients born with either mixed or partial GD. Szarras-Czapnik et al. (2005) assessed 19 patients at a mean follow-up age of 21 years (range, 17-26). Ten were assigned male and nine were assigned female in the newborn period. All 10 male-assigned patients differentiated a male gender identity; of the 9 female-assigned patients, 7 differentiated a female gender identity and two were, although living in the female social role, "ambivalent" about their status as women. Thus, of 19 patients, 17 had an unequivocal gender identity that matched their initial gender assignment. In this respect, the data appear more consistent with the summary reviews for the intersex conditions noted above.

In the current literature, the most direct challenge to the sex-of-rearing hypothesis comes from chromosomal males born with CE and from the much-discussed case of David Reimer, a biologically normal male (and a monozygotic twin), whose penis was burned off during an electrocautery-guided circumcision at the age of 7 months and who was subsequently reassigned to be raised as a girl at around the age of 17 months.

In genetic males with CE of the bladder, the penis is often aplastic and bifid or sometimes entirely absent. Nonetheless, it is believed that the prenatal androgen milieu was normal because the testes are normal. For genetic males with CE who have been raised as girls, in accordance with the optimal gender policy, various reports have noted gender role behavioral masculinization (see Meyer-Bahlburg, 2005b), similar, for example, to what has been observed in chromosomal females with CAH (see Hines, 2004; Zucker, 2005). In this respect, many authors have argued that this represents another line of evidence suggesting that the prenatal hormonal environment influences gender role behavioral development.

More importantly, however, is the recent report by Reiner and Gearhart (2004), who described a high rate of gender change among CE patients raised as female (6 of 14). Along with the marked gender role behavioral masculinization noted in these patients overall, Reiner and Gearhart have made very similar arguments to that of Imperato-McGinley et al. regarding the role of prenatal androgens on gender identity formation.

As summarized by Meyer-Bahlburg (2005b), however, a number of authors have reported variant findings: in the vast majority of other genetic males with CE raised female, a female gender identity has been reported. Thus, there appear to be conflicting data on the natural history of gender identity in CE patients. One must, however, at this point be very cautious in appraising these data because the quality of information on the psychosexual development in these patients is quite varied.

Let us assume that, as more empirical returns become available, the natural history of gender identity differentiation in genetic males with CE will show much variability, along the lines that have been observed in 5-ARD-2 deficiency, in that some patients will retain a female gender identity whereas others will reports gender dysphoria or change from living as a female to living as a male. How might we account for this individual variability? Given that almost all of the female-raised patients appear to show gender role behavioral masculinity, it is quite likely that the normal prenatal exposure to androgen is a causal factor. It might, however, be argued that variations in the psychosocial milieu may work to either accentuate or attenuate this predisposition to masculine psychosexual differentiation.

In the case of CE, the recommendation to raise the baby as a girl has rested primarily on the pragmatic assumption that growing up as a boy without a penis would cause undue social hardship. Parents, in probably the majority of cases, likely realize that their newborn is a "normal" biological male (except for the malformed or absent penis). Thus, for some parents it may be difficult to understand the recommendation and this may create uncertainty or doubt about the underlying rationale and thus affect the psychosocial gendered rearing environment. Until we have more detailed information about parental appraisals, it will be difficult to systematically test this hypothesis.

The David Reimer case has received considerable attention in the literature (Money and Ehrhardt, 1972; Money, 1975; Diamond, 1982, 1997; Diamond and Sigmundson, 1997a, 1997b; Money, 1998; Diamond, 1999; Zucker, 1999; Colapinto, 2000; Hausmann, 2000), so the reader can study the background material in much more detail than space requirements permit here. In many respects, the Reimer case has been gauged as the most rigorous test of the sex-of-rearing hypothesis because he was a completely normal biological male who, because of the traumatic loss of the penis due to the circumcision accident, was reassigned to be raised as a girl (e.g., on the grounds that growing up as a boy without a penis would have induced unnecessary social hardship). Because the decision to reassign Reimer to the female gender was within the window of developmental time that Money and colleagues had deemed acceptable in cases of gender reassignment for patients with physical intersex conditions, it was believed that the gendered social environment would be able to effectively induce a female gender identity (along with the removal of the testes and scrotum, feminizing hormone treatment to induce puberty along female lines, etc.).

It is now well-known that this experiment of nurture failed because by mid-adolescence Reimer switched from living as an unhappy girl to living as a male (sadly, Reimer committed suicide in 2004, at the age of 38, and his twin brother apparently committed suicide in 2002, at the age of 36). For many critics, this social experiment was deemed unwise. It has been argued that it is simply not possible to raise a normal biological male as a girl, for all of the reasons provided by those who believe that sexual biology is the primary determinant of gender identity (particularly, perhaps, the idea that prenatal androgens "imprint" on the brain a male gender identity).

One must recognize, however, some limitations to this analysis. When an experiment fails, the procedural rule is to conclude that one was not able to reject the null hypothesis. When an experiment "fails," there are all kinds of reasons that might account for it (e.g., if a therapeutic drug does not have its desired effect, it could be a dosage problem, it could be non-compliance, it could be that the hypothesized mechanism of action was incorrect, and so on). It is only with further research can one empirically evaluate the various possibilities for why the initial experiment failed. Thus, while the biological argument is plausible, one could just as easily argue that the particular gendered social environment in which Reimer was raised was simply not powerful enough to override his prenatal sexual biology. Perhaps other gendered social environments would have been more effective.

My colleagues and I (Bradley et al., 1998) published a case report on the psychosexual outcome of another case of penile ablation due to a circumcision accident: in our patient, the accident occurred at 2 months and the gender reassignment occurred at 7 months. At the age of 26 years, our patient reported a female gender identity and, in this respect, differed rather markedly from the Reimer outcome. Our patient did, however, share other similarities with Reimer: behavioral masculinity in childhood and adulthood and a predominant sexual attraction to biological females (our patient had had many sexual experiences with both biological males and females and characterized her sexual identity as "bisexual"). Regarding our patient's gender identity, however, the null hypothesis could be rejected, i.e., the gendered social environment appeared to have had an impact (along with, one presumes, the feminizing effects of genital surgery and a feminized puberty induced by exogenous estrogen treatment). Unless our patient was biologically predisposed to develop male-to-female transsexualism, I would argue that the gendered social environment is one of the more plausible explanations to account for why a female gender identity differentiated. Nonetheless, perhaps the main lesson to be drawn is that one has to be cautious in reaching any bold conclusions from just two cases and the other cases of ablatio penis that are available in the published literature are quite lacking in detail about both the gendered social environment and long-term outcome (Meyer-Bahlburg, 2005b).

In closing this section, I would like to make one further remark about the importance in appraising the gendered social environment. Several years ago, Evans et al. (1999) reported on a series of patients with penile agenesis, a physical intersex condition that bears many similarities to the situation with cloacal exstrophy and traumatic loss of the penis. In penile agenesis, one presumes a normal prenatal masculine sexual biology, with the only error in physical sex differentiation being the absence of the penis. One of the patients in Evans et al. was female assigned in the newborn period (and gonadectomized). As it turned out, my group was asked to evaluate this patient at the age of 15 years. She presented as behaviorally masculine and gender dysphoric and we recommended that the patient transition to living in the male social role, to stop taking feminizing hormones, and to begin taking masculinizing hormones.

On the surface, one could again argue that this patient's normal prenatal sexual biology (e.g., male-typical exposure to prenatal androgen) overrode any effect of the gendered social environment. However, based on the clinical data, it was my impression that the patient's social environment (i.e., that organized by the patient's caregivers) was far from unambiguous. The caregivers reported that they never accepted the recommendation that the patient be reared as a girl; hence, in this case, I would argue that the clinical data would result in a "consensus panel" of experts to conclude that the patient's gendered social environment was strongly colored by uncertainty, ambivalence, and skepticism about raising the child as a girl. In my view, the case material was too complex to conclude that the patient's failure to develop an unambiguous female gender identity was simply a function of her prenatal sexual biology.

5. SUMMARY

This brief review of the sex-of-rearing hypothesis vis-a-vis gender identity differentiation in patients born with physical intersex conditions shows that there is considerable variation in outcome across syndromes. In some conditions, such as CAH, PAIS, and micropenis syndromes of unknown etiology, the data appear to show that gender identity differentiates largely in accordance with the sex-of-rearing. In this respect, the original Money et al. (1957) conclusion has been largely substantiated. In other conditions, such as 5-ARD and CE, gender identity differentiation is much more variable. Along with the highly publicized David Reimer case, these data have led many clinicians and researchers to question rather strongly the assumptions that underlie the sex-of-rearing idea. As a result, we can see nowadays a sort of "tilt" towards a biologic, essentialist model of psychosexual differentiation in general and gender identity in particular.

My own conclusion is a more cautious one. I am not convinced that the "sex-of-rearing" baby should be thrown out with the bathwater. The data are too complex to reach this conclusion. We need to continue to study the effects of the gendered psychosocial rearing environment in concert with the biology of physical sex-differentiation to continue our search for the combination of factors that account for gender identity differentiation in people born with physical intersex conditions. On this point, it is obvious that more data are required.

Kenneth Zucker, Professor, Departments of Psychology and Psychiatry, University of Toronto, Ontario, Canada.

REFERENCES

Birnbacher, R., M. Marberger, G. Weissenbacher, E. Schober, and H. Frisch. "Gender Identity Reversal in an Adolescent with Mixed Gonadal Dysgenesis." *J. Pediatr. Endocrinol. Metab.* 12 (1999): 687-690.

Bradley, S. J., G. D. Oliver, A. B. Chernick, and K. J. Zucker. "Experiment of Nurture: *Ablatio* Penis at 2 Months, Sex Reassignment at 7 Months, and a Psychosexual Follow-up in Young Adulthood." *Pediatrics* 102 (1998): E91-E95. (Available at http://www.pediatrics.org/cgi/content/full/02/1/e9)

Cohen-Kettenis, P. T. "Gender Change in 46,XY Persons with 5-Reductase-2 Deficiency and 17-Hydroxysteroid Dehydrogenase-3 Deficiency." *Arch. Sex. Behav.* 34 (2005): 399-410.

Colapinto, J. *As Nature Made Him: The Boy Who Was Raised as a Girl*, New York, N.Y.: Harper Collins, 2000.

Dessens, A. B., F. M. E. Slijper, and S. L. S. Drop. "Gender Dysphoria and Gender Change in Chromosomal Females with Congenital Adrenal Hyperplasia." *Arch. Sex. Behav.* 34 (2005): 389-397.

Diamond, M. "A Critical Evaluation of the Ontogeny of Human Sexual Behavior." *Q. Rev. Biol.* 40 (1965): 147-175.

Diamond, M. "Sexual Identity, Monozygotic Twins Reared in Discordant Sex Roles and a BBC Follow-up." *Arch. Sex. Behav.* 11 (1982): 181-186.

Diamond, M. "Sexual Identity and Sexual Orientation in Children with Traumatized or Ambiguous Genitalia." *J. Sex Res.* 34 (1997): 199-211.

Diamond, M. "Pediatric Management of Ambiguous and Traumatized Genitalia." *J. Urol.* 162 (1999): 1021-1028.

Diamond, M., and H. K. Sigmundson. "Management of Intersexuality: Guidelines for Dealing with Persons with Ambiguous Genitalia." *Arch. Pediatr. Adolesc. Med.* 151 (1997a): 1046-1050.

Diamond, M., and H. K. Sigmundson. "Sex Reassignment at Birth: Long-term Review and Clinical Implications." *Arch. Pediatr. Adolesc. Med.* 151 (1997b): 298-304.

Ehrhardt, A. A., R. Epstein, and J. Money. "Fetal Androgens and Female Gender Identity in the Early-treated Adrenogenital Syndrome." *Johns Hopkins Med. J.* 122 (1968): 160-167.

Evans, J. A., L. B. Erdile, C. R. Greenberg, and A. E. Chudley. "Agenesis of the Penis: Patterns of Associated Malformations." *Am. J. Med. Genet.* 84 (1999): 47-55.

Hausmann, B. L. "Do Boys Have to be Boys? Gender, Narrativity, and the John/Joan Case. *NWSA Journal* 12 (2000): 114-138.

Herdt, G. "Mistaken Gender: 5-alpha Reductase Hermaphroditism and Biological Reductionism in Sexual Identity Reconsidered." *American Anthropologist* 92 (1990): 433-446.

Herdt, G. H., and J. Davidson. "The Sambia "Turnim-man": Sociocultural and Clinical Aspects of Gender Formation in Male Pseudohermaphrodites with 5-alpha Reductase Deficiency in Papua New Guinea." *Arch. Sex. Behav.* 17 (1988): 33-56.

Hines, M. *Brain Gender.* Oxford: Oxford University Press, 2004.

Imperato-McGinley, J., L. Guerrero, T. Gautier, and R. E. Peterson. "Steroid 5-reductase Deficiency in Man: An Inherited Form of Male Pseudohermaphroditism." *Science* 186 (1974): 1213-1215.

Imperato-McGinley, J., R. E. Peterson, and T. Gautier. "Gender Identity and Hermaphroditism." [Letter], *Science* 191 (1976): 872.

Imperato-McGinley, J., R. E. Peterson, T. Gautier, and E. Sturla, E. "Androgens and the Evolution of Male-gender Identity among Male Pseudohermaphrodites with 5-reductase Deficiency." *N. Engl. J. Med.* 300 (1979): 1233-1237.

Kohlberg, L. A. "Cognitive-developmental Analysis of Children's Sex-role Concepts and Attitudes," in: *The Development of Sex Differences*, E. E. Maccoby, ed. Stanford: Stanford University Press, 1966:82-173.

Martin, C. L., D. N. Ruble, and J. Szkrybalo. "Cognitive Theories of Early Gender Development." *Psychol. Bull.* 128 (2002): 903-933.

Mazur, T., "Gender Dysphoria and Gender Change in Androgen Insensitivity or Micropenis." *Arch. Sex. Behav.* 34 (2005): 411-421.

Meyer-Bahlburg, H. F. L., "Gender Assignment in Intersexuality." *Journal of Psychology & Human Sexuality* 10(2) (1998):1-21.

Meyer-Bahlburg, H. F. L., "Gender Assignment and Reassignment in 46,XY Pseudohermaphroditism and Related Conditions." *J. Clin. Endocrinol. Metab.* 84 (1999): 3455-3458.

Meyer-Bahlburg, H. F. L. "Gender Assignment and Psychosocial Management." *Encyclopedia of Endocrine Diseases* 2 (2004): 125-133.

Meyer-Bahlburg, H. F. L. "Introduction: Gender Dysphoria and Gender Change in Persons with Intersexuality." *Arch. Sex. Behav.* 34 (2005a): 371-373.

Meyer-Bahlburg, H. F. L. "Gender Identity Outcome in Female-raised 46,XY Persons with Penile Agenesis, Cloacal Exstrophy of the Bladder or Penile Ablation." *Arch. Sex. Behav.* 34 (2005b): 423-438.

Meyer-Bahlburg, H. F. L., R. S. Gruen, M. I. New, J. J. Bell, A. Morishima, M. Shimshi, et al. "Gender Change from Female to Male in Classical Congenital Adrenal Hyperplasia." *Horm. Behav.* 30 (1996): 319-332.

Money, J. "Hermaphroditism, Gender and Precocity in Hyperadrenocorticism: Psychologic Findings." *Bull. Johns Hopkins Hosp.* 96 (1955): 253-264.

Money, J. "Ablatio Penis: Normal Male Infant Sex-reassigned as a Girl." *Arch. Sex. Behav.* 4 (1975): 65-71.

Money, J. "Gender Identity and Hermaphroditism." [Letter], *Science* 191 (1976): 872.

Money, J. *Sin, Science, and the Sex Police: Essays on Sexology and Sexosophy*, Prometheus Books, Amherst, 1998: 286-326.

Money, J., and A. A. Ehrhardt. *Man and Woman, Boy and Girl: The Differentiation and Dimorphism of Gender Identity from Conception to Maturity.* Baltimore: Johns Hopkins Press, 1972: 118-123.

Money, J., J. G. Hampson, and J. L. Hampson. "An examination of Some Basic Sexual Concepts: The Evidence of Human Hermaphroditism." *Bull. Johns Hopkins Hosp.* 97 (1955): 301-319.

Money, J., J. G. Hampson, and J. L. Hampson. "Imprinting and the Establishment of Gender Role." *Arch. Neurol. Psychiatry* 77 (1957): 333-336.

Phornphutkul, C., A. Fausto-Sterling, and P. A. Gruppuso. "Gender Self-assignment in an XY Adolescent Female Born with Ambiguous Genitalia." *Pediatrics* 106 (2000): 135-137.

Reiner, W. G. "Case Study: Sex Reassignment in a Teenage Girl." *J. Am. Acad. Child Adolesc. Psychiatry* 35 (1996): 799-803.

Reiner, W. G., and Gearhart, J. P. "Discordant Sexual Identity in Some Genetic Males with Cloacal Exstrophy Assigned to Female Sex at Birth." *N. Engl. J. Med.* 250 (2004): 333-341.

Rosenthal, R. "The 'File Drawer Problem' and Tolerance for Null Results." *Psychol. Bull.* 86 (2004): 638-641.

Ruble, D. N. and C. L. Martin. "Gender Development", in: *The Handbook of Child Psychology (5th ed.). Vol. 3: Social, Emotional, and Personality Development*, W. Damon, ser. ed., N. Eisenberg, vol. ed., New York: Wiley (1998): 933-1016.

Russell, D. W., and J. D. Wilson. "Steroid 5-reductase: Two Genes/Two Enzymes." *Ann. Rev. Biochem.* 63 (1994): 25-61.

Schober, J. M. "Sexual Behaviors, Sexual Orientation and Gender Identity in Adult Intersexuals: A Pilot Study." *J. Urol.* 165 (2001): 2350-2353.

Stoller, R. J. "The Hermaphroditic Identity of Hermaphrodites." *J. Nerv. Ment. Dis.* 139 (1964): 453-457.

Swaab, D. F., L. J. G. Gooren, and M. A. Hofman. "Gender and Sexual Orientation in Relation to Hypothalamic Structures." *Horm. Res.* 38 (Suppl. 2) (1992): 51-61.

Szarras-Czapnik, M., Z. Lew-Starowicz, and K. J. Zucker. *A Psychosexual Follow-up Study of Patients with Mixed or Partial Gonadal Dysgenesis*. Unpublished manuscript. The Children's Memorial Health Institute, Warsaw, Poland, 2005.

Thorne, B. *Gender Play: Girls and Boys in School.* New Brunswick, NJ: Rutgers University Press, 1993.

Wilson, J. D. "Androgens, Androgen Receptors, and Male Gender Role Behavior." *Horm. Behav.* 40 (2001): 358-366.

Wilson, J. D., J. E. Griffin, and D. W. Russell. "Steroid 5-reductase 2 Deficiency," *Endocr. Rev.* 14: (1993): 577-593.

Zucker, K. J. "Intersexuality and Gender Identity Differentiation." *Ann. Rev. Sex Res.* 10 (1999): 1-69.

Zucker, K. J. "Evaluation of Sex- and Gender-assignment Decisions in Patients with Physical Intersex Conditions: A Methodological and Statistical Note." *J. Sex Marital Ther.* 28 (2002): 269-274.

Zucker, K. J. "Measurement of Psychosexual Differentiation." *Arch. Sex. Behav.* 34 (2005): 375-388.

Zucker, K. J., and S. J. Bradley. *Gender Identity Disorder and Psychosexual Problems in Children and Adolescents.* New York: Guilford Press, 1995:208-212.

Zuger, B. "Gender Role Determination: A Critical Review of the Evidence from Hermaphroditism." *Psychosom. Med.* 32 (1970): 449-463.

GARRY WARNE AND VIJAYALAKSHMI BHATIA

INTERSEX, EAST AND WEST

1. INTRODUCTION

In Asian countries, approaches towards intersex differ in many ways from the approaches taken in the West. The differences arise partly from the level of poverty in Asia. Poor parents cannot easily access high-quality medical services. The differences also stem from cultural variance; the collective beliefs and attitudes that make up the cultural background inevitably influence the way in which all people, both lay and professional, think about medical management issues. It may be difficult for us to discern cultural influence on our decision-making from "inside" our own culture, but stepping "outside" may give us a glimpse of our culture as others see it.

In the West, the medical profession and intersex patient advocacy groups have been engaged, for over the past decade, in a vigorous and healthy exchange about ethics. The main issues of the exchange relate to the nature and timing of genital surgery and the disclosure of medical information to parents and patients. On the latter subject, there is now widespread agreement that full disclosure is essential. Regarding the first two subjects, the questions remaining are *when* and *how*? Genital surgery performed when the patient is an infant or a young child is still highly controversial because, it is argued, the consent of the person affected cannot be obtained. The alternative is to postpone surgery until the individual is old enough to have a say. Most pediatricians and pediatric surgeons are in favor of early surgery, but most activists oppose it. We have reached a stalemate.

In many Asian countries, however—especially in the poorer ones—children born with ambiguous genitalia grow up with their original anatomy. If such children have surgery at all, they may not have it until they are in late childhood or even adolescence. The culture accepts this because the people see no alternative. Every Asian village has children and adults with deformities and disabilities. People are used to seeing such conditions. How, then, do children with ambiguous genitalia fare in these circumstances? Are they treated with the respect and dignity that would allow them to grow up with intact self-esteem, and are they thereby empowered to make their own decisions about when to undergo surgery, or whether they need surgery at all? In this chapter, we attempt to take a trans-cultural look at the outcome

S.E. Sytsma (Ed.), Ethics and Intersex, 183–205.

for intersexed patients, based on experience the authors have had working in India, Vietnam, and Australia.

Intersex conditions, which are many and assorted, are the postnatal manifestations of significant variations in fetal reproductive tract development. Most intersex conditions stem from aberrant chromosomes or single-gene mutations, and they are often associated with secondary hormonal disturbances that will exert effects throughout life unless treated appropriately. Possible hormonal disturbances include sex hormone deficiency, androgen excess, cortisol deficiency and mineralocorticoid deficiency or excess. The anatomy of the reproductive tract is what draws attention to the presence of intersex conditions, but affected people also usually have to deal with issues related to sexuality, infertility, emotional health, and interpersonal relations. The social dimension often becomes as important as the medical dimension.

In all human societies, Eastern and Western, men and women have different roles. Unless compelled to do otherwise, as in Chairman Mao's China, men dress differently from women. They use language differently, behave differently, and follow somewhat different interests. According to Freud and Foucault, all adult human relationships have a sexual component, one that is recognised by all of the major religions. From a very early age, children usually recognise their genitals as their own and make the association between genital appearance and gender identity. People want to be clearly identifiable as male or female because sex is a fundamental part of personal identity, and uncertainty about sex disturbs other aspects of identity. Transsexual individuals identify strongly with one gender, albeit one that is discordant with their birth sex, and cannot understand why other people cannot see them as they see themselves.

The laws of both civil and religious societies differentiate between males and females. Except in those few places that have recently begun sanctioning same-sex marriages, legal marriage requires that a man marry a woman. The definition of "man" and "woman" comes down to a decision made at the time of the person's birth, a decision based on a cursory inspection of the external genitals by someone who might well have no professional training. Once the birth sex is registered, subsequent records of sex are difficult to change unless it can be shown that an error was made. Inheritance laws are often gender-specific. In Islamic law, ownership of property may only pass from father to son. In matriarchal societies, such as the Mangalore culture in South India, property may only be passed down from mother to daughter. Certain religious occupations, such as the Roman Catholic priesthood and clerical roles in Islam, are restricted to men. Additionally, in traditional Judaism and Islam (religions in which men are more central to worship than women), places of worship are segregated, with separate places for each sex.

In India and Vietnam (and in many other places where there are insufficient public toilets), men commonly urinate in public places without causing offence, but women are required to hide themselves from view for the same function. In many traditional societies, women segregate themselves from their families during menstruation (and may temporarily go to live in a separate dwelling) because they are ritually regarded as unclean.

Indian society places great importance on marriage. For a woman, it is the key to any existence separate from her parents because her husband will support her. If she does not marry, if she is widowed, or worse still, if she is divorced, she may well become unemployable and be reduced to wretched poverty because of the stigma attached to being single. An unmarried man, on the other hand, can find employment and survive independently. Marriages are usually arranged and are considered to be for the purpose of producing children. If the parents know that their son or daughter will never be able to have children—for example, because of irreversible gonadal failure—they cannot offer that child to be married. If the child is female, she will remain unemployed and will be the responsibility of her parents forever. If parents fail to disclose their knowledge of their child's infertility (regardless of gender) to the other family and thereby allow the marriage to go ahead, the marriage can immediately be annulled once the situation is revealed. Once married, men are subject to standards that are different from those applied to women. Unfaithful husbands are tolerated (many men in India and Vietnam have extramarital relationships), but wives are expected to be unwavering in fidelity and are severely punished if they stray.

Societies differ markedly in their tolerance of various forms of sexual behaviour. Residents of India and Vietnam commonly inform Western inquirers that homosexuality is rare in their communities. Homosexuals in India wisely keep a low profile (or opt out of general society and join a fringe group known as *Hijra*, or "hermaphrodites' society" (Nanda, Kucheria, Ammini, and Taneja)) because homo-sexuality arouses intense disapproval. On the other hand, Western societies— which have decriminalised homosexual acts between consenting adults in private— acknowledge that homosexuality is common and increasingly accept it as a normal variation. Many major cities, such as Sydney, London, Toronto, San Francisco, and Copenhagen, hold Gay and Lesbian Festivals. In the Highlands of Papua-New Guinea, *all* adolescent males are encouraged to engage in oral sex with other boys because of religious beliefs that the ingestion of semen is essential for the development of masculinity (Herdt). In Samoa, it is very common for boys perceived as having feminine characteristics to be raised as girls; they are then expected to help the mother as if they were daughters. These boys who live as girls are called *fa'afafine* (Besnier). Although *fa'afafine* are not always effeminate or homosexual, they will live, dress, and behave like females. They are respected, hardworking members of society.

People with intersex conditions are likely to have been the subject of medical and parental confusion concerning their sex when they were born or when the condition was first diagnosed. During childhood and adolescence, they may experience confusion about their gender identity and sexuality. How do they fit into their society, and how does society regard people whose sex is in any way unclear? This chapter will focus on how societies differ around the world in their views about sex and sexual differences and will present evidence from clinical research on the long-term outcome for young people with intersex conditions in three countries, namely, India, Vietnam, and Australia.

In each of these three cultural settings, let us assume that the parents and the health professionals whom they consulted were seeking the best possible outcome for the child. But all of the decision-makers (parents and health professionals alike) were also products of their environment. Their decisions reflected not only the medical facts of the case, but also the cultural setting and belief system in which the problem was being considered. By comparing the outcome for children with intersex conditions living in cultures as different as that of Lucknow in northern India, Hanoi in northern Vietnam, and Melbourne in southern Australia, we have the opportunity to discern some of the cultural influences on medical decision-making. We can also look at differences arising from the timing of genital surgery, because in India and Vietnam, surgery to make the genitalia look male or female is commonly performed in late childhood, adolescence, or even adult life, whereas in Australia, the same surgery is usually carried out when the baby is four to six weeks old.

2. REFLECTIONS OF A NORTH INDIAN PEDIATRIC ENDOCRINOLOGIST

Ethical considerations in the management of intersex disorders in India and similar cultures, as distinct from Western cultures, are, to an extent, highlighted by the evolution of my own philosophy for managing patients with these disorders. I graduated from a pediatric endocrinology fellowship in the USA and returned to my own country to work as a faculty member in a teaching hospital. When I was a trainee in the 1980s, the determining factor for decisions regarding sex of rearing—a factor that determined the protocol for almost all cases except those of virilizing congenital adrenal hyperplasia (CAH)—was, in a nutshell, the size and development of the phallus. If the phallus length and the amount of palpable corporal tissue were generous, a male sex of rearing was advised. If phallus length and tissue were not generous, a female sex of rearing was advised, based on the premise that a neo-vagina with the prospect of satisfactory sexual function could be easily surgically fashioned, whereas the possibility of creating a functional male phallus from a poorly formed pre-existing structure was low (Blizzard). Western thinking has changed since that time. Both the realization that patients with conditions such as 5α-reductase deficiency and 17β-hydroxysteroid dehydrogenase deficiency are often likely to develop a male gender identity (Imperato-McGinley, et al.), and the realization that a somewhat smaller adult phallic length is still compatible with satisfactory sexual function (Reiner et al.), have led to more undervirilized male babies' being considered for male sex of rearing than before.

When I returned to my country in 1989, fresh with the ideas I imbibed during my training, I found a new set of challenging cases in the most populous and backward state of my country. Some were the outcome of late treatment due to economic hardship and scant medical facilities, while others were a reflection of different social mores. I encountered genotypic females, fully virilized from untreated CAH, who had been brought up as boys due to missed diagnosis in the newborn period; they had come to our clinic for the first time at the age of 5, 10, or beyond. To these children, who were unambiguously reared male, I felt that my duties lay in explaining everything to the parents, encouraging them to continue rearing the child as a male, performing necessary supportive surgery, and giving hormonal therapy. Such psychological and social support as could be provided by me and my colleagues in the department was the only source of support for these families, there being no social worker or psychologist trained to provide counseling for these disorders in or near my city.

I often experienced frustration with the families of genotypic females with virilizing CAH who were brought to our attention during infancy. Contrary to my expectations, parents often refused to consider rearing the child as female despite assurances that the child would menstruate and have reproductive capability. I attribute the refusals to ignorance and, in light of the economic and gender issues highlighted below, fear of raising a female child with any hint of a reproductive disorder. Unfortunately, many of these families would discontinue follow-up altogether, despite my assurances that, regarding sex of rearing, theirs was the final decision and it would be respected. My experience was different from an experience reported in southern India. Reporting on 23 genotypic females with CAH, Jini et al. stated that all parents accepted a female sex of rearing (including parents of five patients who had been brought up as boys prior to the clinic visit) if it made fertility possible. In contrast, most parents of 30 undervirilized genotypic male patients preferred a male sex of rearing for their child if in the future, the child would not be able to reproduce as a woman (Jini et al.). It is possible that the advanced literacy rate and progressive society encountered in south and central India allowed for the difference.

The group that brought out the starkest contrast between East and West were undervirilized genotypic males. These babies almost always had a male sex of rearing when brought to us, the visible or palpable external gonad/gonads having given a clue to the parents about the sex of the baby. After explaining the possible disease to the parents, I would emphasize, based on my Western training at the time, that if brought up as male, the future man may not be able to have satisfactory sexual function, whereas the chances were better of sexual function with a feminizing genitoplasty (Blizzard). Invariably, the parents replied that if the daughter they would bring up would not be able to bear children, or worse still, not even menstruate, there would be no chance of her getting married. Any talk of sexual function was therefore irrelevant. She would be all alone in this world with no one to care for her after they, her parents, were no more. On the other hand, if they brought up their baby as a son, he would have a job and survive. God willing, and if the boy wanted it, he would marry. These social considerations were ubiquitous, no matter what the religion of the patient. (Of the eight or so major and minor religions practiced in India, Hinduism and Islam were commonest in my region). It was socio-economic issues, rather than religious preferences, that dictated the parents' course of action. "Doctor, we will have to raise the baby in our society, not yours," was a typical final comment of those who had lengthy discussions with me before making up their minds.

India is a land of great social and economic disparities. The upper class is made up of a fortunate few. Women in that class are educated, though they are still quite traditional compared to women in the West. Their status in society is improving, though it is far from equal to that of men. Although not common, it is possible for a single woman to be a happy, productive member of the society. However, the middle and lower classes, which represent more than 75 percent of India, are highly traditional. Women in these classes have no social status, except through their fathers or husbands. Even if a girl has graduated from college and is employed, a father is not seen to have discharged his duties as a parent if he does not marry off his daughter. Marriage is arranged, and parents or other elders select the marriage partner. Thus a parent is likely to encounter difficulties finding a groom for a daughter who cannot bear children. Many girls with such disorders would be married to a widower with children, or they would be forced to compromise in some other financial or social way. In such a male-dominated society, no one questions whether it would be just if, without first informing the bride and her family, a male with compromised ability to have conjugal relations or procreate were to get married! On the other hand, if it is discovered that a married woman's family has failed to disclose her infertility, and the truth is found out later, she is sent back in disgrace to her father's house, or she faces other, more serious consequences in the house of her in-laws.

The outcome of parental decisions regarding sex of rearing for intersex children in India has been studied. Ammini et al. report on 64 patients for whom sex of rearing had already been decided before the patients arrived at their institution; the majority of the patients were more than 5 years of age at first presentation. The breakdown of cases included 26 patients with virilizing CAH (23 reared as girls and 3 as boys), 10 patients with true hermaphroditism (9 reared as boys), 6 patients with partial androgen insensitivity (5 reared as males), and 8 undervirilised males with disorders other than androgen insensitivity syndromes (5 reared as female). Only the last group showed gender identity discordant with sex of rearing; all 5 of the girls asking for sex reassignment to male.

As I continued to work with and learn from my patients, there was an equally absorbing and sometimes acrimonious debate evolving in the Western world. There had always been, among the giants in the field of intersexuality, differences of opinion regarding the timing and nature of genital surgery. Due to inadequate numbers of long-term outcome studies, the guidelines for surgery had not yet been carved in stone. Physicians and surgeons therefore did what they considered best for their patients, until more data emerged. Now, patient advocacy groups are trying to hasten changes in management practices. As regards the timing of genital surgery in India, considerations in the minds of our patients may or may not be quite different from those in Western cultures. I allude to this issue further in this chapter. But it was the issue of disclosure, also hotly debated at this time, which made me compare the situation in India with that in developed countries.

In India, not just the parents, but often extended family members, and sometimes even all the villagers know about the existence of a disorder in a baby, even if the exact nature of the disorder will become clear only when the baby reaches a tertiary care hospital. Due to the social and economic factors mentioned above, decisions about sex of rearing are dictated as much by social considerations as by medical ones. Obviously, the parents, rather than the doctor, can best interpret the social considerations relevant to the child. Therefore, it is necessary for the specialists caring for the child to place all the facts before the parents so as to enable them to make as informed a decision as possible. Thus, in India, parents have played the primary role in choosing the sex of rearing for their child. In addition, due to the poor state of medical records in our institutions, the poor facilities for communication, and the overwhelmingly large area of our country, it is simply not possible to ensure that information about a patient can be made available to another institution or doctor when the need arises. Therefore the patient's family has to be the vehicle for transfer or safe-keeping of all records.

In contrast to all this, in advanced countries, the first consultation with specialists for intersex disorders has occurred early in the newborn period, when parents have had no time to get over the grief of their baby being born with a serious disease. Doctors, more than parents, have played the primary role of choosing the sex of rearing of the baby (Blizzard). Under these circumstances, doctors use language that will "soften" the shock to the parents rather than speak the blunt language of scientific jargon. The following example is a case in point. I heard a pediatric endocrinologist in an advanced country counseling the parents of a newborn baby with complete androgen insensitivity syndrome thus: "Your baby was never meant to be a boy." Obviously this was an interpretation of the effect that complete lack of androgen receptors has on the body. In my country, no matter how convinced I was of the advisability of rearing a child with complete androgen insensitivity syndrome as a girl (even in the circumstances of my country), I would counsel the parents thus: "Your baby would have been a boy if nature had had its way and no disease had interfered. However, the nature of the disease is such that the child cannot function and may not even look externally or sound like a male. However, if you decide to bring up the baby as a daughter, the following are the advantages…." If, after such counseling, the parents decided to bring up the baby as a boy, I would defer to their decision. The scenario has indeed occurred with a couple of my patients: In one instance the decision for the male sex of rearing was made on religious grounds, and in another, on economic grounds.

Another issue peculiar to India, in connection with intersex disorders, is that of the *hijras*. Specialists in other countries are intrigued by the *hijras* (meaning impotent ones, or, more loosely, hermaphrodites) and want to know what connection, if any, they have with disorders of sexual differentiation. The *hijras* are mainly people with a gender identity disorder or else boys who have been kidnapped and castrated and forced to join the group. Though they wear women's clothes and have female names, they don't look or sound very feminine. Contrary to popularly held beliefs, they are not patients with disorders of sexual differentiation (Kucheria, Ammini, and Taneja). They live in separate close-knit groups and do not like to reveal the details of their lives to "outsiders." Their well-known way of making a living in north India is by singing and dancing at births and weddings (uninvited, of course, but they will not budge until paid handsomely). They also indulge in prostitution. In general, their group is viewed with fear and suspicion and is often subjected to ridicule.

Does their existence have any bearing on the decisions of families with a baby who has a true sexual differentiation disorder? Yes and no. Very few parents have ever asked me whether their baby is *hijra*. Perhaps the very idea and word are too repugnant to them to associate with their child. Those who are concerned word their question this way: "Will my baby grow up to be clearly one sex, after we do the necessary treatment?" To the few parents who have mentioned it, I have had no difficulty answering that their baby is very different from the *hijras*. However, they do have an underlying fear that if a *hijra* group discovers that their baby has genital ambiguity, they will forcibly take the baby away. Obviously, this fear is greater among those of our patients who are at the lowest socio-economic rung. My colleagues and I always bear in mind that the words we use during counseling should alleviate the spoken or unspoken fear in the parents' minds of their baby being *hijra*.

Thus, earning capacity and education, the availability of medical facilities, the status of women in society, and attitudes towards sex and marriage are among the many non-medical factors that play a role in the outcome of disorders of sexual differentiation in India. There is a need to study, more objectively, the long-term psychological, physical, and social outcomes for young people with disorders of sexual differentiation in India; there is also a need for tools to assess these outcomes, validated for our specific culture. One study is ongoing at our center. Summarized here are two preliminary factors considered most and least important by parents while making a decision about sex of rearing for their baby with a disorder of sexual differentiation, and the views of adolescent and young adult patients on the timing of genital surgery.

Seven factors were selected which were thought to represent the common concerns of parents at the time of sex assignment. The factors were: appearance of the genitalia, doctors' advice, ability to bear children, economic independence, religious beliefs, longing for a son or a daughter, and advice of the extended family members. On a Likert scale from 1 to 5, a score of 1 was least important to parents and 5 was the most important. Twenty-eight parents of 25 young patients (median age 3 years) with a disorder of sexual differentiation were administered questions regarding factors affecting decision of sex of rearing. In the parents' opinion, appearance of the external genitalia, medical advice, the ability to bear children and economic independence were listed as the most important factors (scoring 4.9 to 4.3 on the Likert scale), whereas religious beliefs, longing for a son or daughter, and advice of extended family were reported to be least important, scoring 1.6 to 1.2.

Ten patients with ambiguous genitalia ≥12 years who had undergone genital surgery were interviewed regarding the timing of genital surgery. A semi-structured interview was conducted. These were the leading questions: Do you think your genital surgery should have been performed at a younger or older age or the same age? What are your reasons?

Five were adolescents aged 12 to 18 years and 5 were adults (ages 19 to 31 years). Six were reared as boys and 4 as girls. All patients had surgeries late in childhood or adolescence, median age at surgery being 16 years (range 4 years to 19 years). No patient reported being married or sexually active. All patients unequivocally expressed a preference for early surgery, and for it to have been performed early enough so they would not remember the event. Four reasons given in favor of early surgery were that early surgery would (1) decrease the chances of being teased by peers, (2) lead to greater self-confidence because they would not have had to grow up thinking they were different from other children, (3) decrease the chances of discordant gender identity, and (4) have allowed them to avoid the mental trauma of being compared with "normal" children.

The preference of our patients for early surgery cannot be directly extrapolated to the debate on this subject in the Western world, where some patient advocacy groups have been arguing for late surgery based on their sexual experiences. We did not have a comparison group that had had early surgery, nor did we have a group that had had medical and psychological treatment early and surgery later, and whose members already had experience with sexual partners. However, our results do caution specialists working with these disorders in cultures such as ours that late surgery was not preferred by those who underwent it. The results are relevant to the issues confronting the management of intersex patients in India and other countries that share a similar socio-cultural and economic background.

3. OBSERVATIONS ON 29 INTERSEX PATIENTS IN HANOI, VIETNAM

The Socialist Republic of Vietnam is a communist state with a predominantly rural population of 83 million and an average life expectancy at birth of 70.3 years. The literacy rate is 90.3%, but the country is poor, with GDP-per capita of $2500. The religions include Buddhism, Hoa Hao, Cao Dai, Christianity (predominantly Roman Catholic, some Protestant), Islam, and other indigenous religions. The capital city, Hanoi, has a population of approximately 3 million and a surrounding population of perhaps 30 to 40 million.

Medical care is provided by commune health stations and district, provincial, and central hospitals and is on a fee-for-service basis for most citizens except children under the age of 6 years. The percentage of GDP spent on health is 1.29 percent and the per capita funding for health is US$28 per annum. For many people, comprehensive Western-style health care is unaffordable, and they prefer to try cheaper traditional medicines and therapies first. A chronic illness in any member of a poor family is very threatening for economic reasons. The cost of even simple medications, such as estrogen tablets, may place enormous strain on the budget of a Vietnamese family. Hospital stays for children are usually longer in Vietnam than in the West (the average length of stay is between 8 to 10 days) because after-care in the community is lacking. Parents are required to stay with the child in the hospital and provide food, which means that they cannot work and have no income for that period.

The only pediatric endocrinology department in Vietnam is at the National Hospital of Paediatrics in Hanoi. This 500-bed hospital, built with Swedish assistance after the end of the Vietnam War, was opened in 1980. The range of laboratory tests offered there is very limited, and it is not possible to fully investigate intersex conditions. Most patients come from the northern provinces surrounding Hanoi, but some come from very distant provinces in the central and south parts of the country. Mental health issues receive little attention. Although the hospital has a Department of Psychiatry, it is overloaded and cannot provide a counseling service to intersex patients. There are also no genetic counselors or social workers.

The Head of the Endocrinology Department at the National Hospital of Pediatrics, Professor Nguyen Thu Nhan, invited 29 families to attend for interview. Patients were included if they had an intersex condition, were available, and if either they or their parents were willing to speak to the interviewer. Some families were included because their intersexed child was a current in-patient, and others attended expressly to have their child's case reviewed by the visiting expert. The average age of the patients when they first saw a doctor was 3.2 years, and at the time they were seen for this study, 8.9 years, with 6 aged 12 to 27 years. Very few parents spoke English at all, so one of the endocrinologists, Dr. Bui Phuong Thao, interpreted for all interviews. Interviews were unstructured but mainly focused on the experiences of the parents when their child was born and as they sought medical assistance. For many parents, it was the first time anyone had asked them about their emotions. Most parents were asked an open-ended question, without reference to gender, about their child's behaviour, but in answering, most parents related the behaviour to the assigned gender. They were also invited to say what concerned them about the child's future. Older patients were interviewed without their parents if parents and patients consented.

Details for all 29 patients and a summary of the author's contemporaneous notes are recorded in the Table 1 on the next page.

Typically, parents experienced confusion and indecision upon learning of their child's intersex condition. Referral to a specialist was often delayed (patients 1, 3, 5, 6, 8, 9, 10, 11, 12, 16, 20, 24, and 26), and health workers who had no background knowledge of the conditions often gave parents reassurance that was totally inappropriate. Several families were advised to wait until the child was 5 to 6 years old before seeking medical advice.

The child and often the parents were stigmatized in the village because of the child's sexual ambiguity (patients 1, 5, 10, 12, 20, and 24). A particularly pejorative Vietnamese phrase, *ái nam ái nu,* meaning both "hermaphrodite" and "homosexual" was reportedly used in reference to a number of the intersex children by relatives or other villagers (e.g., patients 12 and 20), causing great distress to the parents. Recounting this experience caused the parents to weep. In two cases (patients 25 and 28), a health worker (a radiographer and a midwife) was the first person to use this term when speaking to the parents. The term seems to be used very widely by doctors as well as the lay community.

Some patients (Nos. 3, 9, and 25), on the other hand, were beautifully supported by their local community. One of them (No. 9), a genetic female who became progressively virilized due to undiagnosed non-salt wasting CAH, even negotiated a reversal of gender identity from female to male with the support of school friends but no medical support. He has emerged with high self-esteem and has management responsibilities despite only being 137 cm. tall.

All of the patients with congenital adrenal hyperplasia are members of a CAH Club that was established in 1998. They reported that they found the club to be of tremendous benefit and support. The group currently represents over 200 families.

Genetic counseling is not well developed in Vietnam and several families with multiple children with the same condition (patients 4, 15, 21 and 22) had not been counseled about the risk of recurrence in future siblings. Counseling about the risk

Patient ID	Age when seen	Age at presentation	Genitalia at birth	Assigned sex	Gender behavior	Medical condition	Had genital surgery?	Clinical details and comments
1	4	Birth	Ambig	M	M	46XX/46XY gonadal dysgenesis	N	Microphallus, perineal orifice, R. gonad (2 mL) palp, L. gonad not palp. No mullerian structures. Initially advised to defer investigation and surgery. Risks of surgery & infertility not disclosed to parents yet. Significant social difficulties for child and parents in village already.
2	1.25	Birth	Ambig	M	?	PAIS	N	Phallus 1 cm, perineal orifice, 2 testes, labia-like genital folds. No karyotype. LH 3, FSH 3.8. testosterone 20.6 nmol/L. Ultrasound not done. Surgeon wants to wait until age 3 before operating.
3	7	Birth	Ambig	F	M	No investigations	N	Phallus 2.5 cm, separate genital folds, only L gonad palpable, looks and acts like boy. Probable partial GD. Seen by doctor at birth, parents advised not to worry. When child (girl) started school, teacher urged consultation. Parents then decided to change to a boy's name and are keen to resolve gender question quickly. Other villagers completely supportive.
4	17	Not clear	Ambig	M	F	CAH (SW)	Y (3)	46XX, elevated 17KS, low sodium, high potassium. Short stature, hyperpigmented, voice not deep. Takes hydrocortisone. Repeatedly ill in 1st 2 yrs, not since. Poor surgical result (clitoris removed). Intellectually disabled. Typical female interests but sometimes aggressive. 2 siblings died, probably from CAH (another died of a brain disease). Parents members of CAH Club.
5	0.25	6 wk	Ambig	F	?	CAH (SW)	N	Born with only mild clitoromegaly. Wait and see policy advised. Persistent vomiting started at 10d, doctor not consulted until age 6wk. Then severely salt-depleted and CAH was diagnosed. Came to a hospital 1000 km from home to avoid other villagers finding out.

6	6	2 wk	Ambig	F	F	CAH (SW)	Y (2)	Doctor diagnosed CAH immediately after birth but gave no information or referral. Subsequent vomiting led to dehydration. Seen at 2 weeks and treated with iv fluid and steroids. 46XX. Many adrenal crises before age 3y, none since. Normal linear growth. Still has urogenital sinus. Clitoris is small. Mother belongs to CAH Club.
7	6	Birth	Ambig	F	F	CAH (NSW)	Y (2)	Non-salt loser, diagnosed as neonate. Typical female behavior. Parents concerned about future sexuality. Members of CAH Club.
8	Infant	4 wk	Ambig	M	?	CAH (SW)	N	Initially named as a male. Started vomiting at 2 weeks, village doctor reassured parents. After 2 more weeks, baby was weak and dehydrated. At hospital sodium was 97 mmol/L, potassium "off-scale." Initial karyotype reported 46XY, later repeated and found to be 46XX. Progesterone 56 nmol/L, testosterone 84 nmol/L. Now on hydrocortisone (Cushingoid). Long clitoris and perineal urogenital sinus.
9	27	20	Ambig	F	M	CAH (NSW)	N	46XX, identified as girl until age 14 then independently started transition to male social gender. Never developed breasts or had menses, but knows ultrasound showed uterus. Progesterone 21 nmol/L, testosterone 65 nmom/L. Intelligent and successful in a responsible job. Feels unambiguously male. Attracted to females but no relationships. School friends (including girls) very supportive. Height 137 cm, phallus 5-6 cm, urogenital sinus, hyper-pigmented skin, no palpable gonads. Shaves 2-3 times/wk. Wants surgery to make genitalia male.
10	9	7 mo	Ambig	F	M	46XY, incomplete diagnosis	N	Phallus 4.5 cm, 2 palpable testes, 2 perineal orifices. FSH, LH, testosterone all low. No mullerian structures. Seen by doctor early but advised to do nothing. Still regarded as ambiguous and no decision about gender has been taken. Child wants to be a boy. Cruel and on-going verbal abuse for parents and child in village.

11	4	Birth	Ambig	M	M	46XY, incomplete diagnosis	N	Saw doctor early but advised to wait 2-3 years. Typically male behaviour. Phallus 3.5 cm, peno-scrotal orifice, 2 testes in scrotum. Looks like simple hypospadias but LH, oestradiol and 17KS levels reported to be high.
12	7	6	Ambig	M	?	46XY gonadal dysgenesis	N	At his birth, parents were told he was a hermaphrodite. Grandfather (a doctor) recommended no action, so presentation was delayed 6 years. Parents' relationship suffered and father lives in another town. Child is identified in the village as a hermaphrodite. Has a <2cm phallus with a single peno-scrotal orifice and 2 testes. FSH and LH levels elevated, testosterone undetectable, no mullerian structures.
13	5	2 mo	Ambig	F	M/F	CAH	Y	Diagnosed at 2 months, now on hydrocortisone and fludrocortisone. Parents members of CAH Club. Has a 2-3 cm clitoris buried under skin (clitoris often painful) and 2 perineal orifices. Behaves like a boy.
14	7	7	Ambig	M	M	46XY, incomplete diagnosis	N	Thought to be a girl until testes discovered, then named as a boy. Child is teased but parents have been telling him this is his "fate". Now they want surgery soon. Phallus 2.5 cm, two 2 mL testes, perineal urethra. Male urethra on genitogram. FSH, LH and T all normal, 17KS slightly elevated.
15	21	10	F	F	F	PAIS	Y	Female genitalia but L. testis discovered at age 10y. Not removed until 10y later. Has small breasts, sparse stage 4 pubic hair, a normal clitoris. Wonders if she is a hermaphrodite. Her **brother** (11) has a small (3 cm) penis and two 6 mL testes, no hypospadias.
16	11	4	Ambig	F	F	CAH (NSW)	Y	Ambiguity noted at birth but no attention sought for 4 yrs because mother "knew no better". 46XX, progesterone 49.7 nmol/L, testosterone 10 nmol/L. Now takes prednisolone. Clitoris has been excised, two perineal orifices, pubic hair stage 4, early breast development, not Cushingoid. Reached menarche at 10y.

17	0.9	0.9	M	M	M	?	46XY gonadal dysgenesis	N	46XY, FSH and LH both elevated. Micropenis, impalpable L testis. No mullerian structures.
18	14	?	F	F	F	F	46X9rX)/46XY gonadal dysgenesis	N	Short stature, pubertal delay. FSH 95, LH 37.5, oestradiol 8.3 pmol/L, no mullerian structures seen. No counselling given about risk of gonadal malignancy. Patient does not know diagnosis yet.
19	4.9	1 mo	Ambig	F	M	M	46XY, incomplete diagnosis	N	3 cm phallus, perineal hypospadias, bilateral 2 mL testes. FSH 4, LH 2, T 6.8 nmol/L, oestradiol 67 pmol/L, male urethra on genitogram. No decision on what final sex will be yet.
20	15	14	Ambig	M	M	M	45X/46XY gonadal dysgenesis	Y (2)	Parents first sought advice when he was 14. Called "hermaphrodite" by a relative. Hypospadias, short broad penis, R testis 20 mL, impalpable L gonad. No mullerian structures. Short stature. No endocrine investigations. Has not been counselled about risk of gonadal cancer.
21	7	17 mo	F	F	F	F	CAIS	Y	Hernia containing testis discovered at 17 mo and removed. Referred to Cancer Institute which advised cancer treatment (refused). At another hospital surgeon wanted to operate (again, refused). 46XY karyotype. Female genitalia, R testis (2 mL) in groin, L inguinal scar, no gonad. Prepubertal. Her **sister** (12y, case # 22) has the same condition.
22	12	?	F	F	F	F	CAIS	N	Sister of case#21.Was examined after her sister was found to have testes and she too had testes. No mullerian structures. Female genitalia, bilateral 6 mL testes in inguinal position. Wearing tee-shirt with "Happy Boy" logo. An older sister (14) has breasts, no pubic hair and no menses but she has not been seen by a doctor because she has no lumps in the groin. An aunt (also not seen) is married with no children and she has never menstruated. Family had not been given counselling about CAIS.

23	1.7	1.7	Ambig	M	?	Dysmorphic syndrome, probably Apert's	N	Born with micropenis (<1 cm), hypospadias and bilateral cryptorchidism. 46XY, no ultrasound. Hypertelorism, epicanthic folds, divergent squint, umbilical hernia, developmental delay.
24	5	4	Ambig	M	M/F	46XX gonadal dysgenesis	Y	Extreme poverty. At child's birth, parents were told they had a "hermaphrodite". Initially raised as a boy. Subject of gossip and object of abuse in the village (terrible experience for the mother). Taken to district hospital at age 4, then to children's hospital. Investigations showed 46XX, FSH 5, LH 57 U/L. Mullerian structures present. Was then referred to a surgical hospital. Parents expected surgeon to make child a boy but were told after the operation that he had decided to make genitalia female and that both gonads had been removed. Now has a tiny clitoris, rugose labia and 2 perineal orifices. Parents might not be able to afford oestrogen tablets.
25	5	5	Ambig	M	M/F	Gonadal dysgenesis	N	Tay ethnic minority child. Noted to have atypical genitalia. Other village people completely supportive. At central hospital a technician told mother the child was a "hermaphrodite". Child dresses in a mixture of boy's and girl's clothing. Only wants to play with girls. Phallus 2.5 cm, perineal urethra, R gonad has a hard upper pole and a softer lower pole. L gonad impalpable.
26	10.6	3	Ambig	F	F	CAH (NSW)	Y (2)	Born with darkened and rugose labia but clitoris was considered normal. When later it grew, attention was sought. Serum 17OHP 70.9 nmol/L, 46XX. Now on steroids. Feminine, slender girl. Rugose labia. Clitoris (glans and shaft) completely buried under skin. Two perineal orifices. PH3, breasts stage 1. Parents belong to CAH Club.
27	9	Birth	Ambig	F	F	CAH (SW)	Y	On hydrocortisone and fludrocortisone therapy for CAH. Five adrenal crises in 1st yr, none since. Good cosmetic result from genitoplasty. Parents belong to CAH Club.

| 28 | 5 | Birth | Ambig | F | M/F | ? PAIS | N | Midwife informed parents that child was a "hermaphrodite". Parents thought child was female. Has only very slight clitoral enlargement. Urogenital sinus. Bilateral labial gonads. 46XY, LH 3.5, FSH 7.2, testosterone 0, no mullerian structures. Final gender not regarded as settled. |
| 29 | 4 | 3 | Ambig | F | M/F | 46XY, incomplete diagnosis | Y | Presented with clitoral enlargement and clitoral excision was carried out before any investigations were done. Was then treated for CAH despite lack of investigations. Later referred to Endocrine Unit and found to be 46XY.. When taken off steroids, was found to have elevated 17KS (21 micromoles/d), serum testosterone 24 nmol/L, progesterone 9 ng/mL). Normal electrolytes. Has one palpable gonad (2 mL) and a single perineal orifice. |

of gonadal malignancy in cases of suspected XY gonadal dysgenesis (cases 18 and 20) had not been given.

Several patients (Nos. 5, 6, 8, and 27) had poor general health due to recurrent adrenal crises. Others with CAH became progressively virilized in a way that is rarely seen in more affluent environments. This reflects the high cost of medications that leads some parents to ration the dosage to fit their ability to pay, rather than give the prescribed amount. It may also reflect the inability of the clinic to carry out routine tests to monitor the adequacy of the dosage because the most sensitive test, serum 17-hydroxyprogesterone, is not available in Hanoi and also because the high cost of laboratory tests is prohibitive. No clear diagnosis was available for a number of patients (Nos. 3, 10, 11, 14, 19, 23, 28, and 29) because many tests could not be performed.

Religion did not appear to play a large part in any of the decision-making about the intersex children. One devout Catholic family with two daughters with CAIS had consulted their parish priest who had appropriately advised a medical consultation at NHP.

The quality of the surgery that had been carried out on the patients varied widely, as did the timing of genital surgery. Total clitoridectomy had been performed on two girls (Nos. 4 and 16), while others (Nos. 13 and 26) had an operation that completely buried the glans, causing erections to be painful. The parents of one child (No. 24) were surprised when their child emerged from surgery as a female instead of the male they had been expecting. The surgeon had not sought consent for the sex reassignment, but nevertheless the parents accepted his judgment because he was a professional. One girl with complete androgen insensitivity and healthy inguinal testes was referred to a cancer hospital for chemotherapy, which the parents fortunately refused.

Parents' comments about gender behaviour were obtained in relation to 23 patients. Behavior was considered to be gender-appropriate in 13, gender-inappropriate (i.e., the opposite of what was expected) in 5, and ambiguous (not typical of either sex) in 5. Some parents were quite concerned about their children's behavior. Several patients (Nos. 3, 9, and 24) had changed sexes (in two, from female to male, and in one, from male to female). In four, (Nos. 10, 12, 19, and 28) the gender identity remains uncertain. All parents who continued to feel uncertain about their child's sex said that it caused them great anguish. It is not possible to keep ambiguity hidden for long in Vietnam. Small boys in Vietnam wear either no pants or shorts with the crotch cut out, revealing the genitalia. Gossip in the village soon starts and is hard to stop, once started.

1. A LONG-TERM OUTCOME STUDY OF INTERSEX CONDITIONS IN MELBOURNE, AUSTRALIA

Melbourne is the capital of the Australian State of Victoria, which has a population of 5 million people. Twenty-four percent of the people were born overseas (20.1% from the UK and Ireland, 8.3% from Italy, 5.3% from Greece, and 5.2% from Vietnam, followed by those born in New Zealand, China, India, Germany, Sri Lanka and Malaysia). More recently, significant groups have arrived from Bosnia, Iraq, Ethiopia and Somalia. Victoria's population is predominantly urban. The health system is of a comparable standard to that in western Europe and north America. Australian citizens and permanent residents have universal government-sponsored health insurance as well as optional private health insurance and a pharmaceutical benefits scheme that makes most medications affordable for most people. The Royal Children's Hospital (RCH) is the largest children's hospital in Victoria.

The core team providing care for intersex patients has worked together for over 25 years and has been committed to a policy of disclosing all medical information to the parents of children with intersex conditions since 1984 and to the patients themselves since 1996. Throughout the 25 year-period it has been an advocate of early genital surgery for infants with ambiguous genitalia who are to be female. Surgery at the age of 4 to 6 weeks is advised. The group has also recommended early removal of the testes in cases of complete androgen insensitivity and partial XY gonadal dysgenesis. The group is multi-disciplinary and includes mental health professionals and social workers who are involved with most families. RCH was also involved from the early 1980s in establishing support groups for patients with congenital adrenal hyperplasia and androgen insensitivity syndrome (Warne, 2003). The clinic has published two widely used parent information books (Warne, 1989; Warne, 1997).

The aim of this study was to assess the long-term psychological, sexual, and social outcomes of intersex patients compared with two matched control populations. The original manuscript containing full details was published in the *Journal of Pediatric Endocrinology and Metabolism* in June 2005 (Warne et al., 2005).

Three different aged-matched (18 to 32 years) patient groups completed a self-administered questionnaire of established quality of life and well-being inventories measuring physical health, psychological adjustment, and sexuality, following a mailing to all identified patients. The intersex group (N=50) and the Hirschsprung Disease (HD; a congenital disorder) control group (N=27) were patients who had attended the Royal Children's Hospital, a tertiary center, for their clinical care. The Insulin Dependent Diabetes Mellitus (IDDM) control group was recruited from an adult tertiary hospital. The study was conducted at the hospital-based Murdoch Children's Research Institute and was approved by the Royal Children's Hospital Ethics in Human Research Committee.

The study was planned as an epidemiological study of all patients then aged 18 to 32 years who had had surgery at the Royal Children's Hospital for an intersex condition. One hundred and forty-eight potential participants were identified through a search of specific diagnostic codes in the hospital database. Eleven intersex (IS) patients had died (nearly all from complex congenital abnormalities including heart and/or kidney defects). One patient with a minor genital malformation and five patients with hypospadias had anomalies not severe enough to warrant inclusion in the IS group. Thirty-six patients were not included in the study as they had an intellectual disability (n=2), resided in remote locations (n=3), or could not be located (n=31). Ninety-five individuals were contacted about the study, of which 27 declined to participate, 68 were sent study materials and 50 returned completed questionnaires (participation rate 53%). The final IS sample is representative of the range and frequency of conditions initially identified in hospital records.

Consenting participants received a questionnaire booklet by mail. It was described as a quality of life and well-being survey, investigating the long-term outcomes for people who have been treated for conditions caused by variations in sexual development before birth. The IS group was told that their responses would help provide an understanding of how medical treatment and clinical management has affected different areas of their life. The HD and IDDM groups were informed that their responses would provide a useful comparison. The self-administered questionnaire collected socio-demographic information, along with established inventories measuring physical health, psychological adjustment, and sexuality. The following is a list of the measures used. General Health: Rand-36 Health Status Inventory; Interpersonal Problems: Inventory of Interpersonal Problems (IIPP); Personality: Eysenck Personality Questionnaire Revised (EPQR); Self-esteem: Coopersmith Self-Esteem Inventory (SEI); Anxiety: State-Trait Anxiety Inventory, Form Y (STAI); Trauma Symptoms: Impact of Event Scale – Revised (IES-R); Depression: Beck Depression Inventory, Short Form (BDI); Gender Identity: Personal Attributes Questionnaire (PAQ) and The Bem Sex Role Inventory – Short Form (BSRI); Body Image: Body Parts Satisfaction Scale (BPSS); Sexual Awareness: The Sexual Awareness Questionnaire (SAQ); and Sexual Function and Satisfaction. Individual items were borrowed and modified from various other inventories.

1.1 Results

At the time of data collection, mean age was 25 years (SD 4.0) with a range from 18 to 32 years. In the IS group, there were proportionately more females than in the combined control group (OR = 3.1, 95%CI = 1.3 to 7.2; $p<0.01$). There were no significant group differences on age, education, or socio-demographic variables.

Analysis for measures of psychosocial well being in the intersex and control groups showed no differences on physical or mental health, depression, current anxiety, neuroticism, psychoticism, or stressful life events. The IS group reported lower self-esteem ($p<0.01$) and higher trait anxiety ($p<0.05$) than the HD control group. In the IS group extraversion scores were higher than in the IDDM control group ($p<0.01$). In comparison with the HD group, the IS group reported more interpersonal problems on IIP total score ($p<0.05$).

Analysis based on psychosexual measures showed that the combined control group was more satisfied with size and appearance of their sex organs than the IS group ($p<0.05$). There was a group-by-gender interaction that showed IS males to be the only group reporting that they were "somewhat" dissatisfied with size ($p<0.05$) and appearance ($p<0.01$) of their sex organs. The IS group reported they were satisfied with their overall body appearance, although the HPD control group was more satisfied ($p<0.05$). The intersex group obtained lower scores than HPD on the sexual consciousness subscale of the SAQ ($p<0.05$) and IS females had lower femininity scores than control females ($p<0.05$), but there were no other group differences on the PAQ, BSRI, or SAQ. Sexual activity was defined in the questionnaire as behaviours from self-stimulation or masturbation, to foreplay (arousal with partner), to actual intercourse. The IS group was less likely to experience orgasm than the combined control group ($p<0.05$), tended to experience more pain during intercourse ($p=0.06$), and had more difficulties with penetration ($p<0.01$). In comparison with the IS group, control groups were more likely to have had sexual activity several times or more a week ($p<0.05$). Controls and IS groups did not differ in level of sexual desire or self-reported enjoyment of sexual activities.

1.2 Comments

What these results show is that there were very few differences in the level of psychosocial well-being and psychosexual well-being between a representative group of adults with intersex conditions and two age-matched control populations. Where there were differences, they were mild. The control groups were appropriate in that one group had had major surgery early in life, then long-term follow up, and some subjects had ongoing medical problems. The IDDM group had a long-term medical condition requiring daily attention, frequent contact with endocrinologists over an extended period, and concerns about the effects of the disease on sexual health.

The intersex group included many who had had surgery for ambiguous genitalia. What is significant is that this surgery was carried out when the patients were very young. For nearly a decade, concern has been raised that the policy of performing surgery early denied the individual the right to choose his or her own gender. This is mainly the concern of individuals for whom the long-term outcome has been poor, especially those unhappy with their gender identity (Briffa T, 2004). Such individuals claim, based on their contacts through patient advocacy groups using the Internet, that the proportion of patients with gender identity problems after early surgery is high. In our study population, only two out of 50 people (one with CAH and one with PAIS) changed their gender from female to male, and another person with 17β hydroxysteroid dehydrogenase deficiency, who was assigned female, now wishes to be identified as male, female, transgender and intersex. One person with CAH was assigned female and did not report identifying as male or female. Ninety-six percent of our intersex study population continued to identify as the gender assigned when they were born. Genetic females with CAH rarely develop a male gender identity (Meyer-Bahlburg et al.) and only do so when there has been a delay in the commencement of glucocorticoid replacement and prolonged exposure to androgen excess during childhood. Genetic males with ambiguous genitalia due to PAIS, testosterone biosynthetic defects or gonadal dysgenesis appear to have a higher probability of developing a male gender identity (Melo et al.) than the virilized females with CAH, and the risk of major problems will be greatly reduced if they are assigned as males from the beginning.

Our results indicate the need for improved treatment and sexual counseling for women with intersex conditions to avoid difficulties known to occur with sexual intercourse following vaginal surgery. The surgery required to avoid such difficulties—surgery such as vaginal dilatation or repair of the introitus—is minor. Other reports suggest that difficulties experienced by women with CAH in part appear to relate to lowered libido. The extent to which this can be ameliorated by better counseling and more precise hormone replacement therapy remains to be seen. We also found that intersex patients who were assigned male had a high rate of urological problems (wetting, poor stream, infections) that should be avoidable with the better surgical techniques now available.

2. DISCUSSION

How do parents decide what to do when the sex of the child is uncertain? Under normal circumstances, the decision about the sex of a newborn baby is not a complicated or difficult one: it is based on a fairly cursory inspection of the genitalia. The same applies when the baby has an intersex condition. The parents generally perceive the infant's appearance as being predominantly male or predominantly female and decide accordingly. There may be some bias involved, so if they are hoping for a boy, they may be more likely to interpret any enlargement of the phallus as indicating a male sex. Depending on the training of the birth attendant, any variant anatomy may or may not arouse suspicion of a medical condition needing further investigation and treatment. In Vietnam, some parents with little education saw what in the West would be recognized as ambiguous genitalia as a disorder of the urinary opening rather than as a disorder of sexual development.

How do parents decide what to do when they realize that the child does have ambiguous genitalia? In situations of poverty, they will consult whoever is closest at hand, such as the village's traditional healer, health worker, or elders, and they will receive a wide range of opinions before they proceed and risk incurring expense. The western trained doctor will be the last in line, which means that much of the grieving will have already been done before the family sees the doctor. In underdeveloped countries, referral paths are often lacking and parents can waste much time in following up on incorrect advice.

Is it good or bad to delay surgery to correct ambiguous genitalia? What does the evidence indicate? We have presented some evidence that delaying surgery until late childhood or adolescence leads to greater unhappiness. In India, all patients old enough to have made the decision to have surgery for themselves said they wished the decision could have been made for them when they were infants. In Australia, where early surgery is practiced, only two of 50 subjects changed gender in adult life and two others did not answer the question about gender, for whatever reason. Quality of life for the remaining subjects was good and did not differ substantially from that of two age-matched control groups. We take this as evidence supporting a policy of early surgery, although further modifications to policy are needed to reduce the risk of errors even further.

Is full disclosure of information always in the best interests of the patient? We believe that parents and patients are entitled to the truth, presented to them in a way that they can understand. This is not simple to achieve, and the onus is on the clinicians, who understand the local culture and who are sensitive to the needs of individual parents and patients, to make every effort to communicate in a fully effective way and to ensure that the correct message has been received.

The long-term outcome of intersex conditions is, from our studies, qualitatively different for patients managed in Western vs. Eastern settings. Most of the difference is explained by poverty and poor education. The lack of equity in the availability of medications and services is unacceptable, and strenuous efforts are needed from both the rich countries and the health administrators in the poor countries to achieve better outcomes for the poor.

Is there one ethical framework that applies to all societies, or does each society have its own internal ethical framework? We have only touched the surface of this complex subject, but our view is that people everywhere share similar ethical values. The extent to which these are observed in practice, however, is influenced by poverty. It is difficult to show the same respect for the needs of every individual when there are 200 patients to be seen in a 3-hour clinic; decisions are made on the run, and the chance of making an incorrect decision rises accordingly. The challenge is to ensure that change occurs and that resources are distributed in ways consistent with equity and justice.

The authors gratefully acknowledge the assistance of Professor Nguyen Thu Nhan, Dr. Bui Phuong Thao and Dr. Vu Chi Dung from the Department of Endocrinology, Genetics and Metabolism at the National Hospital of Pediatrics in Hanoi, Drs. Sandeep Julka, Uttam Singh and Preeti Dabadghao at the Sanjay Gandhi Postgraduate Institute of Medical Sciences, and Dr. Ashish Wakhlu at King George's Medical University, both in Lucknow, and the members of the MCRI Sex Study Group (Assoc. Prof. Sylvia Metcalfe, Assoc. Prof. Andrew Sinclair, Dr. Sonia Grover, Prof. John Hutson, Dr. Elisabeth Northam, Mrs. Elizabeth Loughlin, Mr. David Pereira, Prof. Julian Savulescu, Prof. Jeffrey Zajac, Dr. Justin Freeman, Ms. Mary Rillstone, and students Eilis Hughes, Sheri Todd and Juliette Hooper).

Royal Children's Hospital, Melbourne, Australia (Warne)

Department of Endocrinology, Sanjay Gandhi Postgraduate Institute of Medical Sciences, Lucknow, India (Bhatia)

REFERENCES

Ammini, A.C., R. Gupta, A. Kapoor, A. Karak, A. Kriplani, D. K. Gupta, and K. Kucheria. "Etiology, Clinical Profile, Gender Identity and Long-term Follow Up of Patients with Ambiguous Genitalia in India." *Journal of Pediatric Endocrinology and Metabolism* 15 (2002): 423-430.

Besnier, N. "Polynesian Gender Liminality Through Time and Space." In: *Third Sex, Third Gender: Beyond Sexual Dimorphism in Culture and History.* Ed., G. Herdt. New York: Zone Books, 1996, 285-328.

Blizzard, R.M. "Intersex Issues: A Series of Continuing Conundrums." *Pediatrics* 110 (2002): 616-621.

Briffa, T. "Intersex surgery disregards children's human rights." *Nature* 428 (2004): 695.

Herdt, G. "Mistaken Sex: Culture, Biology and the Third Sex in New Guinea." In: *Third Sex Third Gender: Beyond Sexual Dimorphism in Culture and History*. Ed G. Herdt. New York: Zone Books, 1996, 419-445.

Imperato-McGinley, J., R. E. Peterson, T. Gautier, and E. Sturla. "Androgens and the Evolution of Male Gender Identity among Male Pseudohermaphrodites with 5α-Reductase Deficiency." *N Engl J Med* 300 (1979): 1233-1237.

Jini, M., S. Sen, J. Chacko, N. Zachariah, P. Raghupathy, and K. E. Mammen. "Gender Assignment in Male Pseudohermaphroditism: an Indian Perspective." *Pediatric Surgery International* 8 (1993): 500-501.

Kucheria, K, A. C. Ammini, and N. Naneja . "Cytogenetic and Hormonal Aspects of Eunuchs (Hijras)." *J Anat Soc India* 37 (1988): 105-109.

Melo, KF, B.B. Mendonca, A. E. Billerbeck, E. M. Costa, M. Inacio, F. A. Silva, A. M. Leal, A. C. Latronico, and I. J. Arnhold. "Clinical, Hormonal, Behavioural and Genetic Characteristics of Androgen Insensitivity Syndrome in a Brazilian Cohort: Five Novel Mutations in the Androgen Receptor Gene." *J Clin Endocrinol Metab* 88 (2003): 3241-50.

Mendonca, B.B., M. Inacio, I. J. Arnhold, E. M. Costa, W. Bloise, R. M. Martin, F. T. Denes, F. A. Silva. S. Andersson, A. Lindqvist, and J. D. Wilson. "Male Pseudohermaphroditism Due to 17β Hydroxysteroid 3 Deficiency: Diagnosis, Psychological Evaluation and Management." *Medicine* 79 (2000): 299-307.

Meyer-Bahlburg, H. F. L., C. Dolezal, S.W. Bake, A. D. Carlson, J. S. Obeid, and M. I. New. "Prenatal Androgenization Affects Gender-Related Behaviour but not Gender Identity in 5 to 12-year-old Girls with Congenital Adrenal Hyperplasia." *Arch Sex Behav* 33 (2004): 97-104.

Migeon, C. J., A. B. Wisniewski, J. P. Gearhart, H. F. L. Meyer-Bahlburg, J. A. Rock, T. R. Brown, S. J. Casella, A. Maret, K. M. Ngai, J. Money, and G. D. Berkovitz. "Ambiguous Genitalia with Perineoscrotal Hypospadias in 46, XY Individuals: Long-term Medical, Surgical and Psychosexual Outcome." *Pediatrics* 110 (2002): 1-10.9.

Nanda, S. "Hijras: An alternative Sex and Gender Role in India." In: *Third Sex Third Gender: Beyond Sexual Dimorphism in Culture and History.* Ed G. Herdt. New York: Zone Books, 1996, 373-418.

Reiner, W.G., J. P. Gearhart, and R. Jeffs. "Psychosexual Dysfunction in Males with Genital Anomalies: Late Adolescence, Tanner Stages IV to V." *J Am Acad Child Adolesc Psychiatry* 38 (1999): 865-72.

Schober, J. M. "Sexual Behaviours, Sexual Orientation and Gender Identity in Adult Intersexuals: a Pilot Study." *J Urol* 165 (2001): 2350-3.

Warne, G. "Support Groups for CAH and AIS." *The Endocrinologist* 13 (2003): 175-178

Warne, G.L. *Your Child with Congenital Adrenal Hyperplasia.* Melbourne. Department of Endocrinology and Diabetes, Royal Children's Hospital, Parkville, Victoria 3052, Australia 1989.

Warne, G. L. *Complete Androgen Insensitivity Syndrome.* Melbourne. Department of Endocrinology and Diabetes, Royal Children's Hospital, Parkville, Victoria 3052, Australia 1997.

Warne, G, S. Grover, J. Hutson, A. Sinclair, S. Metcalfe, E. Northam, J. Freeman, and others in the Murdoch Children's Research Institute Sex Study Group: E. Loughlin, M. Rillstone, P. Anderson, E. Hughes, J. Hoope, S. Todd, J. D. Zajac, and J. Savulescu. "A Long-term Outcome Study of Intersex Conditions." *J Pediatr Endocrinol Metab* (in press, accepted January 7th 2005).

SARAH M. CREIGHTON

ADULT OUTCOMES OF FEMINIZING SURGERY

1. INTRODUCTION

Intersex conditions usually present in childhood or early adolescence. Where the external genitalia are ambiguous, the diagnosis is made at birth. Presentation can also be later with in childhood with symptoms such as virilization or absent menstruation at puberty (Hughes). Those diagnosed at birth are assessed by a multidisciplinary team, and a sex of rearing is recommended. For the last 50 years or so, standard medical practice in those infants assigned to a female sex of rearing has been to then reinforce that decision by performing feminising genital surgery to align genital appearance with the chosen sex (Money et al.). In those diagnosed later in childhood, it would be unusual to change the sex of rearing. However surgery is usually recommended to treat any external changes such as clitoromegaly or to remove structures not concordant with that sex of rearing such as testes in an XY female.

It is becoming apparent that there is considerable distress amongst patient groups and disquiet amongst some clinicians particularly with regards to genital surgery (Creighton et al., 2002, *BMJ*; Schober, 1998.) Recent debate has focused on all aspects of surgery including indications, timing, and outcomes.

2. SURGICAL PROCEDURES

There are numerous descriptions in the medical literature of surgical procedures used in the treatment of intersex. Selection of the appropriate procedure can be complex and will vary according to many factors including the underlying condition, previous surgery, current indication for surgery, and the surgeon's skills and preferences. For ease of discussion the procedures can be classified into two groups:

1) *Clitoral Surgery*. This is most commonly performed as part of a feminising genitoplasty. Infants with ambiguous genitalia will undergo feminising surgery usually within the first year of life. A genitoplasty comprises clitoral surgery,

S.E. Sytsma (Ed.), Ethics and Intersex, 207–214.

vaginoplasty, and labial refashioning. Clitoral surgery can also be performed without concomitant vaginal surgery.

2) *Vaginoplasty*. This can be part of a feminising genitoplasty but is also performed in those with a shortened or absent vagina but no virilization.

3. ASSESSMENT OF SURGICAL OUTCOME

Although genital surgery for intersex has been widespread for over half a century, collection of longitudinal outcome data has been extremely poor. The policy of feminizing genital surgery to reinforce sex of rearing has been uniformly accepted as appropriate by the majority of clinicians working in this field (Donaghoe, 1991). The assumption that the construction of a functional vagina is technically easier than construction of a functional penis remains unchallenged and leads surgeons to favor female sex assignment (Wilson et al., 1998). Until recently, the only reports in the medical literature were of small series usually published by the operating surgeon, with variable outcome measures and indicators, and with only short term results reported. Collection of data has also been hampered by widespread policies of non-disclosure of diagnosis leaving patients unaware of their diagnosis, unable to access medical or peer support, and unavailable for recruitment into outcome studies. In addition, surgery for ambiguous genitalia has become so universal that it is difficult to recruit those few patients who have not had surgery and their opinion and outcome data largely remains absent (Berenbaum et al., 2004).

Finally, although there has been recent acceptance that surgical outcome data must be collected, there is little consensus on how best to do this. Women have reported not feeling able to discuss sexual matters with their doctors so an absence of complaints in medical records may not mean that sexual experience is positive and experiences relating to elective vaginoplasty in adulthood can be extremely complex (May, et al., 1996; Fausto-Sterling 2000; Boyle, et al.). It is difficult to separate out issues related directly to surgical intervention rather than the underlying difficulties associated with other aspects of an intersex condition.

4. CLITORAL SURGERY

Clitoral surgery is purely cosmetic with the objective of reducing clitoral size. The function of the clitoris is female sexual sensation and enjoyment and this function is unlikely to be enhanced with surgery. Great importance has been placed on achieving a normal female clitoral appearance, as it has been thought this will normalise the psychological development of these children with ambiguous genitals (Money, et al., 1955). Implicit amongst clinicians is the assumption that there is a "normal" size for a clitoris and that the operating surgeon will know what this is and be able to achieve this surgically. There are, however, few reports in the literature regarding overall female genital appearance or the dimensions and positioning of the vagina, clitoris, labia, and urethra, although recent work has confirmed the wide variation in female genital appearance (Lloyd, et al., 2005).

Three main types of surgical procedure for the enlarged clitoris have been described: clitorectomy (or clitoridectomy), clitoral recession, and clitoral reduction. Clitorectomy involves amputation of the whole clitoris including the removal of its innervation and vascular supply. This procedure is no longer practiced in the United Kingdom, but it is still the treatment of choice in some European centers (Riepe et al., 2002). As it is only recently that clitorectomy has fallen out of favor, many adult women will have undergone total clitoral removal as infants. In order to preserve the innervation of the clitoris, various modifications have been reported. Clitoral recession involves burying the clitoral shaft under the pubic bone without removing any erectile tissue. This technique has become unpopular due to reports of pain during arousal (Ansell and Rajfer, 1999). The current most commonly used technique is clitoral reduction. The glans clitoris and neurovascular bundle running along the dorsal aspect of the clitoral shaft are identified and preserved while removing most of the erectile tissue (Baskin et al., 1999).

Concern about the impact of childhood clitoral surgery on future sexual function is of surprisingly recent origin. It would seem disingenuous to assume that extensive surgery to the clitoris would not have an impact on sexual sensation, but pediatric surgeons in the past have been confident that future sexual function would be unimpaired (Rink et al., 1998). Adult patient peer support groups have raised awareness of potential difficulties as a result of clitoral surgery and this has triggered recent work on the effects of clitoral surgery on sexual function. The clitoris is an erotically important sensory organ and its only known function is in contributing to female orgasm. However, sexual response is multifactorial, and the exact contribution of the clitoral glans, clitoral hood, and clitoral corpora to orgasm is poorly understood. Recent work on the anatomy of the clitoris has shown it to more extensive than previously thought, extending behind the pubic bone to reach the anterior vagina (Connel et al., 1998). Further examination of the innervation of the clitoris has demonstrated nerves surrounding the tunica with multiple perforating branches entering the dorsal aspect of the corporeal body and glans (Baskin, 2004). Thus any incision to the clitoral glans, corpora, or hood may damage the innervation.

Attempts have been made to assess the neurological impact of clitoral surgery with varying conclusions. One study demonstrated preservation of a genital electromyographical (EMG) response at the glans clitoris after stimulation of the clitoral dorsal neurovascular bundle in 5 out of 6 children assessed before and immediately after clitoral reduction (Gearhardt et al., 1995). However, preservation of a normal EMG response does not seem to guarantee normal sexual function after clitoral surgery (Chase, 2005). This is likely to be because genital EMG assesses an inappropriate neurological pathway measuring conduction in large myelinated fibers rather than the more appropriate small diameter myelinated and unmyelinated fibres. Sexual function has been compared between adult women with ambiguous genitals who had undergone feminising genital surgery and adult women who had ambiguous genitalia and had not undergone genital surgery (Minto et al., 2003). Overall sexual function scores were poor in both groups when compared to a standard population. However, those who had undergone clitoral surgery were significantly less likely to report experience of orgasm compared with those who had not had surgery. Subsequent work has tested genital sensory thresholds to temperature, vibration and light touch in women with Congenital Adrenal Hyperplasia (CAH). This tests the more appropriate small and unmyelinated nerve fibers and demonstrated marked differences when in compared to normative values (Crouch, et al., 2004). The clitoris and surrounding skin had significantly higher thresholds for all modalities tested and was markedly less sensitive. Sensory input from the genitals is a contributory factor for female arousal and sexual pleasure and is altered adversely by clitoral surgery. Recent studies have been unable to find any significant difference when comparing the outcomes of clitorectomy and clitoral reduction despite the assumption that nerve preservation is beneficial. However, the numbers of patients undergoing reduction who have reached adulthood is small and it may be too early as yet to assess whether nerve-sparing procedures have less of a detrimental effect upon sexual function.

5. VAGINOPLASTY

Vaginoplasty as part of a feminising genitoplasty is most commonly performed for Congenital Adrenal Hyperplasia (CAH). In this condition the internal genital anatomy is normal and a uterus is present with the potential for menstruation. The vagina is fused with the urethra resulting in a single opening on the perineum. The aim of surgery is to create the lower vagina to allow menstrual flow and intercourse.

In women where the vagina is shortened or absent and who have no uterus, such as complete androgen insensitivity syndrome (AIS), vaginal creation with self-dilation is the treatment of choice. This method has few side effects and seems effective although, as with surgery, there is little good data available. The technique is not suitable for children and does not work if there is scarring from previous genital surgery. Numerous surgical techniques have been described for vaginal reconstructive surgery, the two commonest being the McIndoe procedure and intestinal substitution. In the McIndoe procedure a potential neovaginal space is created between the rectum and the bladder and lined with a split-thickness skin graft taken from the thighs or abdomen. The patient however has to continue to maintain her vagina by regular sexual intercourse or dilator use following the procedure to avoid vaginal stenosis (Syed et al., 2001). She will also be left visible scars at the origin of the skin graft site. In intestinal substitution procedures the neovagina is created using a segment of bowel. This requires extensive major abdominal surgery. The main advantage of this procedure is reported to be the avoidance of post-operative stenosis and less need for long term vaginal dilatation. Symptomatic diversion colitis has been reported and can lead to heavy smelly vaginal discharge with bleeding which can be impossible to treat (Alizai et al., 1999).

Newer laparoscopic procedures such as the Vecchietti and Davidov procedures are being increasingly reported. These are less invasive techniques with a quicker recovery period, but as yet outcome data is scarce.

6. OUTCOMES

The aim of vaginoplasty is to allow the passage of menstrual blood flow from an existing functional uterus, if present, and to allow satisfactory penetrative sexual intercourse in adult life. Timing of vaginoplasty is controversial. In children with ambiguous genitalia assigned female, vaginoplasty is commonly performed during the first year of life even though the child will not menstruate for a further 10 or so years and is unlikely to be sexually active until after puberty. Early infant vaginoplasty may be justified if there were good evidence that it produced better long-term anatomical, cosmetic and functional outcomes than later delayed surgery. However, this does not seem to be the case. Most of the follow up studies of vaginoplasty have looked at the exteriorisation of the vagina in congenital adrenal hyperplasia (CAH). High rates of introital stenosis of up to 100% have been demonstrated as well as frequent requirements for repeated reconstructive surgery in adolescence before tampon use or intercourse (Alizai et al., 1999; Creighton, 2001). This is despite the fact most procedures were labelled "one-stage" procedures leading families to assume no further intervention would be necessary for their daughters. Unsatisfactory cosmetic results have been reported in up to 46% of cases although patient opinion on cosmesis has not been sought.

Given that there is no available data to suggest early infant vaginoplasty has a better long-term outcome than later delayed surgery, vaginoplasty in infancy is, then, chiefly to create a reassuring appearance for parents and clinicians. It is true that most of those assigned female will wish to have vaginal intercourse and treatment to produce a vagina will be necessary at some stage. Surgery to the vagina will continue to be performed but delaying this until later in life allows full involvement of the patient in the decision. There may be other practical advantages to delaying vaginoplasty until after puberty. Tissue healing is usually better when vaginal skin is fully estrogenized. Adjunctive treatments to prevent stenosis such as vaginal dilators may be helpful and cannot be used in the young child. Surgical outcomes may therefore be better and the need for repeat surgical procedures should reduce. Vaginal dilators alone may be sufficient to create a vagina in some conditions thus replacing the need for surgery altogether. Early vaginoplasty leaves scarring which precludes vaginal dilation at a later age.

Assessment of the functional outcome of vaginoplasty has focused on women with CAH. Such studies have reported more sexual difficulties in this group of patients when compared to their non-CAH sisters and to women with other chronic medical conditions (Dittman et al., 1992; Boyle et al.). CAH women were less likely to have experienced sexual activity with male partners and were more likely to report pain with intercourse as well as considerable anxiety about sex. It is, of course, difficult to determine the relative contributions of physical and psychological factors in sexual difficulties especially in this group. Lay criticism has also highlighted other factors including poor communication, inadequate follow-up, humiliating encounters with health professionals including medical photography, poor treatment outcome, and inadequate psychological support (Creighton et al., 2002, *BJUI*; Intersex Society). These will of course contribute to patient dissatisfaction and may influence outcome. It is essential that health professionals are aware of these concerns, as many of them are remediable with care and sensitivity.

7. CONCLUSIONS

At present, most intersex patients still undergo feminising genital surgery at diagnosis. This is usually performed at birth in those children with ambiguous genitals or at adolescence in those without ambiguity. In both groups the vagina is an internal organ and is unnecessary until puberty at the earliest. The outcome of early genital vaginoplasty is poor and repeat procedures are common. Complications such as stenosis and persistent offensive vaginal discharge and bleeding are common. Although most women will eventually request vaginal surgery, deferring this to adolescence or later will allow full involvement of the patient and appropriate use of adjuvant treatments such as dilators which may reduce the need for repeat procedures.

It is also increasingly clear that clitoral surgery in childhood is detrimental to adult sexual function. The clitoris is a clear visible external organ and often the focus of parental distress if enlarged. There is great variation in clitoral size amongst children and adults and it is important the family and surgeons recognise this. Clinical management assumes that in normalising the genitals' appearance, psychological and sexual development will likewise be normalized, although the extent to which gender development arises specifically out of the genital anatomy is far from clear. Of course, choosing to defer surgery and leave the genitals unaltered is a difficult decision. It is likely that intersex children and adults are at risk of psychological problems.

However, despite this concern, surgery is not the only possible answer and may not be the best option for every patient. Many adult intersex people with first hand experience of infant genital surgery vehemently condemn this approach and it should be impossible to disregard this view. Our experience is that older children and adult women commonly opt for genital surgery even after a realistic appraisal of the benefit and risks but they have at least had the option of choice. If surgery is deferred, appropriate and long-term psychological and peer support for the patient and their family is crucial. It is important to try and obtain prospective outcome data. Constructive and focused debate between patient groups and health care professionals is needed to determine what information would be most helpful and how to carry out such valuable studies in a way appropriate and acceptable for patients and their families.

Sarah Creighton, Consultant Gynecologist at University College Hospital, London, U.K. and at Great Ormond Street Hospital, London, U.K.

REFERENCES

Alizai, N. K., D. Thomas, R. Lilford, A. Batchelor, and N. Johnson. "Feminizing Genitoplasty for Congenital Adrenal Hyperplasia: What Happens at Puberty?" *Journal of Urology* 161.5 (1999): 1588.

Ansell, J. and J. Rajfer. "A New Simplified Method for Concealing the Hypertrophied Clitoris." *Journal of Paediaric Surgery* 16.5 (1999): 681-694.

Baskin, L., A. Erol, Y. Li, W. Liu, E. Kurzock, and G. Cunha. "Anatomical Studies of the Human Clitoris." *Journal of Urology* 162 (1999): 1015-1020

Baskin, L., "Anatomical Studies of the Female Genitalia: Surgical Reconstructive Implications." *Journal of Pediatric Endocrinological Metabolism* 17.4 (2004): 581-587.

Berenbaum, S., B. Korman, S. Duck, and S. Resnick. "Psychological Adjustment in Children and Adults with Congenital Adrenal Hyperplasia." *Journal of Pediatrics* 144: (2004): 741-746.

Boyle, M., S. Smith, and L. M. Liao. "Adult Genital Surgery for Intersex: A Solution to What Problem?" *Journal of Health Psychology*, forthcoming.

Chase, C., "Re: Measurement of Pudendal Evoked Potentials During Feminizing Genitoplasty: Technique and Applications." *Journal of Urology* 156.3 (2005): 1139-1140.

Connell, H., J. Hutson, C. Anderson, and R. Plenter. "Anatomical Relationship Between Urethra and Clitoris." *Journal of Urology* 159 (1998): 1892-1897.

Creighton, S., C. Minto, and S. Steele. "Objective Cosmetic and Anatomical Outcomes at Adolescence of Feminising Surgery for Ambiguous Genitalia Done in Childhood." *Lancet.* 358 (July 14, 2001): 124-125.

Creighton, S., J. Alderson, S. Brown, and C. L. Minto. "Medical Photography: Ethics, Consent and the Intersex Patient." *British Journal of Urology International* 89 (2002): 67-72.

Creighton, S., and C. Minto, C. "Managing Intersex." *British Medical Journal* 323 (2002): 1264-1265.

Crouch, N., C. Minto, L. M. Liao, C. Woodhouse, and S. Creighton. "Genital Sensation After Feminising Genitoplasty for Congenital Adrenal Hyperplasia: A Pilot Study." *British Journal of Urology International* 93 (2004): 135-138.

Donaghoe, P. "Clinical Management of Intersex Abnormalities." *Current Problems in Surgery* 28 (1991): 519-579.

Dittmann, R., M. E. Kappes, and M. H. Kappes. "Sexual Behavior in Adolescent and Adult Females with Congenital Adrenal Hyperplasia." *Psychoneuroendocrinology* 17.2-3 (1992): 153-170.

Fausto-Sterling, A. *Sexing the Body: Gender Politics and the Construction of Sexuality.* New York: Basic Books, 2000.

Gearhart, J., A. Burnett, and J. Owen, "Measurement of Pudendal Evoked Potentials During Feminizing Genitoplasty: Technique and Applications." *Journal of Urology* 153.2 (1995): 486-487.

Hughes, I. "Intersex." *British Journal of Urology International* 90 (2002): 769-776.

Intersex Society of North America, www.isna.org. Accessed Jan 2005.

Klingele, C., J. Gebhart, A. Croak, C. DiMarco, T. Lesnick, and R. Lee. "McIndoe Procedure for Vaginal Agenesis: Long Term Outcome and Effect on Quality of Life." *American Journal of Obstetrics and Gynecology.* 189.6 (2003): 1569-1573.

Lloyd, J., S. Crouch, C. Minto, L. M. Liao, and S. Creighton. "Female Genital Appearance: 'Normality' Unfolds," *British Journal of Obstetrics and Gynaecology.* Forthcoming 2005.

May, B., M. Boyle, and D. Grant. "A Comparative Study of Sexual Experiences" *Journal of Health Psychology* 1.4 (1996): 479-492.

Minto, C., L. M. Liao, C. Woodhouse, P. Ransley, and S. Creighton. "The Effects of Clitoral Surgery on Sexual Outcome in Individuals Who Have Intersex Conditions with Ambiguous Genitalia: A Cross-sectional Study. *Lancet* 361 (2003): 1252-1257.

Money, J., J. G. Hampson, and J. L. Hampson. "Hermaphroditism: Recommendations Concerning Assignment of Sex, Change of Sex and Psychologic Management." *Bulletin of John Hopkins Hospital* 97 (1955): 284-300.

Riepe, F., N. Krone, M. Viemann, C. Partsch, and W. Sippell. "Management of Congenital Adrenal Hyperplasia: Results of the ESPE Questionnaire." *Hormone Research* 58.4 (2002): 196-205.

Rink R., and M. Adams. "Feminizing Genitoplasty: State of the Art." *World Journal of Urology* 16 (1998): 212-218.

Schober, Justine. "Early Feminizing Genitoplasty or Watchful Waiting." *Journal of Pediatric Adolescent Gynecology* 11.3 (1998): 154-156.

Syed, H., P. Malone, and R. Hitchcock. "Diversion Colitis in Children with Colovaginoplasty. *British Journal of Urology International* 87 (2001): 857-860.

Wilson, Bruce, and William Reiner. "Management of Intersex: a Shifting Paradigm." *Journal of Clinical Ethics* 9 (1998): 360-369.

FRIEDEMANN PFÄFFLIN AND PEGGY COHEN-KETTENIS

CLINICAL MANAGEMENT OF CHILDREN AND ADOLESCENTS WITH INTERSEX CONDITIONS

1. INTRODUCTION

We recently published a monograph on making choices in cases of intersexuality and transgenderism in childhood and adolescence. The monograph covered the wide range of intersex conditions and gender identity disorders and their cultural, legal, diagnostic, and therapeutic implications (Cohen-Kettenis & Pfäfflin, 2003). The following text mainly relies on chapters five, six, and seven of this monograph, cutting down the text to about one tenth of its original length and omitting the large number of references to original research.

2. INTERSEX CONDITIONS

2.1 Why parent counseling is necessary

Parents need adequate information and emotional support when discrepancies among the sex characteristics of their child are discovered. Such discrepancies are obvious when the newborn has ambiguous genitals. Sometimes, however, discrepancies are detected only at a later stage in the child's life when it is discovered that the gonads or chromosomes are discordant with the external genitals and sex of rearing. Parents are usually shocked; they often struggle with feelings of shame, anxiety, and guilt. They may also worry about the child's prospects. Adequate professional support is imperative for helping them to realistically appraise the situation, to cope with needless fears, and to address legitimate concerns. Although some intersex conditions are not associated with any additional impairments later in life, some are. Therefore, teams of clinicians, including psychologists and child psychiatrists, need to monitor the child's development regularly. Fully informed parents will better address their child's treatment needs if they know about the possible developmental problems related to the condition. Thus, parent counseling will help keep additional problems in bounds, will help

S.E. Sytsma (Ed.), Ethics and Intersex, 215–223.

parents address the child's treatment needs, and will support both child and parents as they cope with limitations resulting from the condition.

2.2 Why child counseling is necessary

A child whose intersex condition is diagnosed at birth obviously cannot, at the time of diagnosis, make any decisions for him- or herself. Parents and professionals will have to agree upon when and how to inform and support the child as he or she grows up. Generally, the child should be kept steadily informed according to his or her developing cognitive and emotional capacity. If the child's condition is diagnosed long after birth—for example, at elementary school age—the child is usually already aware of something going on. If that awareness causes distress to the child or the family, the child may need counseling. New developmental stages may necessitate new and more specific explanations. The atypical appearance of the genitals may not have bothered the child during infancy, and the issue of infertility may never have arisen in the child's mind until puberty and adolescence. Having reached these stages, however, the child may want to seek professional help to address his or her new concerns, even if the child was already counseled in childhood.

2.3 Neonatal approach

When a child is born with ambiguous genitals, he or she should be referred to a specialized team as quickly as possible. Such a team can conduct a comprehensive examination and then provide a diagnosis and a prognostic evaluation to determine which sex assignment will most likely result in healthy psychosexual development. It is important that parents not be wrongly informed about the sex of their child or given speculative answers to their questions. Clinicians should refrain from referring to the baby as "he" or "she" before the diagnosis is made because it is very hard for parents to revise their image of the child's sex once a sex has been suggested by such language. If the parents have used a nickname for the unborn, they should be encouraged to continue using that name until the diagnostic procedure has been completed and a decision regarding the sex assignment has been made.

Even if the parents can cope with the initial uncertainty, they usually raise the question of what they should say when relatives and friends ask whether they had a girl or a boy. Both available options—to be open about the condition or to hide it—may be equally problematic, and it is not possible to predict with certainty which parents and children will do better with full openness and which will do better with secrecy. Keeping the condition a secret conveys to the child that there is something shameful about his or her condition, but sharing the information involves a risk that the child will be stigmatized. Once information is released, its spread cannot be stopped, and the social environment is not always tolerant of rare conditions. Most parents nowadays choose to wait for their child to grow old enough to decide for him- or herself whether or not he or she will inform peers and other persons about the condition. Infrequently, however, parents feel a need to share their concerns with others, and professional counseling may then be a supportive way of resolving that conflict.

When a child's life is in danger due to an intersex condition, medical interventions have to be undertaken without hesitation. Whether ambiguous external genitals should be surgically "normalized" in infancy, however, is still highly controversial (see below).

2.4   Giving Information and Support

2.4.1   Parents

If an intersex condition is diagnosed at birth, only the parents should be informed. They should know what they might reasonably expect, but it is not necessary to make them worry about events that may never occur. There is great variation in development, even among children who have the same intersex condition. Parents should be informed right away about every consequence (e.g., infertility) that will certainly occur, but not necessarily about other problems that may not occur. Information about the latter may be communicated later, step-by-step, to allow the parents to raise their child adequately and to prevent potential problems. It is paramount, when the team first provides information and counseling to the parents, that the practitioners proceed in an open, honest, and informative way, and that they convey no contradictory information. Continuity in the content and style of the counseling is helpful. Trust is fostered when the parents' needs to discuss and understand their emotions and concerns are adequately met and their questions are comprehensively answered. Full acceptance of the child's condition is of utmost importance. If parents continue to consider their daughter a "failed son" or, even worse, a "freak," this will obviously harm the child's development.

The issue of disclosure should be discussed tactfully and intensively. Parents should realize that not everybody needs to know all details. Close family members and day-care center caretakers must, of course, be informed about necessary medications. In some cases they should be given an explanation about why the child has scars. Other details, for example, the karyogram, do not usually have to be communicated to others until the child is old enough to decide whom he or she wants to inform.

Albeit less frequently than in the past, some of the children who are brought to specialized teams for a first evaluation are no longer newborn and have already been treated as belonging to a certain gender. Sometimes those children will need sex reassignment. A virilized "baby girl," for instance, suffering from an idiopathic hypospadias but with a 46,XY set of chromosomes may have a much better chance of later functioning socially, sexually, and reproductively as a man than as a woman, if the reassignment is done early enough. Parents confronted with such information may experience additional uncertainty and irritation and may need special attendance and ample time to verbalize their doubts and fears. A legal sex change cannot be kept secret, but the environment usually reacts adequately when there is enough easy-to-understand information about why such a reassignment might be necessary.

2.4.2 Children

Information given to children should be tailored to their cognitive and emotional ability to understand and cope with it. This usually requires step-by-step information at different ages, preferably given by the parents, who, if necessary, can be assisted by the clinicians. It is essential that the information given is consistent and that parents and clinicians convey the same information. Parents may need extra sessions to find a language that both of them can use and that is adapted to the child's developmental stage. Sometimes extra sessions with the parents are also needed to help them cope with their own doubts and uncertainties before they are able to discuss the topic unambiguously with their child.

2.4.3 Topics that have to be discussed

Apart from information about their specific intersex conditions, children should be given adequate and timely information about psychosexual aspects of their development. Children with intersex conditions may also need to be informed about some additional phenomena that they may encounter. These phenomena vary, depending on the specific condition. The most common issues are these:

(1) (Genital) surgery
(2) Medication
(3) Learning and language problems
(4) Social problems (due to lack of social skills, lack of assertiveness, and/or cross-gender-role behavior)
(5) Precocious or delayed puberty
(6) Body growth (too short or too tall)
(7) Absence of menses
(8) Sex hormone substitution at puberty
(9) Non-surgical genital treatment (vaginal dilation)
(10) Infertility
(11) Technical aids for sexual contact
(12) Sex reassignment

Depending on the nature of the intersex condition, one or more of the items listed will become an important issue for the individual child or adolescent. For example, a boy with Klinefelter Syndrome may develop learning and social problems, have a delayed puberty, grow very tall, and be infertile. A girl with congenital adrenal hyperplasia (CAH) may need genital surgery shortly after birth (but see below for the discussion on neonatal genital surgery) and cortisone treatment thereafter to restore the hormonal balance; she may be very tomboyish and remain rather short after a precocious puberty. A child with complete androgen insensitivity syndrome (AIS) may need a gonadectomy, will never menstruate, and may need hormones at puberty to feminize her body; she will have to cope with infertility, and she may need surgical or non-surgical interventions to deepen her vagina.

2.4.4 Obligatory information

Some interventions—for example, medication for girls with CAH—have to be started at birth, without the child being able to comprehend the intervention. At some point, however, children will begin to ask questions, often around kindergarten age. They then need adequate information. Whatever questions the child may raise, parents should be prepared to give correct and comprehensible explanations and should not deny the truth, even about permanent impairments. Even if a candid explanation of the child's condition might be hurtful at the time of disclosure, it would be more painful for the child to realize, at a later age, that his or her parents had been dishonest or secretive.

Intersex-related events that are certain to occur should be discussed with the child in adequate language; others that are not certain may only be hinted at. In this way a child may develop the sense that his or her caretakers really care and can be consulted when the child wants to know more. Issues that may come to the fore as early as the kindergarten years (ages 3 to 5) include early surgery (scars), atypical appearance of genitals, medication, hospital visits, and repeated medical exams. Issues that may surface during the elementary school years (ages 6 to 12) include learning or social problems, onset of puberty, stature, and growth hormone treatment. Still other issues that will have to be dealt with in puberty and adolescence may include the need for feminizing or virilizing hormone treatments, absence of menses, and the choice of what to do about a shallow vagina—either nothing, or dilation, or surgery. (The latter decision can only be made with the adolescent's informed consent.) Around the age of 16 or, at the latest, at the beginning of adulthood, patients must be provided with full information, including information about infertility and karyotype. Sometimes, full information can be conveyed in an appropriate manner much earlier.

In our list, we have appointed the last position to the information about the karyotype. From a historical perspective, the karyotype was, apart from the external genitals, the first additional sex dimorphic factor that was identified, and knowledge about karyotype has become common. It is therefore no surprise that parents usually ask about the karyotype of intersex persons, especially now that the karyotype can be identified prenatally. Although it is certainly an important factor, is it nevertheless only one out of dozens of other factors contributing to adult gender identity and gender role behavior. Clinicians and parents struggle the most with information about the karyotype, and parents often do not want their children to be informed about it. Unfortunately, when this information is given, it is all too often given in a thoughtless manner. For example, girls with complete AIS are told, "You are partly a girl and partly a boy," or "Your origins are male." It would be far more appropriate to emphasize the identity of the child by using language like, "You are what you feel, no matter what chromosomes or gonads you have," or "In daily life, it is not the gonads or chromosomes that define who one really is, but gender identity."

We usually explain that people's feelings about themselves largely depend on how they consider their condition. Well-informed patients can cope much better with whatever condition they have than poorly informed ones.

The ages mentioned above are drawn from clinical experience, and they reflect the ages at which certain questions are usually brought forward by children or adolescents. There are, however, great individual differences, and some children fully understand already, at the age of fourteen or even earlier, the implications of their intersex conditions.

2.4.5 Psychological interventions

When informed adequately and in a timely manner, many children with intersex conditions learn to properly cope, within the context of their families, with their conditions and with any resulting limitations. In the context of their peer-groups, however, they may be exposed to additional stress due, for example, to their extremely short or tall stature or to poorer performance at school, and they may feel less capable of dating and other social behavior. This may lower their self-esteem, and a further result may be social withdrawal or a failure to take care of their health (they may "forget" to take medication, for example, or they may not drink enough liquid in conditions where this is essential for survival). Empathic parents are of great support, but sometimes additional psychological counseling is necessary. This is especially true if a child experiences fear of or conflict about intimacy, a subject that most youngsters would not like to discuss with their parents anyway. Continuity of the persons counseling the child during the developmental process through puberty and adolescence should be granted wherever possible.

In rare cases, adolescents choose to live according to the gender role opposite their sex of rearing. In those cases they will need professional guidance similar to that of transgendered individuals without intersex conditions.

The type of counseling and psychological interventions should be chosen according to the specific needs of the individual child or adolescent. For children, treatment goals may be coping with teasing, establishing a satisfying body image, and enhancing social skills and self-esteem. For adolescents, the focus is frequently on coping with grief or rage resulting from the realization that their bodies will not change. Generally speaking, girls tend to react with depression and hopelessness, whereas boys more often try to deny or rationalize their situation. Sexual education plays an important role and has to include information on how to sexually interact when the genitals have functional limitations (e.g., a very small penis).

2.5 Controversial issues

Until the 1980s, decisions on sex assignment and reassignment in intersex children have almost exclusively been in the hands of medical professionals, and the timing and type of surgery was often decided by the medical staff only. Parents often remained uninformed about short- and long-term outcomes of their child's condition. Little evidence-based knowledge about the influence of hormones on brain development or about other long-term results was available. Fortunately, in many cases, there was (and continues to be) no doubt about the sex assignment. The recent scientific interest in psychosexual and brain development in individuals with intersex conditions will hopefully make assignment decisions easier, as well, in less obvious cases.

Also until the 1980s, information given to the parents and patients was often poor and sometimes totally lacking. This has changed dramatically during the last fifteen years, and this volume collects representative surveys. The better-informed the patients and their parents are, the more favourable will be the expected long-term outcomes.

The demand to leave nearly all clinical decisions to the patients and to delay all surgical interventions until the patients, themselves, are mature enough to request or decline them is based on the unfavourable experience of prior generations of patients and has to be taken seriously. It is, for one, an important reminder of the significance of patient involvement in clinical decision-making. However, such a demand is only partly realistic. Obviously, some decisions cannot be postponed and have to be made early in the interest of the child. When it comes to "normalizing" ambiguous genitals, it is less clear what is in the best interest of the child. Although children would probably not suffer greatly from slightly atypical genitals, we have to acknowledge that it is not always possible to predict whether surgical interventions would enhance the quality of life of children with very ambiguous genitals, and even if an enhanced quality of life were assured, it would still be unclear at what time the surgery should be done. The unfavourable outcomes that most opponents of early surgical interventions now refer to are probably the result of a mixture of poor surgical techniques, feelings of shame due to the message that one's genitals are odd, and multiple traumata (e.g., many painful surgical interventions, insensitive behaviour of doctors, multiple genital examinations usually experienced as humiliating, and negative reactions of parents). As adequate evaluation studies in this field are woefully lacking, the current empirical knowledge does not help clinicians much when they have to decide whether a child will profit from no or late surgical interventions. After all, it is conceivable that late surgery also creates trauma as severe as the trauma derived from early surgery. Presently, the most careful way to proceed, in our view, is to decide on a case-by-case basis, taking into account all information available on the prospective outcomes of specific conditions as well as the critiques of early surgical interventions raised by people who were treated without having given informed consent.

3. GENDER IDENTITY DISORDERS

In children, intersex conditions can always be clearly identified and attributed to certain kinds of biological causes, such as, for example, a specifically identified chromosomal defect. Gender identity disorders in children and adolescents (and adults) have no such clear causes. Instead, there are probably many contributing factors, some of which are more accepted as causes by the scientific community than others. The same holds true for treatment options. As some of the individuals with intersex conditions may eventually develop gender identity disorders, we will now shortly discuss diagnostic and treatment aspects.

When a child is seen because of his or her atypical gender behaviour, the first goal of the clinician is to assess whether the child actually meets the criteria for a Gender Identity Disorder (GID) according to DSM-IV-TR. Although there are no somatic parameters on which the diagnosis of GID may be based, there are now elaborate procedures for establishing the diagnosis (Cohen-Kettenis & Pfäfflin, 2003). Such procedures should preferably follow the recommendations of the *Harry Benjamin International Gender Dysphoria Association's: The Standards of Care for Gender Identity Disorders* (Meyer et al., 2001), which includes special sections on care for children and adolescents.

One of the exclusion criteria for GID is having an intersex condition; consequently, it is difficult for an intersex patient to be diagnosed with GID. Instead, the patient may be seen as displaying "cross-gender behavior," a term that can also describe a transient response to a traumatic life event, the reaction of a child who is unable to assimilate him- or herself among same-sex peers, or a boy's limited interest in wearing female undergarments. Even if the diagnosis of GID is established, the clinician may want to explore what past and present factors may have influenced the cross-genderedness of the child and how the child's behavior may be understood within the broader context of his or her family and social background.

In respect to whether treatment is indicated, there is, as yet, no general agreement. Some therapists treat GID in children to prevent homosexuality; others consider such an intention unethical because becoming or being homosexual is not a psychiatric disorder. Some scientists doubt whether atypical gender behavior in children should even be considered a psychiatric disorder rather than a variant of normal and healthy behavior. Indeed, many authors have criticized the DSM criteria, arguing that they do not sufficiently distinguish between healthy, functional, gender-atypical behavior and cross-genderedness. They claim that when the DSM criteria are applied, a healthy group of children is needlessly pathologized and gets unnecessary treatment. Other scientists think that milder forms of atypical gender behavior may be seen as variants of normal and healthy behavior, but that more extreme forms are a disorder and need treatment.

Treatment options also vary widely. Behavior therapists focus on the enhancement of gender-typical behavior and on the reduction of cross-gender behavior. Psychodynamic therapists focus on the any underlying root pathology, and they expect that the cure of this pathology will establish a gender identity in the child congruent with the child's bodily makeup. Elective therapists may focus on any factor negatively influencing the child's functioning, whether that factor is the child's cross-gender behavior or whether it is another aspect of behavior. Controlled studies are lacking, and despite many treatment approaches it is still an open question whether extreme forms of GID in childhood can be cured, or whether they are unchangeable precursors of adult homosexuality and/or transsexualism.

Unlike children with GID, adolescents with GID usually seek treatment on their own initiative. Some are just uncertain and confused about their gender identity. The majority of adolescents consulting clinical services because of gender identity conflicts, however, straightforwardly demand support for their wish to have sex reassignment.

Friedemann Pfäfflin, Professor of Forensic Psychotherapy and Head of the Forensic Psychotherapy Unit, University of Ulm, Germany.

Peggy Cohen-Kettenis, Professor of Medical Psychology at the Department of Medical Psychology, Free University Medical Center, Amsterdam, The Netherlands.

REFERENCES

Cohen-Kettenis, P., and F. Pfäfflin. *Transgenderism and Intersexuality in Childhood and Adolescence: Making Choices.* Thousand Oaks, CA: Sage, 2003.

Meyer III, W.; W. Bockting, P. Cohen-Kettenis, E. Coleman, D. DiCeglie, H. Devor, L. Gooren, J. Hage, S. Kirk, B. Kuiper, D. Laub, A. Lawrence, Y. Menard, J. Patton, L. Schoefer, A. Webb, and C. Wheeler. *Harry Benjamin International Gender Dysphoria Association's: The Standards of Care for Gender Identity Disorders (6th version).* Düsseldorf: Symposion, 2001. (Also available online in the International Journal of Transgenderism: http://www.symposion.com/ijt/soc2001/index/htm).

LIH-MEI LIAO

PSYCHOLOGY AND CLINICAL MANAGEMENT OF VAGINAL HYPOPLASIA

1. BACKGROUND

The vagina can be shortened as a result of medical treatment (e.g. pelvic irradiation) or as manifestation of certain congenital conditions, some classified in Western medicine as intersex (e.g. androgen insensitivity syndrome, AIS) and some not (e.g. Meyer-Rokitansky-Kuster-Hauser syndrome, MRKH). (See Hughes, 2002 for a review). Scientific and ethical considerations relating to vaginal construction and reconstruction via surgery and pressure dilation for infants and young children are addressed elsewhere. This chapter is limited to discussion of consensual treatment for adolescent and adult women.

I use the term 'reconstruction' to refer to all treatment scenarios, including first treatment episode and repairs or further procedures based on patient requests, all of which are common in my service context. Reconstruction involves either surgery or dilation or both. None of these options is straight forward, medically, or psychologically. Even when anatomical outcome is optimal, psychological barriers to the 'normal sex life' that underpin women's decisions can be considerable. In this chapter, I will discuss some of the complexities relating to process and outcome in vaginal reconstruction and suggest psychological approaches that could be helpful.

2. CLINICAL CONTEXT

Reconstructive surgery followed by dilation has been the main treatment option for vaginal hypoplasia. Reconstructive surgery usually involves dissection and lining of a neovaginal space (Minto & Creighton, 2003). Tissues used to line the neovagina have included skin grafts (usually taken from thigh or buttock) or a section of the intestine. These are major procedures and post-operative complications can include contracture in case of skin graft, persistent bloody and/or offensive discharge in case of intestine, and scarring in both cases (Syed, Malone & Hitchcock, 2001). Malignant change in the neovagina has also been reported (Munkara, Malone, Budev & Evans, 1994). Furthermore, although long-term follow-up studies have reported "normal" sexual function in 80-90% of women following these procedures

S.E. Sytsma (Ed.), Ethics and Intersex, 225–240.
© 2006 *Springer. Printed in the Netherlands.*

(Cali, & Pratt, 1968; Martinez-Mora, Isnard, Castellevi & Lopez-Ortiz, 1992), little information is available as to how this was assessed. Research that does not define outcome from the women's perspectives is not helpful for guiding either the surgeon who has to offer optimal clinical advice or the woman who has to make an informed decision.

In light of the uncertainties surrounding surgical reconstruction, it makes sense to recommend pressure dilation, where appropriate, as the first line approach. First described by Frank (1938), pressure dilation involves insertion into the vaginal space cylindrical shapes that graduate in size. Such shapes are usually made of plastic, glass, or Perspex. As for surgical reconstruction, reliable outcome data for pressure dilation treatment are scant. Studies have claimed 'success' rates of up to 80% (Costa, Mendonca, Inacio, Arnhold, Silva, & Lodovici, 1997), but these studies were retrospective and again offered no information on how success was defined and measured. It is not clear to what extent the women actually carried out the treatment program, or what level of effort was required, and for what period of time. As with the surgical studies, no effort has been made to systematically assess subsequent sexual experiences. A recent report with women with MRKH syndrome suggests that dilation is effective and that the women's sexual function was normal on most of the domains assessed (Nadarajah, Quek, Rose, Edmonds, 2005). However, the study was retrospective and the response rate was low. In the largest study series of women with complete AIS (CAIS) to date (Minto, Liao, Conway & Creighton, 2003), most of the research participants had tried dilation–to create or increase vaginal volume or maintain post-surgical volume, a significant proportion of the sample rated their compliance with treatment as poor, and only a third of the participants expressed satisfaction with dilation treatment. This study did assess sexual function and found that compared to the general population, sexual difficulties were more commonly reported by the research participants.

3. DEFINING TREATMENT SUCCESS

There has been very little debate as to what should constitute 'success' for vaginal reconstruction. Women who seek vaginal reconstruction may not be currently sexually active and chooses to undergo reconstruction in preparation for sexual relationships. In these situations, problems encountered during sexual intimacy may not be identified until some years later. Clinicians are likely to base their own evaluation on anatomical outcome, especially when patients do not complain. However, an absence of complaints in medical records or even in interviews with physicians and surgeons may not mean that sexual experiences are positive (see Kessler, 2002). It is important to bear in mind that not all women feel able to discuss sexual matters with their doctors (Boyle, Smith & Liao, in press; May, Boyle & Grant, 1996). A recent pilot study with women undergoing vaginal dilation provided some support for this contention. Despite a thorough discussion on dilation during their gynaecological consultations, several participants later expressed a desire for the information to be repeated (Liao, Doyle, Crouch & Creighton, submitted).

Shame or embarrassment that may not be obvious during medical consultations can impede communication flow or an understanding of each party's perspective.

Outcome expectancy on the part of the women seems to transcend mere physical changes. A recent qualitative study with intersex women suggests that the participants had expected surgery to transform their 'outsider' (abnormal) status to 'insider' (normal) status, thereby conferring upon them entitlement to relationships and sexual intimacy (Boyle et al., in press). So great was the desire for surgery that the necessity of regular post-operative dilation came to the fore only after surgery, almost as an unwelcome surprise (some women claimed that they simply had not 'heard' the information whilst discussing surgery).

A change in vaginal dimensions will not in itself lead to relationships. Indeed participants in Boyle et al (in press) indicated that surgery per se had not made it easy or even possible for them to subsequently form intimate relationships. On the contrary, post surgery, psychological barriers came into sharp focus, as eloquently expressed by a participant:

> "I felt...like [pause] I hadn't learnt all the social sort of skills that were needed to [pause] you know to-to establish a relationship and that maybe that was the main problem, and having a vagina wouldn't help...there's more going on than just vaginal length." (Boyle et al., in press)

Whilst penetrative sex might now be a possibility, another participant informed us that "hang-ups" about the meanings of the diagnosis now took over as the main barrier to forming relationships.

Women's decision to undergo vaginal reconstruction is, consciously or unconsciously, often driven by gendered aspirations. This raises interesting questions as to what reconstruction is for–a question that becomes important in defining success. Let us consider three examples. If, after reconstruction, a woman is deemed physically capable of vaginal intercourse but has never done so, should she count as a successful 'case'? Consider another scenario where a woman engages in intercourse post-surgery but experiences pain that cannot be explained medically, should she count as a success? For a final example, say a woman is physically and psychologically capable of intercourse but does not do so because she experiences no pleasure, does this represent success? These and many other scenarios common in clinical practice defy neat definitions of success and render any simple counting of cases not especially meaningful.

4.   SURGERY OR DILATION?

Surgery and dilation are of course very different processes. From a woman's point of view, surgery is swift and carried out by experts, whist dilation requires her active management–she would need to, somehow, remain motivated despite the slow progress, discomfort and often pain, and in some situations for an imaginary relationship. It is reasonable to expect many more women to opt for surgery. Indeed in our recent pilot study, only one out of our ten participants cited being able to avoid surgery as an important consideration in weighing up their options (Liao et al., submitted), suggesting that surgery is viewed by the women as low risk and straight forward. Regardless of the accuracy of these ideas of operations to the genitalia, most methods of vaginoplasty need to be followed on by a dilation regime. Thus for many women, the choice is not so much surgery or dilation, but dilation with surgery, or dilation without surgery. An operation could give the woman a 'head start', so that she needs only to maintain the vaginal volume already created, rather than struggle to create the volume first. This said, in my experience, women who have never engaged in a dilation regime are often surprised by the treatment demands after surgery. The result is that many women do not comply with the post-operative dilation regime. Some of the women I see have to live with the end result of stenosis, numbing, and scarring, having derived no real benefit from the vaginoplasty. The absence of benefits for the patient and waste of clinical resources are less of a problem than the fact that where surgery has been unsuccessful because of non-compliance, treatment choice becomes considerably narrower in the future. The presence of scarred tissues is likely to make dilation treatment less effective, even if the woman is ready and willing to take on dilation treatment in future. In many situations then, vaginoplasty is probably best presented not so much as an alternative to dilation, but rather the beginning of the patient's long-term commitment to dilation. In that sense, a woman must be extremely well prepared for any reconstruction involving surgery.

Given such a context, although pressure dilation alone is not particularly rosy as an option, it is a safer first line approach, carries fewer risks, is reversible, and does not compromise future options even if it does not work for the individual. Whichever reconstruction option chosen, however, there are important psychological issues to be addressed.

5. PSYCHOLOGICAL BARRIERS TO POSITIVE OUTCOME

Implied in what I have said up to this point is the idea that anatomical changes must be accompanied by psychological changes if women with vaginal hypoplasia are to fulfil some of the aspirations that underpin their decision to take up reconstruction. I would like to discuss two related sets of issues that could be barriers to positive experiences of sexual intimacy. The first concerns psychological distress associated with vaginal hypoplasia or agenesis and other pelvic anomalies. The second concerns the psychological burden placed upon the sexual act of vaginal intercourse.

5.1 Psychological distress

Recent investigations of psychological well-being of intersex women have reported mixed findings. A small survey by Morgan, Murphy, Lacey & Conway (2004) involved 18 women with congenital adrenal hyperplasia (CAH)–a condition associated with atypical external and internal genitalia for which reconstructive surgery is commonly performed–usually in childhood, reported that these women were psychologically well adjusted. The authors mistakenly equated an absence of psychiatric morbidity with positive adjustment. Overly hasty conclusions are bound to fail to do justice to women's experience of the psychological impact of their conditions. In a retrospective study of 22 women with CAIS (Hines, Ahmed & Hughes, 2003), the authors also found that women with CAIS did not differ significantly with other women in terms of psychological well-being. However, noteworthy is a general observation that a high percentage of research participants have previously sought professional psychological help (see for example Wisniewski, Midgeon, Meyer-Bahlburg, Gearhart, Berkovitz, Brown & Money, 2000). Hines et al. (2003) cautiously conclude: "additional attention to more detailed aspects of psychological well-being in CAIS is needed."

Indeed women born with atypical genitalia have specific concerns including, for example, identity issues and confusion that are not always readily detected in standard surveys with pre-conceived response categories. Research employing standard surveys need to make explicit what dimensions they have assessed as well as what they have not assessed. Women (and men) with stigmatising characteristics who are able to hide their 'difference' and who succeed in avoiding exposure can indeed 'function' well despite a private sense of shame (e.g. Keegan, Liao & Boyle, 2003; Chadwick, Boyle & Liao, in press).

Rather than using standard surveys, a small number of recent studies have made use of in-depth interviews with intersex women, that is, the researchers met with the women and asked them to define challenges in their own terms and tape recorded the interviews for repeated analyses using methods developed in social studies. Whilst the women were 'functioning' well on the whole (keeping up with day to day activities) and did not present major mental health problems, they were deeply concerned about aspects of their condition and the ramifications (Alderson, Madill & Balen, 2003; Boyle et al., in press; May et al., 1996). Their results are corroborated by lay reports by intersex women themselves (e.g. Simmonds, 2004; www.ahn.org.uk). Some of the key themes are briefly mentioned below.

5.1.1. Relationship non-entitlement
Women with a shortened vagina and other congenital pelvic anomalies often talk of feeling like outsiders and of feeling unentitled to relationships (Boyle et al., in press). Some say that they could not imagine 'finding anyone' until they were 'fixed' by experts. At the point of seeking reconstruction, a woman may not be sexually experienced or have tested out their many negative assumptions about themselves and about men in general. I have come across women who would not consider as much as befriending a male colleague in the most general way until they have been 'fixed', even though any friendly social interaction may never have led to sexual intimacy. Avoidance effectively removes opportunities for learning to increase control in social situations and for testing out other people's responses, thereby falsely affirming the negative assumptions held. But does surgical 'fixing' subsequently enable women to explore relationships? In my experience the answer is not obvious; often different barriers emerge and more 'fixing' may be requested. Much more research is needed to clarify in what ways reconstruction affects women's lives positively, or not.

5.1.2. Communication dilemma

Secrecy has been central to the traditional management of congenital pelvic anomalies associated with intersex (see Anonymous, 1994; Simmonds, 2004). Complaints from patients range from inadequate information and non-discussion to outright deception (e.g. being told that the procedure was a hysterectomy when testes were being removed). Where satisfactory answers were not forthcoming, few would press hard for fear of upsetting doctors or family members. As a mid-aged woman with CAIS said, her father "would have walked out of the room" if the remotest reference were made about reasons for the visits to the doctors. Other women have told me that their mother "would just burst into tears", that "all she would say is that she had been through hell."

At the same time, some clinicians had been unable to hide their curiosity about non-typical aspects of the anatomy. A research participant with CAIS once said to me, "I remember being paraded in a lecture, they'd been discussing it and then the door opened and I was put in front of them" (Liao, 2003). Examinations, treatment, and monitoring of the genitalia may be experienced as shaming and may directly or indirectly communicate notions of deformity. These experiences could well have contributed to some women's aversion of their own genitalia (see below), which is often evident in my practice.

Clinical services must make a conscious effort to avoid a sole preoccupation with the patient's sexual apparatus and offer plenty of opportunities for debriefing. Consultations that are skilfully and sensitively conducted would at least not add to the already considerable negative psychological effects on the patient's self-evaluation and sexuality. Criticism from patient forums has indeed led to positive changes in clinical management in intersex, at least in select quarters. Within a new paradigm, collaboration between clinicians and patients is strongly encouraged. But these changes raise new issues and pose different challenges to women. With full diagnostic and treatment knowledge, decisions about disclosure are now the woman's responsibility. But many women do not feel in control of these decisions. Having to explain about vaginal hypoplasia and other atypical genital characteristics to potential partners is often viewed as the most daunting task for those not in relationships. It is frequently cited as a reason for not seeking relationships.

5.1.3. Genital aversion

Pressure dilation, which is so central to reconstruction, puts the woman in regular physical contact with her genitals. Some women may experience a degree of aversion in looking at their genitals, which may be in response to the negative messages discussed above, and/or related to general dislike of their genitals by many women in the general population (Howard, 1997). Preves (1998) reminds us that "being encouraged to keep silent about their differences and surgical alterations only served to enforce feelings of isolation, stigma and shame." Clinical psychologists in the field have observed that deception, evasive answers, and hushed tones by people in authority have had a profoundly negative psychological impact on the body and self perceptions of many intersex women (e.g. Alderson et al., 2004; Boyle et al., in press; Liao, 2003; May et al., 1996).

For some women, negative perceptions of the genitals may also be exaggerated by an idealisation of 'normal'; negative social comparisons may raise anxiety further. Many women that I see, especially those in the younger age groups, have expressed a wish to know exactly how normal their genitals looked, to therefore gauge whether partners would notice anything unusual. Implied in their questions are assumptions that female genitals look the same, that men are highly knowledgeable about the structure, function, and appearance of female genitals, that they are non-accepting of any variation. Research shows that there is tremendous variability in female genital dimensions in the general population (Lloyd, Crouch, Minto, Liao & Creighton, 2005), though there seems to be little awareness of this in the general public.

Female genitalia are now more visible. Images have become much more accessible due partly to increased availability and acceptability of pornography. However, popular images may be highly selective and/or subjected to digital enhancement, so that they are far more likely to affirm to the public an unnaturally narrow range than to celebrate the natural variations between women (as well as men). Relative to the popular, idealized, and in that sense distorted images of female genitals, visual presentations of female genital diversity (e.g. Blank, 1993) are extremely rare. Feminist contributions appear to be drowned out by the powerful messages that are now influencing more and more women to have their standard genitals surgically enhanced (see Braun & Kitzinger, 2001). Hymen reconstruction has existed for a long time, but now 'tidying up' of the labia, injecting or suctioning of fat in different genital regions, and anal bleaching, are only a few of the many newer additions in genital redesigning for the so-called normal woman.

One effect of negative social comparison and aversion is that some women are less likely to allow contact with their genitals for dilation purposes, let alone autoerotic or partnered activities. These women may be less likely to learn to appreciate their body or derive pleasure from it; they are less likely to access opportunities to help them unlearn their aversion or self-disgust. The genitalia become associated more and more with an overwhelming sense of inadequacy and shame–distress that is deemed relievable only through anatomical correction.

5.2 Preoccupation with 'successful' intercourse

I have heard very few women seeking reconstruction spontaneously allude to pleasure as a reason for engaging or wishing to engage in sexual activities. Ironically, intense preoccupation with 'successful' penetration, which invariably means that men cannot 'tell the difference,' could become an obstacle in optimal sexual outcome in vaginal reconstruction. May et al. (1996) compared the sexual experiences of women with CAH and women with diabetes–both groups had been treated in the pediatric services of the same children's hospital. Preoccupation with intercourse was striking for the CAH group, most of whom had undergone genital surgery. The women with CAH were also less sexually experienced and less likely to problem solve for themselves (e.g. initiate the use of a lubricant for vaginal dryness). It is important to appreciate the reasons for the level of preoccupation amongst women with vaginal hypoplasia or agenesis, reasons that are entirely understandable given our social context.

5.2.1 Doing 'normal' through 'sex'

Women generally do not choose reconstruction just to possess a body part. Rather, reconstruction is taken up to also enable the woman to 'have normal sex.' Almost without exceptions, this means engaging in vaginal penetrative sex with men.

As discussed in Boyle et al. (in press), the fact that reconstruction is deemed necessary for women already capable of sex in the sense of sexual arousal, pleasure, and orgasm, can only be understood in light of the strong linguistic and conceptual conflation of 'sex' and intercourse in society. As one of the research participants said, "I'm not going to have sex because I don't want to have plastic surgery." In other words, sex must involve the vagina (and therefore necessitate reconstruction). Another of the participants made it more obvious still by saying that "sex was penetration, full stop."

The desire for a vagina capable of being penetrated by a penis is strongly related to the psychological meanings of vaginal sex, a particular act taken for granted as a yardstick of womanhood (and manhood). Such meanings are, of course, cultural rather than unique to the person. So strong is the conflation of sex and vaginal intercourse in our contemporary culture that, in their general population study, Sanders & Reinisch (1999) found that some sixty per cent of respondents (virtually all heterosexual) would <u>not</u> say they had 'had sex' following oral-genital stimulation. They cited a 1996 survey conducted by a men's magazine in which seventy-five percent of college students said they would not include in a list of sexual partners those with whom they had engaged in oral sex without intercourse.

Intercourse has historically been seen as a psychologically transformative event, particularly for women (Boyle, 1993). A woman is deemed a virgin despite being sexually experienced, provided that her vagina has not been 'used,' as evident in an intact hymen. And, of course, vaginal intercourse resulting in male ejaculation is needed for consummation of marriage.

For the clinical populations in question, the discursive conflation is also reinforced in some medical encounters in which clinicians also take for granted that the woman with vaginal hypoplasia require reconstruction in order to 'have sex'. Many women remember doctors telling them to return for medical reviews when they are about to get married or have a boyfriend or thinking of relationships. 'Successful' intercourse may indeed resolve some of the psychological issues associated with atypical genitalia, but just as intercourse is attributed transformative powers, it also represents high risk. That is, a woman could become a 'normal' woman through the process of 'normal sex,' or they could, conversely, have all their fears of confirmed about their 'freakishness.'

5.2.2. Sexuality on hold

Elsewhere I have discussed how, with so much at stake, wishing for but not looking forward to 'sex' is not uncommon amongst our clinical populations (Liao, 2003). For women who are not currently sexually active, a situation of high stakes and high returns could mean that some are preoccupied with thoughts about relationships and simultaneously withdraw from potential opportunities. Women could remain in this perpetual state of conflict for years. Excessive preoccupation with one particular sexual act has encouraged many of the women that I see to undervalue other forms of sexual expression. Just as hardly any of them alludes to pleasure as the reason for engaging in sex, hardly any of the (heterosexual) women appears to have considered non-penetrative sexual activities as valid forms of sexual expression between people. In men and women magazines as well as orthodox sex therapy manuals, such activities are consistently referred to as 'foreplay', never as sex.

The somewhat magical view of 'being able to have sex like a normal woman,' coupled with negative self-evaluation and a sense of non-entitlement, effectively removes the opportunity for any form of sexual expression for some women. Not engaging in sexual intimacy but not wanting to raise suspicion about her condition, for example, a young woman told me how she would 'laugh it off' when asked about her plans for relationships or become coy in saying 'Oh I don't talk about things like that' (Liao, 2003).

Those who have not taken the risk to experience different levels of sexual intimacy are vulnerable to unrealistic and idealised portrayals of intercourse, so that psychological barriers are further heightened still. In potentially intimate encounters, some of the women describe spectatoring their own performance and their partners' reactions. Problems become self-fulfilling.

5.2.3. Intercourse as treatment

For some decades, the standard sex therapy advice for couples who experience difficulties with intercourse is to first of all abstain from it, on the basis that in removing the pressure, couples would unlearn their anxiety and sense of 'failure' and thereby restore future possibilities of intercourse. Instead, couples are advised to 'sensate focus', or (re-)discover a range of pleasurable activities together (see Masters & Johnson, 1970). And yet, the typical advice to women who have undergone vaginal reconstruction is that they must either engage in regular intercourse or dilate indefinitely. For example, a recent report on a dilation treatment protocol reads "As soon as the vagina was felt adequate for intercourse she was encouraged to have sex" (Nadarajah et al., 2005). Such advice applies not for a restricted period but indefinitely.

The effects of this on sexual experience for the woman and her partner have never really been examined or discussed, but knowledge of sexual difficulties in general and our understanding of some of the specific psychological difficulties associated with atypical genitalia, suggest that the effects may well be counter productive. Because of the way in which clinicians and patients approach reconstruction, where a woman or her partner subsequently report sexual difficulties, it becomes very difficult to ascertain whether the problems are due to (poor) reconstruction, to psychological barriers, or to both.

6. OVERCOMING PSYCHOLOGICAL BARRIERS

As I have discussed, decisions and outcomes relating to vaginal reconstruction are complex. Many questions remain unanswered. What is clear, however, is that clinical services are best provided by a multi-disciplinary team that makes a firm commitment to address the social and emotional dimensions and not just the sexual anatomy. Within such a service context, a psychologist can make useful contributions that go beyond comforting distressed patients or "trouble shooting" sexual problems as they come up for individual woman. Below are a few brief examples of how psychology can be part of the overall approach.

6.1 Education and counseling

In order for patients to have greater control in clinical situations, they would need to become more expert about their condition and treatments. In order for that expertise to develop, women would need to be informed. But, information relating to congenital pelvic anomalies is invariably distressing. Responsible information giving means that patients and families are not left to contemplate the implications without support. Rather than focusing on diagnostic and treatment information, a 'psycho-educational' approach for information delivery will be needed, using richer vocabularies and drawing from alternative discourses to address the social, emotional, and sexual aspects. With some women it might be important to discuss how best to manage the information. With others, the focus of a therapeutic dialogue may be more on identity or existential issues than practical issues. Decision-making regarding (more) genital reconstruction might also be the focus of counselling for some women. Whereas discussion of genital surgery has typically (if not exclusively) emphasised functionality of female genitals as passive receptacle for the penis, in women-centered counseling, female desire, arousal, and choices are emphasized.

Woman should be invited to set their own agenda in counseling. For some of them, an important psychological task may be to distinguish how "living with the condition" might differ from "living the condition." So not to live by a sexual inadequacy narrative, the woman may need to develop a more questioning attitude towards dominant discourses of sex and sexuality and learn to give themselves permission to explore their sexual and sensual likes and dislikes. In time and with appropriate support, I find that many women are able to reconnect with their resourcefulness and to develop new and more positive narratives–sexual and non-sexual–about the future. Practical tasks such as keeping a diary of thoughts and emotions and talking around them, reading a helpful book, creating dialogue within confiding relationships, constructing new life experiences or re-kindling a lost interest, could all go some way towards becoming or returning to a more positive self identity.

Group work can be very helpful for facilitating positive psychological changes. Groups allow the participants to share common concerns and make available to each other different interpretations and alternative solutions. Most of all, participants can make available to each other diverse identities and positions, thereby effectively deconstructing notions of normalcy. Although the literature is small, there is evidence that group work in gynaecological contexts can be an effective intervention for women who experience psychological distress (Hunter & Liao, 1995; Liao, Abramson & Corp, 2000). A recent study reported that a 7-session group intervention for women with MRKH was successful in reducing the participants' psychological distress (Weijenborg & Ter Kuile, 2000).

In the context of counselling and education that target sexual awareness and overall psychological well being, a more positive decision may be reached about vaginal reconstruction based on helpful, even if sobering, information. Sound clinical advice is only possible when account is taken of not just individual gynecological and medical parameters, but also the risks and benefits of vaginal reconstruction options from the woman's perspectives, and in the context of increased self and sexual awareness.

6.2 Optimizing dilation outcome

Whilst it is important to de-focus on penis-vagina intercourse and to discuss sexual intimacy in broader terms, the importance of vaginal sex is culturally reinforced and vaginal reconstruction will remain an important aspect of clinical management for some time. For all the reasons already discussed, in my service context, women are offered vaginal dilation as first line treatment where possible. But, as already discussed, this self-managed treatment regime can bring distressing emotional issues into sharp focus (Liao et al., submitted)–issues that can compromise treatment adherence. Psychological preparation and coping strategies can help patients to overcome some of these barriers.

6.2.1 Informed decision-making

Psychological research in treatment compliance in other medical contexts (e.g. diabetes) suggests that success in self-management relates to some extent to how the perceived benefits of treatment balance against the perceived costs (Horne & Weinman, 2002). Although many benefits may be reaped in accepting treatments, as far as the patient is concerned, there are also costs to bear or losses to suffer. Apparently, only when benefits of complying with the treatment substantially outweigh the costs is the individual likely to sustain their effort. This line of thinking resonates with psychotherapeutic interventions developed in the past two decades that have come to be known as 'motivational interviewing' (Miller & Rollnick, 1992). According to this framework, not only does the cost-benefit balance need to be favorable, but confidence in ability to perform the action also needs to be high. These authors believe that motivation is best viewed, not as all or none, but a question of extent, which can be increased or decreased. Clinicians can then play a more effective role in increasing motivation, for example, by way of giving information that makes the benefits more salient, by helping the patient to problem solve so to reduce the losses and sacrifices involved in performing the treatment regime, and by increasing support to boost the patient's confidence.

Such a model of self-management can offer useful pointers for understanding compliance difficulties with vaginal dilation because, as already discussed, dilation differs from operative procedures in that it has to be actively managed by the patient and that sustained effort is required whilst progress is slow. Although women may be motivated towards achieving greater vaginal volume and its perceived benefits, they may be equally motivated to avoid the perceived or experienced costs of dilation (e.g. time, effort, pain, shame). It is thus important that clinicians appreciate the costs or disadvantages–practical and psychological–as perceived or experienced by the women themselves in relation to regular vaginal dilation.

Within the psycho-therapeutic framework developed by Miller & Rollnick (1992), it would also be important to assess the women's confidence in their ability to carry out the treatment. Where confidence is low, clinicians can work to increase the woman's confidence. In our pilot study for example, the participants on the whole did not express an overriding sense of confidence in being able to successfully carry out treatment (Liao et al., submitted). In order for them to become more confident, some said that definitive medical evidence of high success rates was needed. This highlights the importance of future research in the effects of dilation and in being able to identify gynecological and psychological variables that influence outcome differentially.

6.2.2. Pain management

Some discomfort and/or pain can be expected from dilation. The way in which an individual interprets and reacts to the pain will significantly influence compliance thereby outcome. Some women who elect to undergo dilation treatment express worries about causing damage to existing vaginal tissue (Liao et al., submitted). In general, anxiety can lead to more anticipation of pain, and anticipation can exacerbate pain experience by intensifying muscular spasms, resulting in a vicious cycle. Bergeron, Binik, Khalif, Pagidas, Glazer, Meana & Amsel (2001) provided an example of successful use of psychological pain management techniques in the treatment of dyspareunia associated with another gynaecological condition (vulvar vestibulitis). The effective strategies in this study included helping patients to become more aware of their thoughts and emotions in relation to anticipation and experience of pain. Furthermore, cognitive techniques to modify the elicited thoughts and emotions were also found to be helpful. Techniques involving mental rehearsal, for example in our case that pain or discomfort does not always reflect damage, can help to reduce anxiety and consequently muscular tension. Relaxation training can be a very useful adjunct in pain management and comes in many forms from which patients can choose.

6.2.3. Maximizing social support

Psychological research in chronic disease in general suggests that successful self-management by patients can be enhanced by the availability of social support (DiMatteo, 2004). Thus, ideally, where appropriate, patients should be encouraged to access support from their personal contexts. However, the nature of vaginal hypoplasia means that this is less possible for many of the women, some of whom have expressed a wish to hear about other patients' experience in dilation treatment

(Liao et al., submitted). Support can be provided by clinical services. As already discussed, groups and workshops provide a useful resource for women to share concerns and encourage each other to persevere. Regular appointments with a specialist nurse and/or psychosexual counsellor could provide opportunities for addressing residual anxiety, for problem-solving practical difficulties, and for receiving positive feedback.

6.2 Assisting colleagues

Joint consultations, case discussions, audit and research with colleagues in gynecology, endocrinology, urology, and nursing provide all with opportunities to learn from each other and to learn to function as a team. Psychologists can also usefully contribute to medical research, e.g. in hypothesising about treatment success and failures, in advising on methodology, in interpreting the findings, and in developing and testing new strategies.

Many women make use of patient support forums. It is possible for clinicians to collaborate successfully with consumer groups to create opportunities for important debates (see for example Creighton, Minto, Liao, Alderson & Simmonds, 2004). Contributions to support group literature or meetings are just some of the tangible ways in which psychologists can help to increase awareness of the possibilities and limitations in vaginal reconstruction.

6.3 Psychological research

More research is needed to address gaps of psychological knowledge in this area, for example, to assess the effects of counseling and education, to improve our understanding of partners' perspectives, to delineate factors associated with differential psychological and sexual outcome in vaginal reconstruction, and so on. It is important for all services to audit the effects of reconstruction along a number of dimensions and using improved research methodology. For example, a baseline psychological assessment of emotional well being, psychosexual perceptions, sexual experience and quality of life, will allow post-treatment effects to be calculated in the short, medium and longer term along multiple dimensions and to test for relationships between the different dimensions.

Some women have, quite rightly, pointed out that dilators are 'not made for women,' i.e. they are made for 'patients' (Liao et al., submitted). Indeed dilators tend to have a clinical appearance and could reinforce women's feelings of inadequacy. More research about women's and clinicians' knowledge and attitudes in relation to the use of erotic aids (e.g. vibrators) as substitute for dilators will enable services to offer evidence--based advice (Crouch, Liao & Creighton, 2003).

On the note of research, however, it is worth reminding ourselves that because conditions associated with atypical genital characteristics are relatively rare whilst the number of questions that need answering is large, the same groups of women may have to participate in one research project after another. Our quest for more knowledge in order to assist the women could reinforce the message that they are 'interesting' with all the negative connotations attached. Workers in this sensitive context must assume the additional responsibility to strike a balance between repeatedly investigating the small populations and tangible achievements for those populations. Research that is patient-driven will hopefully give service users greater control and minimise potential negative effects. It will also lead directly to positive changes in clinical services in future.

7. CONCLUSIONS

It is possible that in the not too distant future, sex will no longer be conflated with penis-vagina intercourse, and possession of a vagina that regularly accommodates an erect penis to the point of ejaculation will become less important in defining womanhood. In this future context, women with vaginal hypoplasia or agenesis will experience more of a choice as to whether or not to undergo reconstruction, because they will feel just as able to access sexual pleasure, intimacy and relationships without it. But, while challenges to heteronormative discourses are beginning to be heard in select quarters and will ultimately influence cultural norms, on the whole, our contemporary world is far from ideal, and virtually all heterosexual women with vaginal hypoplasia or agenesis seek reconstruction–sometimes at extremely high personal costs. Reasons for their decision tend to be based on aspirations 'to be able to have sex like a normal woman.'

Even if we all share an understanding as to what that meant or should mean, reconstruction is far more complex than imagined, medically and psychologically. An authoritative evidence base for the effectiveness of surgery and dilation is currently lacking. Despite that, sheer cultural pressure has ensured that both treatments are widely adopted. More research is needed to help women and their clinicians to deliberate thoughtfully on the treatment options as applicable to individual circumstances. Psychological research methods will enrich outcome data and psychologists have an important role in helping their teams to design studies and make sense of findings. Meanwhile, in listening to multiple sources of 'evidence' including patient experiences, psycho-therapeutic approaches can contribute to more effective strategies in preparing women for reconstruction and in helping women to appreciate that their sexuality can to a large extent be their own making. In addition, women and surgeons may need to learn to counter the cultural conflation of sex and vaginal intercourse and to de-emphasise 'successful' intercourse as penultimate achievement for the woman and her partner, not least because such preoccupations may be counter productive, often resulting in 'sexuality on hold.'

In light of the uncertainties, vaginal dilation provides a safer alternative to surgery. Here psychologists have a crucial role in designing a broader service that is also committed to helping women and where appropriate their partners to explore their thoughts, emotions, and behaviour relating to sexual intimacy. Within such a context, certain psychological procedures can be effective for increasing treatment adherence and for enhancing interpersonal effectiveness in social and sexual situations. Above all, reconstruction counseling provides an important opportunity for increasing sexual awareness, for confronting hopes and fears and for learning to value individual choice despite strong cultural pressure to achieve unrealistic goals or conform to prescribed standards. In that sense, whether or not reconstruction is deemed successful on anatomical or mechanical terms, the woman would have gained useful knowledge and skills for negotiating an optimal sexual life.

Lih-Mei Liao, Consultant Clinical Psychologist and Honorary Senior Lecturer, Department of Clinical Health Psychology, University College, London, U.K.

REFERENCES

Alderson, J., A. Madill, and A. Balen. "Fear of Devaluation: Understanding the Experience of Women with Androgen Insensitivity Syndrome." *British Journal of Health Psychology* 9 (2004): 81-100.

Anonymous. "Once a Dark Secret." *British Medical Journal* 308 (1994): 542.

Bergeron, S., Y. Binik, S. Khalif, K. Pagidas, H. Glazer, M. Meana, and R. Amsel. "A Randomised Comparison of Group Cognitive Behavioral Therapy, Surface Electromyographic Biofeedback and Vestibulectomy in the Treatment of Dyspareunia Resulting from Vulvar Vestibuilitis." *Pain* 91 (2001): 297-306.

Blank, J. *Femalia*. San Francisco: Down There Press, 1993.

Boyle, M. Sexual Dysfunction or Heterosexual Dysfunction? *Feminism & Psychology* 3 (1993): 73-88.

Boyle, M., S. Smith, and L. M. Liao. "Consensual Surgery for Intersex Women: A Solution to What Problem?" *Journal of Health Psychology* (In press).

Braun, V., and C. Kitzinger. "The Perfectible Vagina: Size Matters." *Culture, Health & Sexuality* 3.3 (2001): 263-277.

Cali, R.W., and J. H. Pratt. "Congenital Absence of the Vagina: Long Term Results of Vaginal Reconstruction in 175 Cases." *American Journal of Obstetrics & Gynecology* 100 (1968): 752-63.

Chadwick, P. M., M. Boyle, L. M. Liao. "Size Matters: Experiences of Atypical Genital and Sexual Development in Males." *Journal of Health Psychology*. (In press).

Costa, E. M., B. B. Mendonca, M. Inacio, I. J. Arnhold, F. A. Silva, and O. Lodovici. "Management of Ambiguous Genitalia on Pseudohermaphrodites: New Perspectives on Vaginal Dilation." *Fertility & Sterility* 67 (1997): 229-32.

Creighton, S. M., C. L. Minto, L. M. Liao, J. Alderson, and M. Simmonds. "Meeting Between Experts: Evaluation of the First UK Forum for Lay and Professional Experts in Intersex." *Patient Education & Counselling* 54 (2004): 153-157.

Crouch, N.S., L. M. Liao, and S. M. Creighton. "Dilators or Vibrators; Breaking Down the Barriers." Abstract in *Royal Society of Medicine Section of Obstetrics and Gynaecology Annual Conference* (2003).

DiMatteo, M. R. "Social Support and Patient Adherence to Medical Treatment: A Meta-Analysis." *Health Psychology* 23.2 (2004): 203-218.

Frank R.T. "The Formation of an Artificial Vagina Without Operation." *American Journal of Obstetrics & Gynecology* 35 (1938): 1053.

Hines, M., S. F. Ahmed, and I. A. Hughes. "Psychological Outcomes and Gender-related Development in Complete Androgen Insensitivity Syndrome." *Archives of Sexual Behavior* 32.2 (2003): 93-101.

Horne, R., and J. Weinman. "Self-regulation and Self-management in Asthma: Exploring the Role of Illness Perceptions and Treatment Beliefs in Explaining Non-adherence to Preventive Medication." *Psychology & Health* 17 (2002): 17-32.

Howard, B. "Your Sexual Landscape." *American Health for Women* 16 (1997): 58-61, 108.

Hunter, M.S., and L. M. Liao. "Problem Solving Groups for Mid-aged Women in General Practice." *Journal of Reproductive & Infant Psychology* 13 (1995): 147-151.

Hughes, I.A. "Intersex." *British Journal of Urology International* 90 (2002): 769-776.

Keegan, A., L. M. Liao, and M. Boyle. "Hirsutism: A Psychological Analysis." *Journal of Health Psychology* 8.3 (2003): 311-329.

Kessler, S. J. "Questioning Assumptions about Gender Assignment in Cases of Intersexuality." *Dialogues in Pediatric Urology* 25 (2002): 3-4.

Liao, L. M., Z. Abramson, Z., and C. Corp. "Self-help and Support Groups." (2000) In D. Singer, & M. Hunter (eds.) *Premature Menopause: A Multidisciplinary Approach*, 202-231. London: Whurr.

Liao, L. M. "Learning to Assist Women Born with Atypical Genitalia: Journey Through Ignorance, Taboo and Dilemmas." *Journal of Reproductive & Infant Psychology* 21 (2003): 229-238.

Liao, L. M., J. Doyle, N. S. Crouch, and S. M. Creighton. "Dilation as Treatment for Vaginal Agenesis and Hypoplasia: A Pilot Exploration of Benefits and Barriers as Perceived by Patients." (Submitted).

Lloyd, J., N. S. Crouch, C. Minto, L. M. Liao, and S. M. Creighton. "Female Genital Appearance: Normality Unfolds." *British Journal of Obstetrics & Gynaecology* 112 (2005): 643-646.

Masters, W.H., and V. E. Johnson. *Human Sexual Inadequacy.* Churchill, 1970.

Martinez-Mora, J., R. Isnard, A. Castellevi, and P. Lopez-Ortiz. "Neovagina in Vaginal Agenesis: Surgical Methods and Long-term Results." *Journal of Pediatric Surgery*, 27 (1992): 10-14.

May, B., M. Boyle, and D. Grant. "A Comparative Study of Sexual Experiences: Women with Diabetes and Women with Congenital Adrenal Hyperplasia Due to 21-hydroxylase Deficiency." *Journal of Health Psychology* 1 (1996): 479-492.

Miller, W.R., and S. Rollnick. *Motivational Interviewing: Preparing People to Change Addictive Behaviour.* Guildford Press: New York, 1991.

Minto, C. L., and S. M. Creighton. "Vaginoplasty." *The Obstetrician & Gynecologist* 5(2) (2003): 84-89.

Minto, C.L., K. L. M. Liao, G. S. Conway, and S. Creighton. "Sexual Function in Women with Complete Androgen Insensitivity Syndrome." *Fertility & Sterility*, 80.1 (2003): 157-164.

Munkara, A., J. Malone, H. Budev, and T. Evans. "Mucinous Adenocarcinoma Arising in a Neovagina." *Gynecologic Oncolog* 52.2 (1994): 275.

Nadarajah, S., J. Quek, G. L. Rose, and D. K. Edmonds, "Sexual Function in Women Treated with Dilators for Vaginal Agenesis." *Journal of Pediatric Gynecology* 18 (2005): 39-42.

Preves, S. E. "For the Sake of the Children: Destigmatising Intersexuality." *Journal of Clinical Ethics* 9.4 (1998): 411-420.

Sanders, S. A., and J. M. Reinisch, J. M. "Would You Say You 'Had Sex' If...?" *Journal of the American Medical Association* 281 (1999): 275-277.

Simmonds, M. "Patients and Parents in Decision Making and Management." In A. Balen, S. Creighton, M. Davies, J. MacDougall, R. Stanhope (Eds.) *Multi-disciplinary Approach to Paediatric & Adolescent Gynaecology*. Cambridge, UK: Cambridge University Press, 2003.

Syed, H. A., P. S. J. Malone, and R. J. Hitchcock. "Diversion Colitis in Children with Colovaginoplasty." *British Journal of Urology International* 87 (2001): 857-860.

Weijenborg, P. T. M., and M. M. Ter Kuile. "The Effect of a Group Programme on Women with the Mayer-Rokitansky-Kuster-Hauser Syndrome." *British Journal of Obstetrics and Gynaecology* 107 (2000): 365-368.

Wisniewski, A.B., C. J. Migeon, and H. F. L. Meyer-Bahlburg, J. P. Gearhart, G. D. Berkovitz, T. R. Brown, and J. Money. "Complete Androgen Insensitivity Syndrome: Long-term Medical, Surgical, and Psychosexual Outcome." *Journal of Clinical Endocrinology & Metabolism* 85 (2000): 2664-2669.

SHARON E. SYTSMA

THE ETHICS OF USING DEXAMETHASONE TO PREVENT VIRILIZATION OF FEMALE FETUSES

1. INTRODUCTION

The practice of administering dexamethasone to pregnant women at risk of having children with congenital adrenal hyperplasia in hopes of reducing or eliminating virilization of their female children's genitals began in the late 1970's and has become not only increasingly prevalent, but also increasingly controversial. Because sexual differentiation occurs early in pregnancy, treatment with dexamethasone (hereafter DEX) begins as soon as an at-risk woman knows she is pregnant, ideally around six weeks of gestation. Treatment is discontinued if screening tests later reveal that the fetus is male and therefore unaffected by the disease, but if the fetus is female and affected, treatment continues throughout pregnancy. Although DEX has been administered to adults to treat various conditions for over forty years, it has never been approved for prenatal use, and there has been growing evidence that such use may not be appropriate. This chapter will briefly document the history of DEX use to prevent virilization in fetuses with congenital adrenal hyperplasia and will call attention to some of the problems involved. I will defend the view that, at minimum, prenatal DEX administration should be considered an experimental treatment rather than the standard of care, but that, even as an experimental treatment, prenatal DEX administration requires further justification. I agree with those researchers who have argued that any further experimentation with DEX should take place in the context of long-term, multi-centered, and, preferably, international clinical studies. However, the primary purpose of this examination is not to make proclamations about the propriety of prenatal DEX use, but rather to identify ethical issues involved in prenatal DEX use, to identify criteria that must be met in order for such issues to be resolved, and, to the extent that current practices might be ethically suspect, to speed up the awareness of ethical problems among members of the relevant professions. In order to set the stage for this examination, I begin with some facts about congenital adrenal hyperplasia (CAH) and the traditional clinical approaches to its treatment.

CAH is an autosomal recessive genetic and congenital disease that causes overproduction of androgens, which in females leads to virilization of the genitals. Whereas nonclassic CAH does not become apparent until later in life and poses no

S.E. Sytsma (Ed.), Ethics and Intersex, 241–258

real medical emergency at birth, the classic forms (salt-wasting and non-salt wasting) are apparent at birth, and the salt-wasting form is a potentially fatal medical problem requiring immediate medical intervention.

Virilization is typically classified by five stages commonly referred to as Prader Stages (Prader, 1954). Whereas a female infant with CAH-P1 will have only a slightly hypertrophied clitoris, an infant with CAH-P3 will have ambiguous genitalia (a clitoris that is indistinguishable from a small penis), and an infant with CAH-P5 will have apparently male genitals. Since the 1960's, aberrations in genitalia have been treated as medical and psychosocial emergencies. Doctors have thought it imperative to perform tests to determine which gender an affected child should be assigned to, and then to surgically alter the child's genitals to conform to expectations for that gender. In the United States and England, the surgery for masculinized female genitals used to involve clitorectomy, but more recently, physicians have been using less drastic procedures to normalize the appearance of the genitals. In other European countries and elsewhere, clitorectomy is still a prevalent practice. In the United States, Europe, and elsewhere, vaginoplasty might also be performed.

Such traditional practices regarding infant genital surgery have been called into question, and there is heated controversy over whether the procedures should be performed in infancy, whether they should be delayed until the child can participate in the decision to have them, or whether they should even be performed at all. Some opponents of early surgery have argued, for instance, that surgeries involving clitoral recession have a mere cosmetic function and that infants don't require vaginas. Some have also observed that genital surgeries, whether masculinizing or feminizing, can be followed by significant complications and often need to be repeated (see chapters by Creighton and Liao). Nevertheless, it will probably be many years before there are studies available that conclusively show whether children are better off not having had infant genital surgery. Thus, a method of preventing virilization and thereby obviating any question of surgery is highly desirable. The disease cannot be diagnosed at the embryonic stage, so *in vitro* fertilization followed by embryo transfer is not a viable alternative.

2. HISTORY OF THE USE OF DEXAMETHASONE FOR CONGENITAL ADRENAL HYPERPLASIA

Experimentation with prenatal dexamethasone to prevent virilization of female fetuses began in France in the late 1970's. In their initial reports, the French researchers claimed that the treatment "appears safe for the mother and the child and is effective in preventing virilization of CAH affected females" (David and Forest, 1984; Forest and David, 1989; Forest et al., 1993, 1998; Nivelon et al., 1993). While the researchers noted that the prevention of virilization was not always complete and that a few mothers experienced complications, they nevertheless concluded that the advantages of DEX treatment outweighed the risks and disadvantages.

During the 1990's, articles published in scientific journals began to document a more mixed set of results and attitudes. In the early 1990's, researchers obtained a 75% success rate at preventing or reducing genital virilization, but they voiced concerns about the safety of prenatal DEX treatment both for mothers and for fetuses (Pang et al., 1992; Kelnar, 1993; Levine and Pang, 1994). Nevertheless, the practice of administering DEX to pregnant women was spreading around the world, and articles appeared documenting the practice in Canada (Quertia et al., 1988), Australia (Couper et al., 1993), Germany (Wudy et al., 1994), Spain (Rodriguez et al., 1997), Poland (Malunowicz et al., 1998), Sweden (Lajic et al., 1998), Greece (Spiliotis, 2001), and India (Mathur and Kabra, 2000). The reports from Germany, Canada, Spain, Poland, and India indicated unequivocal success—or at least unsceptical attitudes—but they were based on single cases or small samples. Reports from the United States were also favorable, and they began to involve increasing numbers of pregnant women and infants (Speiser and New, 1994; New, 1995; Mercado et al., 1995; and Carlson et al., 1999). In all of the favorable reports, no concern about future neuropsychological consequences is mentioned.

Sobering studies also appeared. A Swedish study documented "several adverse events" (defined as events requiring hospitalization during the first year) in 8 out of 44 infants prenatally treated with DEX, compared to 1 from the control group. The events included delayed psychomotor development, hydrocephalus, agenesis of the corpus callosum, mental retardation, physical abnormalities, and cryptorchidism (Lajik, 1998). Other studies appeared claiming that children treated prenatally with DEX showed "significantly higher Internalizing and Total Behavior Problems scores. They were more shy, emotional, and less social" (Trautman, 1995; Spiliotis, 2001). Animal studies showed that prenatal DEX led to renal problems, decreases in brain size and short-term memory, and increases in morbidity and blood pressure (Secki et al., 1997; Uno et al., 1994; Celsi et al., 1998; Spiliotis, 2001). (The relevance of these studies for DEX use in human fetuses to prevent virilization, it is true, is not entirely clear. See New, 2001).

Given these results, several doctors and researchers argued that DEX should not be administered unless as part of multi-centered (and preferably multinational), long-term, clinical studies (Miller, 1999; American Academy of Pediatrics, 2000; Brook, 2000; Kelnar, 2000; and Ritzen, 2001). They noted that in order to prevent virilization in any one fetus with CAH, seven other fetuses must also be treated who, because they are male or because they are unaffected females, do not benefit from the treatment—a point glossed over in more favorable accounts. For those seven fetuses, there are no beneficial consequences to outweigh any possible adverse effects.

The same mixture of favorable and uncertain reports continues into this decade. One center in the United States still reports having not witnessed any adverse affects in children treated prenatally with DEX (New, 2001, 2003; Meyer-Bahlberg, et al.; New, 2004). Researchers in the United States have yet to take up the call to participate in multi-centered, multinational, coordinated studies of prenatal DEX treatment. Eight European countries are collaborating on research, but they have yet to release information because of the early stage of the studies (Ritzen, 2001).

Recently, however, the European Society for Pediatric Endocrinology published a study showing significant levels of adverse effects: 53% of pregnant women who began taking DEX at around 6 weeks of pregnancy had adverse effects, as did 8% of treated fetuses (Riepe et al., 2002).

Other significant concerns regarding the safety of DEX relate to its use in treating other conditions. DEX has been widely administered to premature infants to prevent lung disease since the early 1970's (Casper, 1998). In 2000, however, the NIH called attention to follow-up studies showing that infants who perinatally received DEX manifested adrenal suppression, neonatal sepsis, psychomotor delay, behavioral problems, chronic lung disease, decreased somatic and brain growth, and mortality (NIH, 2000). Further recent studies comparing premature infants who received DEX with those who did not have, among the former group, documented increased incidences of abnormal brain growth, poor neurodevelopmental outcome, and behavioral problems in early childhood (Newnham, 2001); lower IQ (Yeh, 2004); increased somatic problems (Stoelhorst et al., 2003); increased incidences of cleft lip and palate (Ozbey, 2002); and increased incidences of cerebral palsy (Murphy, 2001; Doyle, 2001; Barrington, 2001a, 2001b, 2002; Neonatal Formulary, 2002; and Yeh, 2004).

In 2003, researchers conducted a retrospective study of the use of DEX to prevent congenital heart block. The researchers identified 13 fetuses at risk for the condition, 6 of which were treated with 4 to 5 mg of DEX a day from the time pregnancy was diagnosed. Among those six cases, there were two spontaneous abortions, two stillbirths, and two babies born with intrauterine growth restriction and mild adrenal insufficiency. The researchers concluded that using DEX prenatally to prevent congenital heart block was "questionable" because it did not lead to improved outcomes (Costedoat-Chalumeau et al., 2003).

There have also emerged newer and more relevant animal studies suggesting that prenatal DEX treatment might lead to predispositions (some of them gender specific) towards hypertension, reduced cardiac function, glomerulosclerosis, and diabetes in adults (Newnman, 2001; Ortiz, 2002; O'Regan, 2004; Neal et al., 2005; and Burlet at al., 2005). McArthur argues that his studies of rats "have significance for the increasing use of [glucocorticoid dexamethasone] in prenatal medicine and indicate potential mechanisms whereby perinatal distress may predispose to the development of a range of psychiatric conditions in later life" (McArthur, 2005).

Despite the worrying evidence from both animal and human studies, articles asserting the safety of prenatal or perinatal treatment with DEX are still being published (Warne et al., 2005; Nimkarn, 2005). The sheer number of articles that unhesitatingly assert the safety of prenatal DEX treatment encourages many doctors to adopt the practice. However, while I was serving as an ethics consultant at a workshop on intersexuality sponsored by the National Institute of Child Health and Human Development (NICHD) in 2001, several doctors shared their personal uneasiness with me about prenatal DEX therapy. The above review of the published literature seems to vindicate such uneasiness. On the basis of that literature, it is premature to claim that prenatal DEX administration is both effective in reducing virilization *and safe.* The focus of favorable follow-up studies has been on the reduction of virilization of external genitals and on early childhood effects. No detailed studies of the effects of the drug on the formation of the vagina have been forthcoming, nor have there been studies examining the effects of prenatal DEX treatment on sexual orientation. We have yet to determine conclusively whether prenatal DEX treatment affects cognitive ability or whether it predisposes people to adult onset diseases.

3. ETHICAL ISSUES PERTAINING TO USE OF DEXAMETHASONE AS PRENATAL THERAPY FOR CONGENITAL ADRENAL HYPERPLASIA

There are many reasons why prenatal treatment for CAH is desirable and attractive. The virilizing effects of untreated CAH can obviously be traumatic for both the parents and the children. If a case of CAH is severe enough to cause complete virilization, treatment could reduce the possibility that a CAH-affected child might be assigned to the wrong gender. If the case is less severe, the parents can be spared the agonizing choice of subjecting their children to surgery or raising them with ambiguous genitalia. Effective treatment could also spare children the risks and complications of cosmetic normalizing surgery, which often leads to a diminution of sensual and orgasmic capacity. The children could also be spared the adverse effects of either corrected genitalia or uncorrected, ambiguous genitalia on sexual and social development; in particular, they could escape being teased by peers or being isolated to prevent such teasing. Where CAH might otherwise lead to an insufficient vagina or an absent vagina, children treated prenatally could be spared the trauma, pain, and discomfort of vaginoplasty, which often needs to be repeated in adolescence, requires life-long dilation procedures, and is susceptible to many complications.

No one doubts that prenatal DEX treatment is tremendously successful at reducing virilization. The questions that remain, however, are whether it is safe enough, all things considered: (1) to be considered standard treatment, (2) for doctors to recommend it in the clinical setting, and (3) for continued research to be justified, given our present state of knowledge. Some pediatric endocrine societies have collaborated in publishing a consensus statement that DEX treatment should neither be regarded as the standard of care, nor be undertaken independently by physicians outside of centralized studies (Joint LWPES/ESPE CAH Working Group). In this section, I will defend this conservative stance. I will begin with some practical considerations and then proceed to objections based on moral principles.

3.1 Practical Considerations

3.1.1 There Is No Medical Need.
The first practical consideration is that there is no medical need to prevent virilized genitalia. Granted, growing up with ambiguous genitalia would be much more difficult that growing up with normal anatomy. Nevertheless, prenatal DEX treatment is not required for the future, *physical* well-being of the child. And

although escaping surgery might seem to be of medical benefit, infant genital surgery, itself, is not a medical need.

To be sure, medical interventions are often morally permissible when there is no medical need for them. They can be justified by emotional, psychological, or social reasons, whether those reasons constitute actual needs or mere preferences. But medical and surgical interventions should be undertaken only when the benefits are likely to outweigh the risks and when the interventions are consistent with the rights of others. Thus, otoplasty to prevent the psychologically harmful consequences of being teased because of very prominent ears poses no moral problem, since the risks of surgery are minimal and the benefits are obvious. Smile-surgery for those suffering from Moebius Syndrome or other causes of facial paralysis involves greater risks than otoplasty. Nevertheless, those risks seem to be outweighed by the benefits of being able to smile; because facial expressions play an exceedingly important role in communication and relationships, there is an even weightier reason for smile-surgery than for otoplasty. On the other hand, if otoplasty eliminated or compromised hearing capacity, the justification for performing that surgery on children unable to give informed consent would be far more tenuous, as the life-long negative effects of hearing loss could be worse than negative effects of being teased for having large ears.

Infant genital surgery involving clitorectomy, clitoral recession, or clitoral reduction can have life-long negative effects including pain during intercourse, reduced or eliminated capacity for orgasm, and reduced or eliminated capacity for sensual pleasure (see Creighton), effects which could, in turn, form obstacles to sexual intimacy as great as those caused by unusual genitalia. Such surgical interventions cannot accurately be characterized as simple "nip and tuck" procedures with only minor risks—and they are therefore neither moral nor medical requirements. But if infant genital surgery is not a medical need, then prenatal DEX treatment cannot be justified on the grounds that it spares the child the "need" for such surgery.

Prenatal exposure to DEX might also lead to life-long results that outweigh the benefits of decreased virilization. Some of the complications noted in research studies suggest the possibility of consequences that would be significantly more harmful than virilization. Further, even fetuses with CAH may not develop genitals so virilized as to justify the risks of surgery, or by extension, the risks of DEX treatment. As others have argued, there is significant variation in female genital appearance even in non-intersexed individuals (See Creighton). It doesn't make sense to provide treatment to a child before it is even known whether the child has CAH, or before it is known to what the extent the CAH might cause virilization.

3.1.2 There Is a Safer Alternative

A second practical consideration is that the psychological trauma that might occur as a result of ambiguous genitalia can very likely be avoided by a safer alternative that has, to this point, been largely untried: education and counseling. Unlike other physical aberrations or deformities, unusual genitalia do not compromise physical functioning for the child, and they can be easily covered up. Even the difficulty of taking showers in the schools or in gyms is largely exaggerated (Caffrey, 1997). When difficult situations do arise, however, education and counseling can help children and families learn to deal with them. Counseling can also help the child to build self-esteem strong enough to block the sting of offensive remarks by peers and others.

As an alternative to DEX treatment or surgery, counseling has the advantage of not inflicting potentially irreversible, life-long harm as a way of dealing with a delicate situation. Too often we choose short-term advantages over long-term ones. Struggling with physical defects can lead to the development of inner strength serviceable in all areas of life. It is not uncommon for people with physical defects to attest that, in some ways, they feel better off than others because of their defects. Further, it is not even clear that micropenises and hypertrophied clitorises are *defects*.

Although children who are not subjected to surgery or prenatal DEX treatments will face the difficulties of growing up with ambiguous genitalia, parents can explain to them that they chose against surgery and pharmaceuticals because they were worried about long-term consequences. The parents can explain that they didn't want to do something the child would not be able to correct, or could not correct without inflicting more damage. They can say that their love for their child was so strong that they felt confident that they could help the child overcome any painful hurdles on the way to the child's reaching an age at which he or she could decide his or her own gender identity and priorities.

3.1.3   We are Ignoring Other Conflicting Obligations

A third extremely important consideration is that, since CAH is a recessive disease and since male fetuses do not require prenatal treatment, only one out of eight fetuses at risk for CAH will stand to benefit from the treatment. Furthermore, since DEX only reduces virilization enough to prevent the "need" for surgery in 50% of cases, DEX treatment will ultimately obviate surgery for about 1 in 16 children (Brook, 2000). The degree of virilization cannot be predicted even when a woman's previous daughter has been severely virilized due to CAH; thus, even if a fetus is a female affected with CAH, the degree of virilization that would result may not be significant enough to require surgery anyway.

Additionally, there is some empirical evidence that fewer surgeries are being performed on infants with Prader Stage 1 or 2. Responding to the reports of intersexuals who wished they had never had genital surgery, and also responding to research indicating that surgery yields neither normal-appearing nor normal-functioning genitals, fewer doctors are recommending genital surgery in cases of mild masculinization (NICHD Workshop, 2002). Moreover, Peter Lee reports that over the last fifty years, parents of female infants with CAH have decreasingly opted for surgery (Lee, 2002). Two factors have affected the parents' decisions: first, they are more aware of variability in genital appearance; and second, they realize that the relative size of the clitoris will regress as the child grows. According to Lee, these changes occurred independently of complaints by intersex support groups that genital surgery is associated with scarring and desensitization of the genitals. Therefore, if DEX only prevents the "need" for surgery in 50% of cases, but if surgery for more and more of those cases will be declined, anyway, due to the above factors, then the 50% figure further exaggerates the number of surgeries prevented by prenatal DEX therapy.

Finally, while the difficulties of growing up in cultures that do not welcome intersexes should not be downplayed, we should still be asking whether it is intersex children who should be modified to fit the cultural standards, or whether it is the cultural standards that need to be changed. Cultural standards that are based on falsehoods are more susceptible, anyway, to both change and criticism. Those that needlessly cause suffering are morally objectionable. It often appears that truth, by its nature, has an emergent quality. We have passed the time when we can pretend ignorance about intersex being a natural fact of animal and human life.

3.1.4 Research Ethics and Nonvalidated Practices

While the distinction between *therapy* (medical treatment that is provided for the benefit of the patient), and *research and experimentation* (medical treatment designed to increase our body of medical knowledge) is conceptually clear, in actual practice, the distinction between them tends to blur (Levine, 1988). Physicians are free to treat patients using innovative practices, provided they have the informed consent of the patients and reason to believe that the practices will be salutary. Many practices develop without ever having been tested, or without adequate testing, because there seems to be no need for such studies. Further, physicians might use standard medications or procedures for purposes other than those for which they were designed when they have good reason to believe that the treatments will be of therapeutic value for the patient. Such freedom is important because it allows the physician to individualize treatment and can lead to improved healthcare in general. Physicians' freedom to draw from experience also paves the way for official clinical trials that demonstrate the superiority of certain techniques, methods, drugs, or dosages. Innovative practices, untested or insufficiently tested practices, and practices used for something other than their approved use are all examples of *nonvalidated practices*. Their use in the clinical setting is justified if there is reasonable hope of success and if the patient has given informed consent. All promising nonvalidated practices that have been used in the clinical setting and that involve an element of risk should lead to formal research studies that can determine the safety of such practices (Belmont Report).

Since DEX has not been sufficiently tested for prenatal use generally—and never for the purpose of preventing virilization—and since there is now significant evidence that it may cause serious harm, its use to prevent virilization in CAH-affected fetuses should be considered a nonvalidated practice. While there may have been sufficient reason to think prenatal DEX use for preventing virilization was safe when it initially began, and while subsequent causes for concern may not have been based on relevant studies, the newer research since the turn of the millennium imposes, at the very least, a moral obligation, even if not a legal one, to restrict DEX use for preventing virilization to scientific, multi-centered research studies approved by ethical review boards, as Pang and Levine (1994), Lajik (1998), Miller (1999), Ritzen (2001), and others have argued. The integrity of the studies depends on cooperation and coordination with many centers because of the rarity of intersex conditions; international cooperation is highly desirable. Furthermore, efforts need to be taken and documented that the women choosing prenatal DEX therapy have given fully informed consent.

3.2 Objections Based on Major Medical/Moral Principles

The previous objections to prenatal DEX use as the standard of care were based on practical considerations; however, objections to such DEX treatment can be deepened by an application of major moral principles. Such principles give further support to the claim that all DEX use to prevent virilization should take place only under the surveillance of clinical trials carefully scrutinized for scientific and ethical integrity. The principles are also relevant to our last project—that of determining whether continuing clinical trials, at all, is morally permissible.

3.2.1 Nonmaleficence

Given the aforementioned safety concerns, it would appear that DEX use to prevent virilization seems to violate the most basic and central medical professional dictum, "First (or above all), do no harm," (*Primum non Nocere*), also commonly referred to as the Principle of Nonmaleficence. The goal of prenatal DEX use in the minds of practitioners and parents, to be sure, is to prevent the harms of ambiguous genitalia to the child. However, this defense misses the point of the importance of distinguishing between the Principle of Nonmaleficence and the Principle of Beneficence (Beauchamp and Childress; Levine and Lebacqz), and of the significance of the word "*Primum.*" It also overlooks the reason why the principle of "First, Do No Harm" plays such an essential role in medical ethics.

It is important to distinguish between beneficence and nonmaleficence because if they are taken as one principle, the prima facie priority of refraining from harming "gets lost" among the other aspects of beneficence: removing harm, preventing harm, and promoting the good. The prima facie priority of refraining from harm is grounded in the principle that all things being equal, it is worse to actively bring about harm than to let harm occur. The principle that it is worse to actively harm than to let harm occur is vital to the medical profession because of its role in protecting trust. Without that trust, the medical profession's attempts to remove or prevent harm, or to help patients, is severely threatened. Trust is not so easily undermined when nature inflicts physical hardships on people.

3.2.2 Respect for Persons

This principle is also known as the Principle of Autonomy. The principle is rooted in the conception of the intrinsic worth and inherent dignity of persons. Respect for the dignity of other persons requires respecting their rights and allowing them to be self-determining. In familiar Kantian terms, respecting persons means that we ought to always refrain from "treating others as a means only." In the case of human beings who have not developed the capacity for self-determination or whose capacity for self-determination has been diminished, respect takes the form of protection (Levine, 15). While the moral status of the fetus, in general, is a major source of contention, and while some have argued that respect for persons is not required for fetuses, these issues need not be solved here because the fetuses that are being treated are fetuses that are going to term. Therefore, they are subjects in need of protection.

Prenatal DEX therapy to prevent virilization requires subjecting at least seven out of eight fetuses—or perhaps more accurately, fifteen out of sixteen—to the risks of DEX treatment even though they do not stand to benefit from it. They are being subjected to those risks in order to prevent a child from being born with ambiguous genitalia and to spare the parents the burdens of raising such a child. Therefore, they are being treated as a means only.

One might argue that we allow some children to be used as means to help their siblings, and if that is permitted, prenatal DEX treatment should also be allowed. For instance, we permit parents to allow one of their children to be a bone marrow donor to save another one of their children. It has been argued that this is morally permissible because the donor children have an interest in saving the lives of their siblings (Ross, 1994). It might then be suggested that a sibling could have an interest in helping another child who would otherwise be virilized because of CAH. Such an interest is surely not as compelling as an interest in the continued existence of a sibling. Nevertheless, given that there will likely be difficulties for a virilized girl, it is not unthinkable that another child would be willing to take risks to prevent those difficulties, *depending on the risks involved*. If the risks included cerebral palsy, hypertension, cognitive defects, a lowered IQ, or even only a tendency towards shyness, the chances of such willingness would be slight. Yet that is precisely the information we need to have, and this information can only be efficaciously and expeditiously gathered from multi-centered clinical trials.

3.2.3 The Principle of Precaution (The Precautionary Principle)

The Precautionary Principle is a principle that captures the conventional wisdom articulated in such slogans as "look before you leap," "better safe than sorry," or "an ounce of prevention is worth a pound of cure." Some view it as a principle for the risk-averse that has the effect of impeding technological progress, while others, including many European biomedical ethicists, view it as a needed correction to a deficiency in the American view of major biomedical ethical principles (Häyry, 2003). The principle of nonmalificence only prohibits actively and directly inflicting harm. It says nothing explicit about avoiding risks.

Under its most meaningful interpretation, the Principle of Precaution can be defined as the principle urging us to either take appropriate action in order to prevent harm, or to refrain from engaging in standing practices due to uncertainty about the risks they pose. The principle of precaution, then, is relevant in situations in which:

(a) decisions must be made in the face of uncertainty,

(b) there is something valuable at stake,

(c) there is some evidence indicating that the risk of harm is plausible, and

(d) the value in question is sufficient to shift the burden of proof from those who have some evidence of impending danger, albeit incomplete, to those who support the status quo.

Some worry that the Principle of Precaution could have the effect of stifling the development of technology or pharmaceuticals that could save lives or bring about great advantages, and thus, that the principle could backfire on the goal of protection (Engelhardt, 2004). However, precaution can also promote creative resolutions to present problems. Careful judgment is required to determine which envisionment of possible harms is more plausible or serious. Thus, it might be argued that continued research on DEX treatment to prevent virilization in females with CAH is required by the Principle of Precaution, since there are obvious risks involved in not attempting to prevent virilization. That argument, however, fails to attend to the risks involved with prenatal DEX use, and especially to the seven out of eight fetuses or more that will be treated, and subjected to risks, without incurring benefit.

The Precautionary Principle is applicable to our issue because there is uncertainty regarding DEX treatment, and some plausible evidence seems to suggest that DEX use may lead to adverse effects either in the short or the long term. The burden of proof lies with the defenders of prenatal DEX use to provide sufficient evidence of its safety, which can only be determined by long-term, multi-centered clinical trials.

We have seen that the mixed outcome of previous studies involving animals and humans strongly suggests the need for more research. To dismiss negative reports would violate the moral imperative to respect persons and to take precautionary measures to avoid inflicting harm. Prenatal DEX use cannot be regarded as the standard of care. Physicians convinced of the treatment's overall benefit should recommend its use only if the case it is used in can be part of a multi-centered investigation meeting the requirements of ethical review boards.

4. FEDERAL GUIDELINES PERTAINING TO THERAPEUTIC RESEARCH FOR FETUSES

We turn now to the question of whether research should continue on prenatal DEX therapy. Federal guidelines for therapeutic research on fetuses stipulate that no such research should be conducted unless the following general conditions apply:

(1) Appropriate studies on animals must have been completed.

(2) The purpose of the research is to rectify the needs of the particular fetus.

(3) The research must involve only minimal risk for the fetus.

(4) The risk must be the least possible for the purposes of meeting those needs.

Further guidelines are listed, such as the stipulation that researchers must not be involved in decisions to abort the fetus or to determine its viability, but those guidelines are irrelevant to the question at hand. All four relevant requirements pose difficulties for prenatal DEX use. We will examine each in turn.

4.1   Animal Studies

As we have seen, some researchers expressed concern over prenatal DEX use early on because of findings from animal studies (New, 2001). Defenders of prenatal use argued, in response, that the studies were inconclusive because they made use of a higher dosage of DEX than is used for virilization prevention. Further, some animal studies suggest that DEX use in animals is innocuous. For instance, Australian researchers very recently have published a report showing that low-dose, early gestational DEX treatment does *not* lead to renal problems or adult hypertension (Dodic, 2001). However, that study was small, and it does not address any risks to neurological, psychological, or cognitive function.

As we have also seen, newer animal studies have highlighted further possibilities that fetuses subjected to DEX treatment in utero may be predisposed to adult-onset diseases. And while some of the newer studies were structured to study the perinatal effects of administering DEX to premature infants to prevent lung collapse, it is not unreasonable to suspect that early, prenatal exposure to DEX—exposure that is simultaneous with the development of the brain, and that continues throughout pregnancy in the fetuses affected by CAH—would pose more danger, rather than less. Whether prenatal DEX use to prevent virilization of female fetuses with CAH is permissible therefore depends on whether sufficient animal studies have been done. If animal studies are for some reason not relevant, arguments should be provided to show this.

Thus, the requirement that animal studies be performed before research on fetuses is performed raises three questions about prenatal DEX treatment: (1) Are animal studies likely to shed light on this issue? (While there is always an epistemic leap from animal to human studies, at least some animal studies must be able to yield meaningful information. Otherwise, doing them would not be morally required.) (2) Do the published studies showing adverse consequences to fetuses indicate cause for concern, and if not, why not? (3) If some of the published studies are scientifically relevant to the question of the safety of DEX to prevent virilization, have enough of those studies been done?

4.2   Health Needs of the Particular Fetus

This requirement poses two major problems for ethical research on prenatal DEX use. First, as discussed earlier, it is questionable whether reducing virilization constitutes a health need. Genital surgery for infant girls with CAH is normalizing surgery, normalizing in a purely cosmetic sense. Though some would argue that the psychological trauma of growing up with abnormal or ambiguous genitalia constitutes a mental health need, even this is not obviously true, since that trauma may possibly be overcome with education and counseling for the parents and for the child.

Second, as we have noted, the status of CAH as an autosomal recessive genetic disease means that seven out of eight fetuses will be treated before it can be determined whether they are proper subjects for DEX use. If we factor in the information that DEX use, while effective, only diminishes virilization sufficiently to remove the "need" for surgery in 50% of cases, and that fewer surgeries are being performed for minor degrees of virilization, we find that the number of fetuses subjected to treatment that do not stand to benefit from it is significantly higher than 7 out of 8, but perhaps 15 out of 16, or 31 out of 32. Therefore, most of the time, it is not the "particular fetus" that is being subjected to risk. Even if it is, the urgency of the surgery would be dubious, and thus, the effort to prevent virilization could be unnecessary, or at least not worth the possible risks associated with DEX use.

However, there is an exception to the federal regulation that research must address the health needs of the particular fetus, so the fact that some fetuses do not stand to benefit from the studies does not, by itself, imply that ongoing studies are unethical. According to 45CFR46.208, which specifically pertains to activities directed toward fetuses in utero, the requirement that the fetus subjected to risk must also be the fetus that stands to benefit is modified so that allowable research can address either the health needs of the particular fetus *or* the attainment of important biomedical knowledge. If the latter justification applies, the risk to the fetus must be minimal. Knowing whether virilization can be prevented by early gestational DEX treatment would qualify as important biomedical knowledge because even if having abnormal genitals is not a health problem, most parents would probably choose to prevent it if they could do so without undue risk to the fetus. Nevertheless, the problem of whether the risks are minimal remains.

4.3 Minimal Risk

Two obstacles seem to prevent a conclusive determination of whether DEX use involves greater than minimal risk to the fetus: (1) Disparities between the conclusions of some follow-up studies to DEX treatment and incompleteness or deficiency of other studies (as discussed above), and (2) the lack of conceptual clarity inherent in the concept of "minimal risk." The second of these problems needs further discussion.

According to 45CFR 46.102i, minimal risk means "the probability and magnitude of harm or discomfort anticipated in the research are not greater in and of themselves than those ordinarily encountered in daily life or during the performance of routine physical and psychological examinations or tests." The description provides an inclusive disjunction that compares the research risks to everyday risks or to risks of routine medical examinations. Both disjuncts are themselves subject to a variety of interpretations.

Interpreting minimal risk as risks we encounter daily is problematic because it is difficult to know what our "everyday" risks actually are (Kopelman, 2004). For instance, we don't know what the chances are of being hit by a bus or being the victim of a terrorist attack. Also, it is difficult to know which risks, among all the risks that are in fact taken in daily life, constitute "everyday" risks (climbing a ladder or speeding on a country road). Some people may face daily risks that would be unacceptably high in research on children or fetuses.

On the other hand, interpreting minimal risks as comparable to those involved in a routine medical examination seems to provide a clearer and more acceptable guide, at least as long as by "routine" examinations we mean the ones most people have on a regular basis, rather than those a person with a serious disorder might have to endure (Kopelman, 204). Applying this standard to prenatal DEX research might first appear to suggest a prohibition because in the course of routine exams we are not subjected to chemical compounds which at certain doses or at certain stages, or for certain purposes, have been associated with adverse consequences in the past. Those convinced of its safety, however, would counter perhaps that the risks of prenatal DEX are well within the limits of what constitutes "minimal risk," if not altogether negligible. Nevertheless, in order to demonstrate the permissibility of prenatal DEX research, it needs to be shown, empirically or at least by cogent argumentation, that the risk is negligible.

4.4 Least Possible Risk to Meet Health Needs

Normally, it makes sense that in situations where there are two or more ways to meet a health need, we ought to choose the way that involves the least amount of risk. However, this requirement may be difficult to apply to our problem since having abnormal genitalia is not a physical disease, and so there is no physical health "need" to meet. If the "need" to be met is psychological health, it may be that the psychological harms associated with having ambiguous or hypertrophied genitalia would be better dealt with through counseling and education. On the other hand, counseling and education have not been studied for their efficacy in securing the psychological well-being of women with virilizing CAH. We do know that some individuals who did not receive normalizing surgery as infants or children have been able to adjust to their unusual bodies, but we don't know what factors helped them to make these accommodations. We can easily predict that different people will have contradictory opinions about whether prenatal DEX therapy is the least risky measure.

Therefore, whether research on DEX use is ethically justified comes down to the question of whether the risks involved qualify as minimal and whether there have been sufficient animal studies to pave the way.

5. CONCLUSIONS

The review of available empirical evidence yields a mixed verdict on the safety of prenatal DEX therapy to prevent virilization of female fetuses. The negative evidence is both substantial and varied enough to impose a moral obligation to conduct long-term, multi-centered studies. The positive evidence is not based on sufficiently large, long-term study samples and does not address important, possible, long-term effects. Such positive evidence therefore does not provide enough assurance to offset the worries generated by the negative reports and to cancel the moral obligation for further study. We have demonstrated that:

(1) DEX treatment should not be considered or promoted as "standard of care" until it has been shown not to exceed the standard of minimal risk.

(2) DEX treatment should not be recommended in the clinical setting without being part of a large research endeavor.

(3) Women considering participating in prenatal DEX treatment trials should be aware that DEX use is controversial, and that it has led to adverse effects in animals, women, infants, and fetuses, and that some of those effects are serious.

(4) All research on prenatal DEX treatment should include long-term follow-up because of the possibility that adverse effects might not become evident until adulthood.

(5) Continued research on DEX use for preventing virilization should continue only if: (a) animal studies are shown to be irrelevant for determining whether its use poses only minimal risk to the fetus, or (b) researchers can provide arguments against the plausible possibility that, since perinatal DEX use has been shown to be dangerous, prenatal exposure to the drug while the brain and other organs are developing is even more so.

To continue without answers to these questions would be to shirk the epistemic humility that befits the "track record" that Silverman reports: Of 25 unproven treatments in neonatology "introduced during his professional lifetime, four have led to improved practice, 12 have misled into fruitless byways, and nine have led to disaster" (Silverman, 1980; cited by Brook, 2000). Following the above recommendations will protect trust in the studies needed to determine the safety of medical treatments, and in the medical profession in general. This trust is essential to the continued participation of research subjects, and to the ability of medicine to fulfil its goal of beneficence.

Sharon Sytsma, Associate Professor, Philosophy Department, Northern Illinois University, DeKalb, Illinois, U.S.A.

REFERENCES

American Academy of Pediatrics: Section on Endocrinology and Committee on Genetics (Ad Hoc Writing Committee). "Technical Report: Congenital Adrenal Hyperplasia." *Pediatrics* 106.6 (Dec. 2000): 1511-1518.

Barrington, K.J. "Postnatal Steroids and Neurodevelopmental Outcomes: a Problem in the Making." *Pediatrics* 107 (2001): 1425-1426.

Barrington, K.J. "The Adverse Neurodevelopmental Effects of Postnatal Steroids in the Preterm Infant: a Systematic Review of RCTs." *BMC Pediatr* 1 (2001):1; Barrington, KJ. In Reply, Letters to the Editor, 2002; 109(4): 717.

Beauchamp, Thomas. L., and James Childress. *Principles of Biomedical Ethics,* 2nd ed. New York: Oxford University Press, 1983.

Belmont Report, http://www.med.umich.edu/irbmed/ethics/belmont/belmontr.htm#basic

Brook, C. G. D. "Antenatal Treatment of a Mother Bearing a Fetus With Congenital Adrenal Hyperplasia" *Arch Dis Child Fetal Neonatal Ed* 82 (2000): F176-F178.

Burlet G., B. Fernette, S. Blanchard, E. Angel, P. Tankosic, S. Maccari, A. Burlet. "Antenatal Glucocorticoids Blunt the Functioning of the Hypothalamic-pituitary-adrenal Axis of Neonates and Disturb Some Behaviors in Juveniles." *Neuroscience* 133.1 (2005): 221-30.

Carlson, A. D., J. S. Obeid, N. Kanellopoulou, R. C. Wilson, M. I. New. "Congenital Adrenal Hyperplasia: Update on Prenatal Diagnosis and Treatment," *J. Steroid Biomchem Mol Biol* 69.1-6 (1999): 19-29.

Caffrey, Brynn. "Showering Sans Penis." *Chrysalis (Special Issue on Intersexuality)* 1997.

Capelanes, Angela, and Philippe Jeanty. "Congenital Adrenal Hyperplasia," (2000) *http://www. thefetus.net/page.php?id=2631.*

Casper, Monica. *The Making of the Unborn Patient: A Social Anatomy of Fetal Surgery.* (New Brunswick, New Jersey, Rutgers University Press); 1998.

Celsi, G., A. Kistner, O. Aizman, et al. "Prenatal Dexamethasone Causes Oligonephronia, Sodium Retention, and Higher Blood Pressure in the Offspring." *Pediatric Res* 44 (1998): 317-322.

Codes of Federal Regulations.

Costedoat-Chalumeau, N., Amoura, Z., Le Thi Hong, D. Weshsler, B. et al. "Questions about Dexamethasone Use for the Prevention of Anti-SSA Related Congenital Heart Block." *Annals of Rheumatic Disease* 62 (2003): 1010-1012.

Couper, J. J., J. M. Hutson, and G. L. Warne. "Hydrometrocolpos Following Prenatal Dexamethasone Treatment for Congenital Adrenal Hyperplasai (21-hydroxylase deficiency). *Eur J. Pediatr.* 152.1 (1993): 9-11.

David, M. and M. G. Forest. "Prenatal Treatment of Congenital Adrenal Hyperplasia Resulting from 21 Hydroxylase Deficiency." *The Journal of Pediatrics* 105 (1984): 799- 803.

Deaton, Michael, et al., "Congenital Adrenal Hyperplasia: Not Really a Zebra," *American Family Physician* 59.5 (1999) 1190-1199.

Dodic, Miodrag, Chrishan Samuel, Karen Moritz , Marely Wintour, John Morgan, Leeanne Gigg, James Wong. "Impaired Cardiac Functional Reserve and Left Ventricular Hypertrophy in Adult Sheep after Prenatal Adult Sheep After Prenatal Dexamethasone Exposure." *Circ Res* 89 (2001): 623-9.

Doyle L.W., P. G. Davis, C. J. Morely. "Does Postnatal Corticosteroid Therapy Adversely Affect Long-Term Outcome?" Abstract of a presentation at the "Hot Topics in Neonatology" Conference in Washington, 9-11 December 2001.

Engelhardt, Tristram H. *The Foundation of Bioethics*. Oxford: Oxford University Press, 2004.

Engelhardt, Tristram H. "The Precautionary Principle: A Dialectical Reconsideration". *The Journal of Medicine and Philosophy* 29.3 (2004): 301-312.

Forest, M. G., H. Betuel, M. David. "Prenatal Treatment in Congenital Adrenal Hyperplasia Due to 21-Hydroxylase Deficiency: Update 88 of the French Multicentric Study. *Endocr. Res.* 15(1-2) 1989: 277-301.

Forest, M. G., M. David, Y. Morel. "Prenatal Diagnosis and Treatment of 21-Hydroxylase Deficiency." *J. Steroid Biochem Mol Biol.* 45.1-3 (1993) 75-82.

Forest, M. G., Y. Morel, M. David. "Prenatal Treatment of Congenital Adrenal Hyperplasia." *Trends Endocrinol Metab.* 9 (1998): 284-9.

Hallisey, P. L. "The Fetal Patient and the Unwilling Mother: A Standard for Judicial Intervention." *Pacific Law J* 14 (1983): 1065-1094.

Häyry, Matti. "European Values in Bioethics: Why, What, and How to be Used?" *Theoretical Medicine and Bioethics* 24 (2003): 199-214.

Joint LWPES/ESPE CAH Working Group, "Consensus Statement on 21-Hydroxylase Deficiency from the Lawson Wilkins Pediatric Endocrine Society and the European Society for Paediatric Endocrinology," *The Journal of Clinical Endocrinology* 87.9 (2002): 4048-4053.

Kant, Immanuel. *Groundwork for the Metaphysics of Morals.*

Kelnar, C. H. "Congenital Adrenal Hyperplasia (CAH)—the Place for Prenatal Treatment and Neonatal Screening." *Early Hum. Dev.* 335.2 (Dec. 1993): 81-90.

Kelnar, C. H. "Commentary." *Arch Dis Child Fetal Neonatal Ed* 82 (2000): F180-181.

Kopelman, Loretta. "Minimal Risk as an International Ethical Standard," *The Journal of Medicine and Philosophy* 29.3 (2004):3 51-378.

Lajic, Svetloana, Wedellen, Anna, Bui, T-H, Ritzen, M,, and Holst M. "Long-Term Somatic Follow-Up of Prenatally Treated Children with Congenital Adrenal Hyperplasia." *J Clinical Endocrinology and Metabolism* 83.11 (1998): 3872-3880.

Lee, Peter. "Genital surgery Among Females with Congenital Adrenal Hyperplasia: Changes over the Past Five Decades."*J Pediatr Endocrinol Metab* 15.9 (2002): 1473-77.

Levine, Robert, and Karen Lebacqz. "Some Ethical Considerations in Clinical Trials. *Clin Pharmacol Therapeutics* 25 (1979): 723-741.

Levine, Robert. S., and Sonya Pang. "Prenatal Diagnosis and Treatment of Congenital Adrenal Hyperplasia." *J. Pediatric Endocrinology* 7.3 (1994): 193-200.

Levine, Robert. *Ethics and Regulation of Clinical Research*: 2nd ed. (Urban and Schwartzenberg, December 31, 1988).

McArther, S., E. McHale, J. W. Dalley, J. C. Buckinham, G. E. Gillies. "Altered Mesencephalic Dopaminergic Populations in Adulthood as a Consequence of Brief Prenatal Glucocorticoid Exposure." *Journal of Neuroendocrinoly* 17(8) (Aug., 2005): 474-82.

Malunowicz, M., Ginalska Malinowska, et al. "The Influence of Prenatal Dexamethasone Treatment on Urinary Excretion of Adrenocortical Steroids in Newborns." *Eur J. Pediatr.* 157.7 (1998): 539-43.

Mathur M. and M. Kabra, "Prenatal Diagnosis and Treatment of Steroid 21-Hydroxylase Deficiency," *Indian Journal of Pediatrics* 67.11 (2000): 813-818.

Mercado, A. B., R. C. Wilson, K. C. Cheng, J. Q. Wei, M. I. New. "Prenatal Treatment and Diagnosis of Congenital Adrenal Hyperplasia Owing to Steroid 21-Hydroxylase Deficiency." 80.7 (July, 1995): 2014-20.

Meyer Bahlburg, Heino, Curtis Dolezal, Susan Baker, Ann Carlson, Jihad Obeid, and Maria New. Cognitive and Motor Development of Children With and Without Congenital Adrenal Hyperplasia after Early-Prenatal Dexamethasone. *The Journal of Clinical Endocrinology and Metabolism* 89.2 (2004): 610-614.

Miller, W. L. "Dexamethasone Treatment of Congenital Adrenal Hyperplasia in Utero: an Experimental Therapy of Unproven Safety." *J Urol* 162 .2 (Aug. 1999): 537-40.

Murphy, Brenden P., Terrie Inder, Petra Huppi, Simon Warfield, Gary Zinetara, Ron Kikinis, Ferenc Jolesz, and Joeseph Volpe. "Impaired Cerebral Cortical Gray Matter Growth After Treatment with Dexamethasone for Neonatal Chronic Lung Disease." *Pediatrics* 107.2 (2001): 217-221.

Nass, R., L. Heier, T. Moshang, S. Oberfield, A. George, M. New, P. Speiser. "Magnetic Resonance Imaging in the Congenital Adrenal Hyperplasia Population." *J. Chil. Neurol.* 12 (1997): 181-186.

Miller, W. L. "Dexamethasone Treatment of Congenital Adrenal Hyperplasia in Utero: An Experimental Therapy of Unproven Safety. *Journal of Urology* 162.2 (1999): 537-40.

Neal, C. Jr., G. Weidemann, M. Kabbaj, and D. Vazquez. "Effect of Neonatal Dexamethasone Exposure on Growth and Neurological Development in the Adult Rat." *Am J Physiol Regul Integr Comp Physiol* 287 (2004): R375-R385.

New, Maria. "Prevention of Ambiguous Genitalia by Prenatal Treatment with Dexamethasone in Pregnancies at Risk for Congenital Adrenal Hyperplasia." *Pure Applied Chem* 75.11-12 (2003), 2013-2022.

New, Maria. "Prenatal Treatment of Congenital Adrenal Hyperplasia: Author Differs with Technical Report." *Pediatrics* 107.4 (Apr., 2001): 804.

New, Maria, et al. "Prenatal Diagnosis for Congenital Adrenal Hyperplasia in 532 Pregnancies." *Journal of Clinical Endocrinology Metab* 86.12 (2001): 5651-7.

New, Maria. "Antenatal Diagnosis and Treatment of Congenital Adrenal Hyperplasia." *Curr Urol Rep* 2.1 (Feb., 2001): 11-8.

New, Maria. "Steroid 21-Hydroxylase Deficiency (Congenital Adrenal Hyperplasia) *American Journal of Medicine* 98.1A; (Jan., 16, 1998): 2S-8S).

Newnham J.P. "Is Prenatal Glucocorticoid Administration Another Origin of Adult Disease?" *Clin Exp. Pharmacol Physiol.*; 28.11 (Nov., 2001): 957-61.

Nimkarn, Saroj. "Prenatal Diagnosis and Treatment of Congenital Adrenal Hyperplasia Owing to 21-Hydroxylase Deficiency 31.4 (2005): 91-96.

Nivelon, J., M. Chouchane, M.G. Forest, Y. Morel, F. Huet, A. Nivelong-Chevallier, C. Francois. "Prenatal Treatment of Congenital Adrenal Hyperplasia Due to 21-Hydroxylase Deficiency: 9 Treated Pregnancies." *Ann Pediatr* 40.7 (Sept., 1993): 421-5.

NIH Consensus Statement Online. "Antenatal Corticosteroids Revisited: Repeat Courses." 17.2 (Aug. 17-19, 2000): 1-10.

O'Regan, D., C. J. Kenyon, J. R. Seckle and M.C. Holmes. "Glucocorticoid Exposure in Late Gestation in the Rat Permanently Programs Gender Specific Differences in Adult Cardiovascular and Metabolic Physiology." *American J. Physiol Endocrinol Meta* 287 (2004): E863-E870.

Ortiz, Luis, Albert Quan, Arthur Weinberg, and Michel Baum. "Effect of Penatal Dexamethasone on Rat. Renal Development." *Kidney International* 59.5 (May, 2001): 1663-69.

Ortiz, Luis, Albert Quan, Francisco Zarzar, Arthur Weinberg, Michel Baum. "Prenatal Dexamethasone Programs Hypertension and Renal Injury in the Rat." *Hypertension* (2003): 328-334.

Ozbey, N. "Prenatal Treatment of Congenital Adrenal Hyperplasia and Fetal Malformations." *J. Endocrinol. Invest.* 25 (2002): 91-92.

Pang, S. and A. T. Clark, et.al., "Maternal Side Effects of Prenatal Dexamethasone Therapy for Fetal Congenital Adrenal Hyperplasia." *J. Clin. Endocrinol. Metab.* 75.1 (July 1992): 249-53.

Prader, A. *Helv. Paediatr. Acta* 9 (1954): 231.

Quercia, N., D. Chitayat, R. Babul-Hirji, M. I. New, D. Daneman. "Normal External Genitalia in a Female with Classical Congenital Adrenal Hyperplasia Who Was Not Treated During Embryogenesis." *Prenatal Diagnosis* 18.1 (1988) 83-5.

Riepe, F. G., N. Krone, M. Viemann, C. H. Partsch, W. G. Sippell. "Management of Congenital Adrenal Hyperplasia: Results of the ESPE Questionnaire." *Hormone Research* 58.4 (2002): 196-205.

Ritzen, E. M. "Prenatal Dexamethasone Treatment of Fetuses at Risk for Congenital Adrenal Hyperplasia: Benefits and Concerns." *Semin Neonatol* 6 (2001): 357-362.

Rodriguez, A., B. Ezquieta, J. M. Varela, M. Moreno, and E. Dulin. "Prenatal Molecular Genetic Diagnosis and Treatment of Congenital Adrenal Hyperplasia Due to 21-Hydroxylase Deficiency." *Med Clin (Barc)* 109.17 (1997): 669-72.

Ross, Lainie. "Justice for Children: The Child as Organ Donor." *Bioethics* 8.2 (1994): 105-126.

Secki, J. R., and W. L. Miller. "How Safe is Long Term Prenatal Glucocorticoid Treatment?" *The Journal of the American Medical Association* 277 (1997): 1077-1079.

Silverman W.A. "Retrolental Fibroplasias: a Modern Parable. Monographs" in *Neonatology*. New York: Grune and Stratton, 1980.

Speiser, P. W., and Maria New, "Prenatal Diagnosis and Treatment of Congenital Adrenal Hyperplasia." *J Pediatr Endocrinology* 7.3 (Jul. – Sept., 1994): 183-91.

Spiliotis, B. E. "Prenatal Diagnosis and Treatment of Congenital Adrenal Hyperplasia and Consequences in Adults." *J Pediatr Endocrinol Metabolism* 14 Suppl. 5 (2001): 1299-302, discussion 1317.

Stoelhorst, G. M., S. E. Martens, M. Rijken, P. H. van Zwieten, A. h. Zwinderman, J. M Wit, S. Veen, et al. "Behavior at 2 Years of Age in Very Preterm Infants (Gestational Age < 32 Weeks). *Acta Paediatr*; 92.5 (2003): 595-601.

Trautman, P. D., Heino Meyer-Bahlburg, Jill Postelnek, and Maria New, "Effects of Early Prenatal Dexamethasone on the Cognitive and Behavioral Development of Young Children: Results of a Pilot Study" *Psychoneuroendocrinology* 20.4 (1995): 439-449.

Trautman, P. D., Heino Meyer-Bahlburg, Jill Postelnek, Maria New. "Mothers' Reactions to Prenatal Diagnostic Procedures and Dexamethasone Treatment of Congenital Adrenal Hyperplasia," *J Psychosom Obstet Gynaecol* 17.3 (Sep., 1996): 175-81.

Uno, H. S. Eisele, A. Sakai, S. Shelton, E. Baker, O. DeJesus, J. Holden. "Neurotoxicity of Glucocorticoids in the Primate Brain. *Hormones and Behavior* 28 (1994): 336-48.

Warne, Gary, Sonia Grover, and Jeffrey Zajac. "Hormonal Therapies for Individuals with Intersex Conditions: Protocol for Use." *Treatments in Endocrinology* 4.1 (2005): 19-29.

Wudy, S. A., J. Homoki, W. M. Teller. "Successful Prenatal Treatment of Congenital Adrenal Hyperplasia Due to 21-Hydroxylase Deficiency." *Eur. J. Pediatr* 153.8 (1994): 556-9.

Yeh Tsu F., Yuh J. Lin, Hung C. Lin, Chao C. Huang, Wu S. Hsieh, Chyi H. Lin, Cheng H. Tsai. "Outcomes at School Age after Postnatal Dexamethasone Therapy for Lung Disease of Prematurity." *The New England Journal of Medicine* 350.13 (Mar 25, 2004): 1304-13.

SHARON E. SYTSMA

INTERSEXUALITY, CULTURAL INFLUENCES, AND CULTURAL RELATIVISM

1. INTERSEXUALITY, CULTURAL INFLUENCES, AND CULTURAL RELATIVISM

In the following, a difficult case involving intersex is examined. Although intersexuality is somewhat rare, leading pediatric urologists and endocrinologists involved in the treatment of intersexuality report all having dealt with similar cases.[1] Since the case involves a conflict of cultural values, physicians have tended to resolve the issue by an appeal to the duty to respect the values of other cultures.[2] Published commentaries on the case have also framed the issue in terms of cultural relativism.[3] The aim of this paper is to show that the justification for the resolution of the case need not, and should not involve either subscribing or succumbing to cultural relativism.[4] The argument clarifies the role of cultural considerations in ethical decision-making. I argue that understanding the appropriate role of cultural values in ethical decision-making is vital to the integrity of the medical profession. The paper begins with a description of the case, followed by an account of how it would have been addressed according to previous practices for dealing with intersexuality. Then a description of our revised practices and the factors that led to them will be provided, along with an application of those practices to the case. In the second section, evidence of cultural disparities in the medical treatment of intersexuality will be canvassed. The third section addresses the question of what is entailed by the duty to respect the values of other cultures, stressing that respecting the values of other cultures does not require condoning, accepting, or acceding to those values. In the fourth section, I provide a resolution of the case based on empirical studies on the intersexual condition involved and a realistic confrontation with all morally relevant circumstances of the case.

S.E. Sytsma (Ed.), Ethics and Intersex, 259–270.

2. THE CASE

Parents from a middle-eastern country brought their 13-year-old son to a large metropolitan hospital.[5] The boy had noticeable breast development, which caused him to be the victim of taunting and teasing by his peers. He also had hypospadias, an abnormality of the penile structure such that the urethral opening is somewhere other than at the tip of the penile shaft. He had experienced unexplained bleeding through the penis. Tests revealed that the boy had a 46XX karyotype, ovaries, a partial uterus, and congenital adrenal hyperplasia (CAH), a condition that leads to the varying degrees of masculinization of the genitalia in affected females. The levels of masculinization are referred to as "Prader-stages" one (CAH-1; least severe) through five (CAH-5; most severe). Females with the least severe forms of CAH are born with somewhat enlarged clitorises. More severe cases result in ambiguous genitalia. Sometimes, as in our case, the genitals are so masculinized that the newborn appears to be male. CAH can go undetected until puberty, when breast development and menstruation occurs.

Psychological tests showed that the boy manifested a propensity toward masculine gender behavior, although he was unusually fond of children. The parents came from a culture in which the parents, in particular the father, are regarded as being responsible for medical decisions for their children. Reflecting this cultural outlook, the parents wanted to make medical decisions for their son without involving him in the decisions. The parents desired that he continue to be raised as a male, despite his female procreative capacity, perhaps largely because they come from a society where the male sex is preferred, and only men have rights. Removing the ovaries was necessary to prevent the production of female hormones, and the boy would have to be put on a regimen of male hormones for the rest of his life. Further, they did not want to traumatize their son by returning to their country and declaring that their child is really a female. When asked how they would react if their son became a homosexual, the parents responded that they and their society viewed homosexuality as an abomination deserving of death. In the event the child became a homosexual, he would likely be killed.

Unfortunately, the boy was also in need of a kidney replacement. So the parents requested that the boy have a double mastectomy, hypospadias repair, hysterectomy, oopherectomy, and nephrectomy all at the same time. Limited resources required that they return to their own country in the not too distant future. They insisted that the boy not be informed of his karyotype, female reproductive capacity, or of the removal of his gonads. The request created a conundrum for the medical team: The psychologist felt strongly that the boy should be informed of his medical condition and that he should be able to participate in the decision of whether to eliminate his female procreative ability and to continue to live as a male.

In the United States and other western countries, the practice has traditionally been to assign neonates with Congenital Adrenal Hyperplasia to the female sex, even if severely or completely masculinized. This practice was based on the "optimal-gender policy", developed in the middle 1950's.[6] The policy was rooted in a quasi-Aristotelian notion that flourishing requires the exercise of essential potentialities or functions, along with the belief that gender identity is neutral at birth and is developed by social conditioning. Females with CAH have (or can have, with surgery and hormonal treatment) reproductive capacity, so even those with completely masculinized genitals have been "assigned" as females, undergoing feminizing surgery of the genitals as infants. Surgery was thought to be required in infancy in order to facilitate the inculcation of a female gender identity, both because phenotype was thought to be a determinant of gender identity, and because it would encourage the parents to relate consistently to the child as female. The goal was to preserve reproductive function. Similarly, males born with Androgen Insensitivity Syndrome (AIS) or other conditions leading to ambiguous, feminized, or undermasculinized genitals were assigned as females, since they would be incapable of procreation or of sexual penetration.

In some cases, parents of intersexual children were not fully informed of their child's condition. In other cases, the parents were informed, but were advised not to inform the children. Yet in others, parents were advised to disclose information to the child in a manner appropriate to their cognitive development, but many failed to do so. Physicians thought that failures of disclosure were justified by beneficent concerns to ensure parent/infant bonding and to spare unnecessary psychological trauma.

Recognition of the harms of secrecy for intersexed children have come to light, and physicians now understand, or ought to, that full disclosure to the parents is required for appropriately informed consent, and disclosure to children by parents is required for psychological health and family stability. Indeed, several lawyers at medical research ethics and medical ethics conferences have pointed out that physicians could be liable for any failures to extend information regarding the child's intersexual status.[7] Members of the North American Task Force on Intersexuality were all urged to practice full disclosure in the clinical setting.[8] The change in disclosure practices in cases dealing with intersex has been largely effected by the efforts of intersex advocacy groups.

Another change is that female sex assignment is no longer the unquestioned response to CAH involving significant degrees of masculinization. Some have argued that 46XX infants with completely masculinized genitals (CAH-5) should be raised as males because of "prenatal hormonal imprinting"—that is, the masculinization of the brain and behavior that occurs because of the effects of androgens on fetal development.[9] The infamous John/Joan/John case has been thought to provide evidence of prenatal gender imprinting.[10] Some have not subscribed to the theory of prenatal imprinting, but nevertheless recognize that further masculinization occurs during and after birth, and that in cases where CAH is undiagnosed until later in the child's development, male assignment should be continued. Others have objected to all but medically necessary genital surgery for sex assignment or normalizing purposes because of the ill effects of surgery on genital function and sensitivity, the unpredictability of gender identity, and the rights of children to choose their own genders.[11] As a result, severely masculinized females are now often (but not always) raised as males.

If a child has approached puberty before being diagnosed with a female karyotype and CAH, the physicians would explain the condition and options first to the parents and then to the child, and the child would be involved in the decision as to the course of action to follow. This practice respects the emerging autonomy of the child and helps to ensure a concordant gender assignment. Further, since parents and physicians did not impose the decision, the child would less likely be resentful towards their parents or physicians in the event of an incongruent gender assignment.

In our case, however, the parents are adamant in their refusal to involve the child in the decision-making. What should the medical team do? Does the duty to respect other cultures require that they perform the surgeries requested? Exactly what cultural beliefs are at play here? And are they cultural beliefs we ought to respect?

3. CULTURAL DIVERSITY IN ATTITUDES TOWARD INTERSEX

Attitudes toward intersexuality are clearly tied to cultural values. Most cultures subscribe to the idea of sexual dimorphism—the belief that human beings are, or ought to be, either male or female. That belief is an historical accident promulgated by Christianity, but it is not rooted in biological facts.[12] Anthropological studies show that some cultures have not only recognized that some humans are "in between," but have accommodated them into the social structure, according them specific roles and even conferring on them specials powers and privileges.[13]

In cultures that accord preference to the male gender, there are more sex assignments to the male gender, just as there are fewer cases of male infanticide or abortion of male fetuses. A recent Saudi Arabian study of 14 intersexuals born with male chromosomes, but undervirilized (ambiguous) genitals, revealed that ten out of eleven of those who were assigned to the female gender at birth requested surgical sex reassignment, and thereafter affirmed their decisions, cherishing their male societal status even while expressing some dissatisfaction with their small penises. The author states: "The male genotype is a more important factor than phallic adequacy in determining the gender of rearing in the Kingdom of Saudi Arabia, an observation attributable to the financial, social, and cultural benefits that the male gender confers in Saudi society."[14] In Turkey, two physicians report that children born with genital abnormalities, including ambiguous genitalia, are not diagnosed until very late and surgical sex assignment is not performed until puberty or even later.[15] The society, then, must be more tolerant of sexual ambiguity than ours. A report on medical practices for gender assignment for intersexual children in Egypt attests to the "several social, cultural and religious factors related to [the] local area influencing gender assignment."[16]

Ursula Kuhnle and Wolfgang Krahl, working at the largest children's hospital in Malaysia found that while Chinese and Indian segments of the population were averse to female sex assignment of intersexed children with ambiguous genitalia, "it was never difficult to convince a Muslim family to assign a severely virilized girl or an undervirilized boy to the female gender."[17] The authors explain that the difference in gender assignments were a reflection of the superior economic and social status of women in Malaysian culture. In Kuhnle and Krahl's observation, gender identity appears to develop independently of how children are raised and educated; however, they recognized that more study is needed before a final conclusion is reached on the nature/nurture influences on gender identity. Kuhnle and Krahl have come to see that our own practices have been based on cultural biases rather than biological fact, and they are no longer think that patient satisfaction with assigned gender necessarily indicates that whatever sex assignments have been made have been correct.[18] Rather, they entertain the idea that other cultural responses that allow for flexible gender roles might be best. While they suggest "cross-cultural studies might allow a new approach in dealing with intersexed persons, their families and their social backgrounds," it is unclear whether they believe that cultural attitudes ought always to be the determining factor in gender assignment.[19] They state that "the ideal that cultural background should guide medical decisions is nowhere generally accepted."[20] However, they do not explicitly claim that they believe it should. Their overall thesis seems to be that noting variations in cultural valuations in response to intersexuality may help us to recognize cultural bias in our own responses, and may motivate open-mindedness regarding the possible acceptability or even superiority of other responses.

Our case requires us to make a decision regarding whether cultural values *ought to be* the determining factor in surgical gender assignment, since the request of the parents is based on cultural attitudes towards child-raising and gender bias. We need to ask whether we ought to defer to other cultures' values when making these medical decisions. If doing so is morally correct, is it always so? Are there limits to how far we should accede to medical requests judged to be morally inappropriate in our own? Trends toward multiculturalism in higher education, while laudably encouraging respect for the values of other cultures, lend little guidance on these matters.

4. THE DUTY TO RESPECT OTHER CULTURES

That we have a duty to respect other cultures is obvious, and education promoting multiculturalism that is geared toward expressing and furthering that duty serves a useful and a moral function. The duty to respect other cultures can be understood as a corollary of our duty to respect persons. After all, all of us have been "thrown" into a culture as an essential aspect of our being in the world and with others. We neither have any control over having been introduced into a culture, nor over the particular culture into which we have been thrown. Rather, all of us belong to a culture, or even to several subcultures, as part of the "givenness" of our existence. We can come to realize the extent to which our culture affects our values and world views; and so, just as we would want others to appreciate the role of our culture in understanding us, we know we ought to appreciate the role of other cultures in understanding and interacting with others. The duty is an application of the Golden Rule on a larger scale. Diversity of cultures need not be regarded as a threat, but as

264 SHARON E. SYTSMA

an opportunity for education and even celebration of the richness of human social expression. Also, respect for other cultures has obvious utilitarian benefits, as it instills a mindset that is conducive to open-mindedness, generosity, and tolerance, and antithetical to ethnocentricity, provincialism, intolerance, conflict, and war.

However, it is not always clear exactly what respect for other cultures requires. We need to consider more carefully what the duty to respect other cultures means in the medical setting—and in the difficult case under consideration. Indubitably, there are limits to what is demanded by our duty to respect other cultures. Respecting other cultures does not require allowing them to use force against us, nor does it imply that all cultural norms and practices are morally permissible. Recognizing the duty to respect other cultures does not commit one to the acceptance of cultural relativism--the view that actions are right or wrong only in reference to their coherence or incoherence with prevailing cultural values. Resolving or managing cultural conflicts requires impartiality, careful balancing, and discernment. On a personal level, when a friend is planning on committing an act that you think is immoral, your respect for the friend requires you to explain why you think the friend's plans are objectionable--not to condone, and certainly not to abet the act. An attitude of indifference toward our friend's views would make personal integrity impossible. Similarly, when cultural values clash, cultural integrity requires, not that we relinquish our values, but that we attempt to explain our views. Professions, too, can possess or fail to possess integrity. The medical profession is distinctly at risk of facing cultural conflicts which demand resolution, given that it is concerned with health, life, and death, which are key structures involving values.

Just as respecting persons requires us to transcend egotism, to understand the naturalness of the development of personal values and idiosyncrasies, and to accept and celebrate the uniqueness of others, respecting other cultures requires us to transcend the tendencies to ethnocentricity and provincialism, to understand the naturalness of diversity in the origination of values, to accept and celebrate a wide diversity in the expressions of values, and to refrain from condemning individuals whose values have been molded by socialization. Further, we can agree that most of the time, even when we regard the practices of another culture as immoral, we nevertheless ought to refrain from using violence in order to impose our own values. Just as when differences exist in morals on an personal level, it is better to explain, provide reasons, and demonstrate (where possible) the superiority of our own views, it is better to encourage change from within the culture than to impose it from without, because values forcefully imposed are not authentically held, and relapse is likely to occur. If the differences are severe, the best response might be a parting of ways, either on the personal or the cultural level. On the cultural level the parting of ways could consist in a decision to boycott or to refuse opportunity for commercial trading. It may simply involve a refusal to comply with or accede to wishes.

There is some evidence that, in dealing with cases of intersexuality, the duty to respect other cultures might be being interpreted in a way that threatens the integrity of the medical profession. For instance, one psychologist writing on intersexual issues makes the following claim: "*The clinician's role* is not to superimpose her/his cultural values on those of others, but to come to a decision that likely minimizes potential harm to the patient in her/his cultural environment."[21] David Diamond, in his commentary on the case here presented, concluded that: "the parents' own value system must be the guide."[22] These claims are surely motivated by beneficence, and indeed possess certain plausibility. Superimposing our cultural values on those of others may nearly always be inappropriate or even immoral, but is it the *clinician's role* to make medical decisions based on whatever values another culture might possess? It would seem to matter what the value is, how deeply ingrained it is, and whether acting in compliance with the culture's values would involve treatment that is tantamount to a violation of human rights. In light of such concerns, Alice Dreger and Bruce Wilson quite appropriately express a disapproval of the "idea that sexual anatomies are an acceptable locale for cultural relativism."[23] Focusing only on cultural values in the medical setting fails to consider the intrinsic worth, rights, and well being of the patient. Disregarding them altogether can have the same effect.

5. OUTCOMES OF GENDER ASSIGNMENT IN INDIVIDUALS WITH CONGENITAL ADRENAL HYPERPLASIA

All parties to the controversy surrounding surgical sex assignment or normalizing procedures agree at least on one thing: there is a dearth of long-term retrospective studies on such surgeries. The lack of sufficient empirical studies leads some critics to claim that infant genital surgery is "experimental."[24] On the other hand, of all intersex conditions, congenital adrenal hyperplasia has been studied the most. The empirical findings must be regarded as preliminary, since the studies are not large enough or designed well enough to provide conclusive evidence. Given the empirical evidence we have to date, can we determine what the *likely* outcome of performing the surgeries on the 13-year-old in terms of gender identity and sexual orientation would be?

Heino Meyer-Bahlburg reports in 2001: "Most 46, XX CAH patients who have been reared in the male gender until late childhood/early adolescence, elect to stay males once they are correctly diagnosed and informed in late childhood/adolescence, although occasional patient-initiated reassignments to the female gender have been reported."[25] A nation-wide study in Germany in 2002 canvassed 16 genetic females with CAH associated with complete virilization who had received a male sex assignment at birth. Six were diagnosed within the first month and five of those immediately received female surgical assignment surgery, the sixth did so at 19 months. Ten of the original 16 patients were not diagnosed until later, between 3.4 and 7 years of age. Seven of those ten retained their male sex assignment, though one of these later expressed some gender dysphoria. Three of the ten were reassigned as females, but one has poor female gender identity and another is considering reversing that procedure.[26] These empirical findings, therefore, together with our 13-year-old boy's self-expressed desire to shed female characteristics and with his consistent manifestation of predominantly masculine behavior, strongly suggest the biological likelihood that his gender identity will continue to be male. Furthermore, he has reached the age where gender identity is *normally* fixed. While it is still controversial whether prenatal hormones masculinize not only external genitals, but also the brain and gender identity, we do know that postnatal hormones and postnatal rearing combine to further solidify a male gender identity.[27]

If it is likely that the boy has a stabilized gender identity, the concerns about removing his reproductive potential pale in significance. Studies have indicated that women with CAH have significantly decreased rates of childbearing, "particularly among the more severely affected women, i.e., those who were prenatally more severely masculinized."[28] This finding is confirmed more recently in a study in the Netherlands.[29] Given the further masculinizing effects of both androgens and having been reared as a male, it would seem to follow that among 46 XX individuals raised as males until adolescence, the reduction would be even more pronounced.

The loss of reproductive capacity is further balanced by considerations of sexual functioning. Remaining male spares—him any need for surgery other than oopherectomy, and all the problems including desensitisation—of genital surgery and vaginoplasty.[30] Intersex advocates and physicians alike challenge the success of such surgery.

Furthermore, Meyer-Bahlburg reports that: "46XX individuals raised as males— thus combining pre/perinatal elevated androgens with postnatal and pubertal elevations of 'activating' androgens—usually appear to be gynecophilic."[31] In a society that condones persecution of homosexuals, then, it would be far safer to adhere to a male gender assignment, and safety considerations would plausibly influence the boy's decision were he to be making it, and would likely further mean that he would be understanding, even if not completely grateful, for his parents' decision to continue his male gender assignment.

Regardless of intersex conditions, it seems that the majority of people surgically assigned to a gender continue to accept that gender assignment, even while perhaps exhibiting behavior typical of the opposite gender.[32] One plausible explanation for this widespread satisfaction is that gender identity is somewhat flexible. Just as there is a range of degrees of femininity and masculinity in the appearance and behavior of both men and women, there may be degrees of masculine and feminine gender identity. Some people may be in the middle of the continuum between extremely masculine or feminine gender identities and therefore be able to accommodate whatever sex assignment is given to them at birth. Others who have gender identities towards either extreme would have more trouble growing up with an incongruent gender assignment. Experiential factors may play a role in strengthening or weakening an inherent flexibility. Further, some people are bi-gendered and experience the need to express themselves in both feminine and masculine modes, and are not satisfied with a unisex life-style.

True, at this point, gender flexibility is but a theory, and a critic might at this point argue that all the empirical studies to date are inadequate, not being based on large enough sample populations. Even if we did have larger, more reliable studies, it could still be argued that gender identity cannot always be predicted, either in intersexuals or in the general population, so we should refrain from any surgical means of imposing gender except for those chosen by the individual in order to avoid harm. In response, it is helpful to remember that morality does not demand omniscience. Often morally responsible choices must be made only on the basis of probability.

Regarding surgery for hypospadias repair, Dr. Justine Schober reports "currently, we can correct severe hypospadias and provide a very good masculinized appearance, with less reoperation."[33] If this were true, performing the surgery would likely make the boy more comfortable with his male identity image. Furthermore, Schober claims that sexual sensitivity would not be adversely affected, since tissue is not removed. Schober is fully acquainted with the drawbacks of feminizing surgery, and is forthright in her reporting of these; hence, her assertion regarding hypospadias repair gains credence, even though she cites no studies.

6. CONCLUSIONS

In an ideal world, all societies would be flexible regarding gender identities so that every individual would feel free to express their gender identities even when discordant with chromosomes, gender of rearing, or sexual orientation. Those who do not identify either with the masculine or feminine gender identity, as is the experience of some intersexuals, or those who do not identify exclusively with either, as those who are bi-gendered, would be accepted without prejudice or bias. Such a world would be ideal because it would be most in keeping with our duty to respect persons, since respecting persons requires allowing them to live authentically. Living authentically requires being true to oneself, and our gender identities are vital to our overall personal identities. Framed in utilitarian concerns, humankind would be "greater gainers" since everyone knows their own gender identity best, and because everyone is most motivated to be able to express their gender identity or identities freely.[34] Since most of us are heterosexual, single-gendered, and have an orientation toward the opposite sex, there is no worry about the human population dwindling beyond repair.

While our country falls short of this ideal, at least there is a growing awareness that gender identity is not something that can always be molded by social and parental forces. Also, at least there is some availability of psychological counseling for those experiencing gender dysphoria. We have come to see the importance of the child's input into gender assignment when being reassessed at puberty. Finally, we have learned the dangers of secrecy surrounding intersexuality.

The child's parents, buoyed by cultural norms, adamantly refuse to engage in deliberation with their son regarding his gender assignment, and share their culture's preference for the male sex. They are ill-prepared to deal with a sex change in their son. We are not privy to their motives, but it is certainly plausible that they request the operations out of concern for the child.

I have argued that the decision should not be made on the basis of cultural relativism alone. There are numerous considerations independent of cultural values that suggest that it would be morally permissible for the doctors to accede to the parents' wishes. Based on empirical evidence from several different countries, we know that the child's apparent male gender identity is probably fixed, that it is unlikely that he would want to reproduce even if a sex change were to occur, and that he most likely would be gynecophilic. We know that given the pervasive social preference for males, however skewed, flexibility in the formation of gender identity will likely help the child deal with ambivalence he might experience, and compensate, in the child's experience, for the loss of having an alternative gender assignment opened to him.

These findings become especially relevant, given that the child has demonstrated male pattern behavior, even though sometimes gender behavior and gender identity are discordant. Further, the child articulates a desire to have the mastectomies performed—a plausible sign that he is rejecting any expression of a female gender identity. These indications suggest that he would likely be grateful for the parents' frankly paternalistic decision.

Consider the trauma the boy and the family would have to face if the doctors refuse to perform the surgeries. The boy would continue to develop breasts and to menstruate, and the female hormones might incline him to be attracted to males, which would be dangerous in his society. He would become a more visible target of teasing that could very well escalate to social ostracism. That ostracism could extend to the entire family, and the fear of it could keep them from returning to their own home.

Dreger's proposal that the boy take leuprolide to delay puberty until he has been fully informed about his condition and alternatives does not seem realistic. First, the boy is already suffering from the taunting of his peers. Second, the boy has already expressed a desire for the mastectomies, and all things considered, would not likely desire delaying hormonal treatment necessary to begin masculine development. Secondly, counseling would be unavailable to him in his own country to help him through the process of digesting what would be bewildering and psychologically challenging information. To be sure, if empirical evidence were not available that strongly supported the prediction of a firm male gender identity in cases of individuals with 46XX CAH, Prader level 5, who were reared as males, these conclusions would be hasty and unjustified.

Two possible objections need to be considered. First, it might be contested that even though the evidence suggests probable male gender identity, we cannot be certain of it. We cannot even be certain about gender identity in nonintersexuals. The possibility cannot be denied that the boy would come to identify as female and regret the loss of his reproductive functioning. However, it is only because of the dire situation the boy and family face that the decision can be justified on the basis of strong probability.

Second, if the boy is not provided with a proper explanation of his medical condition, he may not be compliant in taking the masculinizing hormones. Many intersexuals have stopped taking hormones because they have not fully understood their importance. In general, compliance is greatly enhanced by patient understanding and participation in medical decisions. So the boy could be harmed in the future by not having been informed. In response, it could be argued that if the boy were willing to take the drastic steps of having his breasts removed, he is obviously anxious to appear male, and if it were explained that the medication was necessary for that, he would be motivated to comply.

Given all the evidence and facts available to us, the boy would probably be better off returning to his country as a male. This judgment is not a matter of respecting or rejecting cultural values. To approach the case on that basis involves taking a shortcut that fails to accord proper respect for the boy and fails to consider his overall best interests. Taking into consideration cultural values does not imply deferring to them, nor does it imply an abdication of our own values. The case clearly involves conflicts of duties, and such conflicts by definition do not allow of completely satisfactory solutions. Nothing has been said to call into question the duty to procure informed consent for surgeries that may conflict with gender identities, sexual functioning, and the capacity to live an authentic existence.

Sharon Sytsma, Associate Professor, Department of Philosophy, Northern Illinois University, DeKalb, Illinois, U.S.A.

---

[1] The National Institute of Child Health & Human Development (NICHD) Research Planning Workshop on Intersex, May 19-20, 2002, Tempe, Arizona, 2002. (The author was present at this meeting serving as an Ethics Consultant.)

[2] Heino Meyer-Bahlburg, "Gender and Sexuality in Classical Congenital Adrenal Hyperplasia," *Endocrinol Metab Clin North Am* 30.1 (2001): 155-71, viii.

[3] Diamond David, Sharon Sytsma, and Alice Dreger and Bruce Wilson. "Case Study: Culture Clash Involving Intersex," *Hastings Center Report* 33.4 (July-August 2003): 12-14.

[4] By cultural relativism, I refer specifically to the moral theory that cultural values determine what is moral or immoral.

[5] This case has been published in the Hastings Center Report, with commentaries by this author, David Diamond, and Alice Dreger and Bruce Wilson.

[6] Heino Meyer-Bahlburg, "Gender Assignment in Intersexuality," *J Psychol Hum Sex* 10 (1998): 1-21.

[7] Gordon Burton, Esq., "General Discussion of the Legal Issues Affecting Sexual Assignment of Intersex Infants Born with Ambiguous Genitalia," *Third National Symposium: Bioethical Considerations in Human Subject Research*, Clearwater, Florida, March 2000; Julie Greenberg, Esq., "Legal Aspects of Gender Assignment," *Hormonal and Genetic Basis of Sexual Differentiation Disorders*, Tempe, AZ, May 16-18, 2002; Hazel Beh and Milton Diamond, "An Emerging Ethical and Medical Dilemma: Should Physicians Perform Sex Assignment Surgery on Infants with Ambiguous Genitalia? *Michigan Journal of Gender and Law* 7.1 (2000): 1-63; L. Hermer, "Paradigms Revised: Intersex Children, Bioethics & The Law," *Annals of Health Law* 11 (2002): 195-236.

[8] North American Task Force Meeting, November 18th, 2000, Columbia University, New York.

[9] Milton Diamond and H. K. Sigmundson, "Management of Intersexuality: Guidelines for Dealing with Persons with Ambiguous Genitalia," *Arch Pediatr Adolesc Med* 151 (1997): 298-304.

[10] John Colapinto, "The True Story of John/Joan," *Rolling Stone Magazine* (Dec. 11, 1997): 56-97; John Colapinto, *As Nature Made Him: The Boy Who was Raised a Girl*, New York: Harper Collins, 2000. Also, Kenneth Kipnis and Milton Diamond, "Pediatric Ethics and the Surgical Assignment of Sex," *The Journal of Clinical Ethics* 9.4 (1998): 398-410.

[11] See literature by the Intersex Society of North America located on their website: http://www.isna.org/. See also Sarah Creighton and Catherine Minto, "Managing Intersex," *BMJ* 323 (Dec., 2001): 1264-65; and Justine Schober, "A Surgeon's Response to the Intersex Controversy," *The Journal of Clinical Ethics* 9(4): 393-97.

[12] See Alice Dreger, *Hermaphroditism: The Medical Invention of Sex;* Suzanne Kessler, "The Medical Construction of Gender: Case Management of Intersexed Infants," *J. Women Culture Society* 6 (1990)

3-26; Heino Meyer-Bahlburg, "Gender Assignment in Intersexuality," *J. Psychol. Hum. Sexuality* 10 (1998): 1-21.

[13] G. Herdt, *Third Sex, Third Gender* (New York: Zone Books, 1994); W. Roscoe, *The Zuni-Man Woman* (Albuquerque: University of New Mexico Press, 1991); W. Williams, *The Spirit and the Flesh: Sexual Diversity in American Indian Culture* (Boston: Beacon Press, 1986).

[14] S. A. Taha, "Male Pseudohermaphroditism: Factors Determining the Gender of Rearing in Saudi Arabia," *Urology* 43.3 (1994): 370-4.

[15] B. Yücel, A. and A. Polat, "A Late Sex Reassigment in 5-apha Reductase Deficiency: Case Report," *International Journal of Psychiatry in Medicine* 33.2 (2003): 189-93.

[16] N. M. Dessouky, "Gender Assignment for Children with Intersex Problems: An Egyptian Perspective," *Saudi Medical Journal* 24.5 (2003): S51-2.

[17] Ursula Kuhnle and W. Krahl, "The Impact of Culture on Sex Assignment and Gender Development in Intersex patient," *Perspectives in Biology and Medicine* 45.1 (2002): 85-103.

[18] Kuhnle, 90.

[19] Kuhnle, 65.

[20] Kuhnle, 87.

[21] Heino Meyer-Bahlburg, *Gender and Sexuality in Classical Congenital Adrenal Hyperplasia* 2001(emphasis added).

[22] David Diamond, "Culture Clash Involving Intersex: Commentary," *Hastings Center Report* 33.4 (July-August 2003): 12-13.

[23] Alice Dreger, Bruce Wilson, "Culture Clash Involving Intersexuality: Commentary," *Hastings Center Report,* 33.4 (July-August 2003): 14.

[24] Kenneth Kipnis and Milton Diamond, "Pediatric Ethics and the Surgical Assignment of Sex," *Journal of Clinical Ethics* 9 (Winter 1998): 398-410.

[25] Heino Meyer-Bahlburg, "Gender and Sexuality in Classic Congenital Adrenal Hyperplasia," *Endocrin Meta Clin North Am* 30.1 (2001): 155-171.

[26] J. Woelfle, W. Hoepffner, et al., "Complete Virilization in Congenital Adrenal Hyperplasia: Clinical Course, Medical Management and Disease-related Complications," *Clinical Endocrinology* 56.2 (2002): 231-8.

[27] Meyer-Bahlburg, 2001.

[28] Heino Meyer-Bahlburg, "Gender Identity and Congenital Adrenal Hyperplasia," *Dialogues in Pediatric Urology* 25.7 (2002): 2-3.

[29] N. M. Stikkelbroeck, A. R. Hermus et al., "Fertility in Women with Congenital Adrenal Hyperplasia Due to 21-hydroxylase Deficiency." *Obstetrical and Gynecological Surgery,* 58.4 (2003): 275-84.

[30] Meyer-Bahlburg, 2002.

[31] Meyer-Bahlburg, 2002. See also Peter Lee, "Care of the Intersex Patient: Changing Guidelines," *Dialogues in Pediatric Urology,* 25.7 (2002): 7-8.

[32] Heino Meyer-Bahlburg and Robert Blizzard, "Research on Intersex—Summary of a Planning Workshop," 14.2 (2004): 59-69.

[33] Justine Schober, "A Surgeon's Response to the Intersex Controversy," *The Journal of Clinical Ethics* 9.4 (1998): 393-97.

[34] John Stuart Mill, *On Liberty* (Indianapolis: Bobbs-Merrill Co, 1956) 17.

HERMAN E. STARK

AUTHENTICITY AND INTERSEXUALITY

Ich wollte ja nichts als das zu leben versuchen, was von selber aus mir heraus wollte. Warum war das so sehr schwer?

(I wanted only to live in accord with the promptings of my true self.
Why was that so very difficult?)

Demian, Hermann Hesse

1. INTRODUCTION

One is struck, in reading intersexual self-assessment literature, at how often phrases such as "my true self," "the real me," "being a genuine person," and "the inner self" arise. It seems that a common intersexual problem, in other words, is grappling with the haunting sense that one is not living as a true human self—or not living as the self truly is. Perhaps this is really a universal and even defining human experience, but in the case of intersexuals the self–estrangement seems peculiarly aggravated. The traditional medical treatment of infants born with ambiguous genitalia, for example, involves "deciding" what sex the intersexual should be, and then to perform sex assignment or normalizing surgery and administer hormones accordingly. The problem is not only that incorrect decisions about sex can be made, or that the resulting genitalia can fail to be "normal," but that a number of intersexuals claim that they would have been more truly themselves if they had been left "in between." As it is, however, these outspoken intersexuals, and presumably others shy of the public glare, are bitter about the preemptive surgeries and the accompanying secrecy, deceit, and shame. They are moreover burdened by the sense that somehow they are failing at existence, and feel unnecessarily hindered from the outside in the struggle to be themselves.

The twentieth century German philosopher Martin Heidegger, in his magnus opus, *Being and Time* (which for better or worse stands as prime contender for *the* philosophical book of the twentieth century), draws attention to both the possibility and the problems of achieving truthfulness about one's own self. His key concept is authenticity (*Eigenlichkeit*), and his analysis of it can fruitfully be brought to bear on intersexual experience. Heidegger's insistence on separating authenticity from moral

S.E. Sytsma (Ed.), Ethics and Intersex, 271–291.

concepts allows him to articulate neglected, *existential* dimensions of human experience, including, I suggest, some hinted at in the growing discussion of the traditional treatment of intersexuality.

In recent years there has been a growing movement that advocates rethinking the standard medical response. While a radical alternative is to abandon the male/female dichotomy, intersex advocates suggest giving a preliminary but defeasible sex assignment at birth, and postponing surgery until the child is capable of articulating his or her preferences on the matter. (See the Mission Statement of Intersex Society of North America, www.isna.org). While the tendency in philosophy is to start thinking about these matters in terms of ethics or biomedical ethics, I want to sidestep these issues and concentrate on another dimension of the intersexual issue. My focus is on a specialized, existential, or even ontological philosophical concept: authenticity. I suggest that a discussion of authenticity might serve to articulate both *universal* and *particular* issues at stake, including what might be imperilled for infants through the traditional treatment, why autonomy matters, why some intersexuals doggedly track down medical information, and just what it is that despairing adult intersexuals might be seeking. I suggest also, in what turns out to be a philosophically worthwhile payback, that thinking about authenticity in terms of intersexuality raises questions about the content and range of Heidegger's notion of authenticity.

This essay, then, is intended for at least three audiences: those interested in intersexuality, those interested in Heidegger, and those interested in the study of concepts and their applications. For instance, with respect to intersexuality we might ask: What does it means to be either male or female (especially in the face of stark ambiguity)? Does the application of the male/female dichotomy to intersexuals force the mutually–exclusive binary to be now seen as the ends of a continuum? In the same way, a problem with Heidegger's analysis is that it is not clear what authenticity covers and what it does not cover. How integral, in other words, is our gender–identification to our authentic self? Also, can authenticity be subject to external threats? And, are there degrees of authenticity? Moreover, there are multiple senses of self, and thus of self–estrangement, and so a caveat and provisional idea here is that just as Heidegger's analysis might illuminate the intersexual's homelessness, so also might thinking through the intersexual's lament illuminate Heidegger's analysis of authenticity.

2. BIOLOGICAL, PSYCHOLOGICAL AND SOCIOLOGICAL CONSIDERATIONS

The single term "intersexuality" actually refers a number of conditions that belie our habits of thinking about sex in dimorphic terms, that is, as male or female. A number of factors contribute to sexual differentiation, and these factors can affect each other. Intersexuality can be caused at the chromosomal level by mosaicism, at the genetic level by the presence or absence of gene sequences, at the gonadal level through aberrations in the development of the gonads, and at the hormonal level. We can speak of chromosomal sex, genetic sex, gonadal sex, phenotypic sex; we can talk about sex of rearing, gender identity, and sexual orientation. All these can line up in consistent or in inconsistent ways. Chromosomal males can appear typically female, and chromosomal females can appear typically male, and some intersexual conditions are marked by ambiguous genitalia. Determining—or assigning—the sex of a child at birth can be a highly complex matter.

Consider all that can hinge on gender assignment: name, manner of dress, male or female bathroom, way of using the bathroom, education, occupation, inheritance, being a husband or wife, a mother or a father, a heterosexual or a homosexual. The consequences of making a sex–determination are staggering—even if the person (for example, the attending physician) making the determination is not around a decade or two later to witness them. The choice of assigning a sex of male or female, then, is not merely a matter of looking, or identifying chromosomes, or examining gonads, or testing hormones.

Given, then, that decisions on sex assignment are of the sort that William James (1899) called "momentous," it behooves us to ask whether they are also, to borrow further from James, "forced." A forced decision is one that cannot be realistically avoided. For example, at some point Othello has to make a decision between trusting Desdemona or trusting Iago. Though sometimes intersexuality is associated with conditions in need of immediate medical treatment, such as Salt-wasting Congenital Adrenal Hyperplasia, it does not seem that there is any *medical* reason for regarding the sex assignment decision on newborns as a forced decision.

Perhaps it is rather that there are social/psychological factors that make newborn sex determination decisions a forced decision. It must be horribly traumatic, after all, to go through childhood years as "neither a boy nor a girl," to say nothing of those already horribly traumatic teenage years. But the evidence here is not straightforward; with more intersexuals speaking out in recent years one sees that past actual sex assignment decisions created some hells of their own. Even those intersexuals satisfied enough with the correctness of the male or female choices made for them can still harbor regret, shame, misery, and *a longing to have been left alone, that is, left to live with their bodies as they were.*

It might be objected here that while exceptions are inevitable, on average sex determination decisions on newborns promote the greatest good for the greatest number, whether the number reckons society as a whole or is restricted to the patients themselves. Moreover, it might be that soon enough cosmetic surgery will be safe, convenient, and affordable enough so that unhappy adult sex–reassigned intersexuals can simply opt to go back to their "original" condition. The relative allure of these objections will depend, in part, on how utilitarian one is, how much faith one has in cosmetic surgery, and on how redeemable those intervening "lost" years are.

There have been several strands of concern in the literature on our traditional medical practices in dealing with intersexuality. One strand of discussion has to do with the psychological possibility that the child will not accept the assigned gender. Another strand discusses psychological harms of medical treatment other than that of the surgically induced gender dysphoria, for instance, feelings of shame or fear resulting from secrecy. Yet another strand has to do with physical matters such as whether the surgical approaches are successful. An ethical strand of the discussion concerns whether infant genital surgery violates the future autonomy of the child. We are in position now to isolate an *existential strand* motivating the worry with the traditional treatment: the existential concern that the traditional treatment of intersexuality poses a unique, or at least unnecessary, problem for achieving *authenticity* in one's existence.

3. INTERSEXUALITY AND PROMPTINGS FOR AUTHENTICITY

In this section I want to highlight aspects of intersexual experience that bespeak the philosophical notion of authenticity. I will draw on a collection of essays by intersexuals edited by Alice Domurat Dreger (1999). Admittedly, these are narratives by individuals for whom sex-assignment or genital normalizing surgery has led to a negative, even traumatic, experience, and hence, may not be objectively representative of the majority of intersexuals. Dreger admits as much (in Dreger, ed., 1999, p. 20), but notes that her requests for contributions from proponents of the older model were met with either "silence" or "lack of time" replies ("Quiet! Surgery in progress!") Nevertheless, listening to these intersexuals helps to isolate more deeply what might have been "lost" in those intervening years during which intersexuals lived as sex–assigned individuals.

The experiences to which I draw attention result from the practice of imposing a male or female sex assignment on a person who either is not one or the other (that is to say, is an intersexual), or who is not able to function in ways expected of their sex. The general approach is the "Optimal Gender Approach" of determining whether the child's physical condition is more conducive to the kinds of functioning thought to be most essential to being male or female. Thus, any child having female reproductive potential is assigned to the female sex, even if born with a normal appearing penis. If no female reproductive capacity exists, then male assignment is given providing that the phallus is substantial enough to penetrate (perhaps with some surgical assistance) a vagina. Otherwise, a female assignment is made. In practice, the policy means that nine out of 10 intersex sex assignments are to the female sex. ("It is easier to make a hole than build a pole.") (*Redefining Sex*, 2000).

The policy is based on numerous assumptions, including that there are and ought only to be two sexes, that male successful functioning requires a substantial penis, that female functioning requires a vagina, and if possible, reproductive capacity, and that gender identity is so malleable that sex assignment will be (almost always) successful. But why should one suppose, *even if sex is malleable,* that surgical alteration or sex assignment would make life easier than leaving the child alone? In the case of David Reimer (Colapinto, 2000), for example, *perhaps too much concern was given to potential future socialization problems and not enough to the overall process of becoming a self;* it may turn out, in other words, that an authentic self can be achieved only by the self learning and struggling to forge an identity from how it was thrown into the world (barring, of course, genuine medical emergency).

All these presuppositions have been called into question as a result of the experience of intersexuals, as indicated by the following passages:

On Father's Day I decided that I had had enough of the [testosterone] patches…I no longer feel "caught between." I am a unique blend of my female and male essences, and I expect to continue evolving on that level (Cameron, in Dreger, ed., p. 96).

I feel in between male and female. I don't really know what "masculine" feels like, but I don't feel like the "feminine" that I see in my Mom and my sisters, either (Walcutt, in Dreger, ed., 1999, p. 200).

I have become accepting of my intersexuality…and I have an awareness of myself as a valuable and unique person, an intersexed person who is feminine (Triea, in Dreger, ed., 1999, p. 143).

There are a lot of things that could have happened to me that would have been a lot worse. My physical condition has not stopped me from enjoying the truly wonderful things in life—a perfect sunset, a sumptuous meal, the laughter of a close friend, or the softness of my lover's kiss. I am glad to be who I am (Hawbecker, in Dreger, ed., 1999, p. 113).

These quotes force us to ask what exactly is wrong with leaving intersexed people intersexed? If no medical threat is present, then the primary justification would seem to be to help people "fit" into the binary constructs of our society. But the above quotes are from people who were not able to fit in, either during or after completion of the traditional treatment, and who moreover managed to fit in, somewhat at least, only after they accepted themselves as intersexuals. It appears that at least some intersexuals do better, psychologically, socially, and physically, when left or returned to their intersexed status.

David Reimer, the man behind the infamous John/Joan case recounted by John Colapinto (2000), expresses similar experience. Though not an intersexual by nature, David became one through surgery undertaken after he had lost his penis during circumcision to correct phimosis. David, the boy who was supposed to have been successfully raised a girl, we later found out, did not at all embrace his female sex assignment. (See chapter by Murphy). After a miserable, unhappy, lonely, uninformed childhood and early adolescence of acting and feeling utterly like a boy, his father finally reveals to him the story of his birth, medical mishap, and surgical female sex assignment. Colapinto reports that besides the "anger, disbelief, and amazement" David experienced at the moment of truth, the overriding emotion was relief. In David's words:

"I was *relieved*," he says. "Suddenly it all made sense why I felt the way I did. I wasn't some sort of weirdo. I wasn't *crazy* (Colapinto, 2000, p. 180).

If I was raised a boy, I would have been more accepted by other people. I would have been way better off if they had just left me alone, because when I switched back over, then I had *two* problems on my hands, not just one, because of them trying to brainwash me into accepting myself as a girl. So you got the *psychological* thing going on in your head (Colapinto, 2000, p. 262).

You know, if I had lost my arms and my legs and wound up in a wheelchair where you're moving everything with a little rod in your mouth—would that make me less of a person? It just seems that they implied that you're nothing if your penis is gone. The second you lose *that*, you're nothing, and they've got to do surgery and hormones to turn you into something. Like you're a zero. It's like your whole personality, everything about you is directed—all pinpointed—toward what's between the legs. And to me, that's ignorant. I don't have the kind of education that these scientists and doctors and psychologists have, but to me it's very ignorant. If a woman lost her breasts, do you turn her into a guy? To make her feel "whole and complete" (Colapinto, 2000, p. 262).

The institutionalized degree of paternal deception and secrecy intrinsic to the traditional practices would be surprising even to Kremlinologists. This paternal secrecy spreads beyond intersexuality, as some who have dealt with American hospitals and healthcare have learned, but with respect to intersexuality, it has profound implications:

> The primary source of harm described by former patients is not surgery per se, but the underlying attitude that intersexuality is so shameful that it must be erased before the child can have any say in what will be done to his or her body (Chase, in Dreger, ed., 1999, p. 147).

The existential slant of these passages remind us of our sometime yearning for *authenticity,* and that moreover reminds us of Aristotle's remark that even dearer than Plato is…truth. The practice of sex assignment, with all of the attendant hushing up, is not only a threat to honesty, informed consent, and autonomy, but it is *treating someone as incapable of hearing their own truth.* Sherri A. Groveman writes,

> It is disorienting when you have always considered yourself female to learn that you have XY chromosomes and once had testes. It is equally disorienting when you have always considered yourself loved and cared for to discover that your parents and doctors have lied and left you to your own devices to discover this truth (in Dreger, ed., 1999, p. 26).

Sharon E. Preves, in interviewing forty–one adults born sexually ambiguous, records,

> According to the participants, lacking information about their bodies and medical histories was far more difficult than actually knowing the truth (in Dreger, ed., 1999, p. 57).

Angela Moreno:

> I am horrified by what has been done to me and by the conspiracy of silence and lies (in Dreger, ed., 1999, p. 139).

This is not to say that one must be crass or brutally direct, for as Coventry reports, "coming out as a hermaphrodite has its own precious timing (in Dreger, ed., 1999, p. 76), that is, even those who already know still have difficulty:

> But I'm kind to myself when I can't quite tell the whole truth, as all intersexuals should be. We have lifetimes of shame to overcome and, for most of us, this has been a secret that we have guarded with our lives and at great expense (in Dreger, ed., 1999, p. 76).

This last remark has a distinctly Heideggerian ring to it, for it illustrates the thesis that we slide back and forth between authenticity and inauthenticity, that is, not only cannot one be continuously authentic, one does not want to be.

I propose that a philosophical lesson to learn from these intersexual experiences is that both their number and content points to authenticity, or rather the call for authenticity, as a fundamental concern. That is, in these narratives one can find, it seems, a call from intersexuals to let them suffer the truth of who they are. They show how authenticity is linked to truth, or more precisely a respect for, a reverence for, and a courage about truth. The tough drive for truth—the quest for a meaningful, based–in–reality, existence—is the underlying unifier for the various moments or modes of authenticity, including, as will be explained below, authentic projection (of one's existence) and anticipatory resoluteness (about one's existence).

4. TRANSITION TO HEIDEGGER

What may have been lost in the traditional treatment of intersexuals? Above I spoke of authenticity in terms of willingness to suffer the truth, but now I offer a different entry: what may have been lost is the sense that one's life is one's own project, one's own projection, and instead is a following out of another's projection. Authentic existence means, in part, living out our own life, not the life others have foisted upon us (I hasten to admit that all authentic projection is circumscribed, pardon the pun, by our "thrownness"; see Heidegger, 1962, p. 183, H144, and Golomb 2001). The opening quote of this essay underlined the *universality* (intersexuals may well be peculiarly plagued but they are not alone) of this struggle, and apropos Hesse, let me add another revealing line about the *process* of becoming an authentic self:

> Der Vogel kämpft sich aus dem Ei. Das Ei ist die Welt. Wer geboren werden will, muß eine Welt zerstören (Hesse, 1974, p. 91).

> The bird struggles out of the egg. The egg is the world. Who wants to be born must destroy a world (mine).

Psychoanalyst Alice Miller, using Hesse's troubled childhood as an example of the drama of the gifted child and his search for the true self, notes:

> Many people suffer all their lives from this oppressive feeling of guilt, the sense of not having lived up to their parents' expectations. This feeling is stronger than any intellectual insight that it is not a child's task or duty to satisfy his parents' narcissistic needs. No argument can overcome these guilt feelings, for they have their beginnings in life's earliest period, and from that they derive their intensity and obduracy.

> That probably greatest of narcissistic wounds—not to have been loved just as one truly was—cannot heal without the work of mourning. It can either be more or less successfully resisted and covered up (as in grandiosity and depression), or constantly torn open again in the compulsion to repeat (p. 85).

Miller's main theme is the repression of the true self in gifted children (defined in terms of sensitivity, alertness, and range and depth of feeling), rooted in the children's recognition of and adoption to their parents' needs, thereby blocking access to authentic individual feelings (healthy narcissism), and confining the true self within the prison of the false self (narcissistic disturbances). But her insights seem applicable also to intersexuals. Miller's psychoanalysis might extend beyond gifted children to intersexual children in that the latter are almost perforce intensely sensitive and also probably vaguely aware of not having met expectations.

To continue on this path of thinking about intersexuality in terms of authenticity, we again look at some psychological insight, this time from Kipnis and Diamond, who under a section heading "Psychosocial Life" write:

> While it remains to be seen how deeply our gendered behavior is neurologically hard–wired, there are at least three aspects of it that deserve consideration. The first calls attention to one's *sexual identity*. How does one see oneself at the deepest level? In addition to female and male, some now self–identify as intersexed (in Dreger 1999, p. 185).

It is a weighty and fascinating question that they ask: How does one see oneself at the deepest level? But it is precisely here that we can finish off the transition to Heidegger, for he raises a question about this very question: what is the most fundamental way that we can address this question? His ensuing treatment of these questions, and his answers, do not involve (primarily) psychological introspection but a different, allegedly deeper, plane than we have come to expect. And the same goes with respect to Miller's work; her psychoanalysis might indeed be as astute as one can get on that level, but she also does not address the question of self as Heidegger does. For Heidegger, the way to address how one should see oneself at the deepest level is not psychoanalytically, psychologically, sociologically, or anthropologically, but *ontologically*.

A caveat, however, about talk of the authentic self: the aim here is not to twist or stretch authenticity so that it fits our purposes. I have thus limited myself to Heidegger's analysis to lessen the chance of authenticity running away on us. I am worried, in other words, about *ad hoc* stipulations to "the" notion of authenticity (Whose notion? Is there just one?) so that it "fits" someone's intuitions about a phenomenon. I am worried also by the conflation between authenticity and autonomy; the latter is the concept really required, I suggest, in a number of biomedical ethical arguments that needlessly, if not improperly, make authenticity their cornerstone. Arnason (1994), for example, admirably sets out to apply "the existential notion" of authenticity to the patient–professional relationship, but ends up both with an alternative idea of authenticity and one that sounds too "ethical" to be, at any rate, Heidegger's. (How many notions of authenticity are out there? For surveys, see Taylor 1992 and Guignon 2004). From my vantage point, I will see at best a spectral notion of authenticity in Heidegger, to say nothing of the different, sometimes intriguing but usually less ontological, that is, less anchored in reality and thus more makeshift, concepts of authenticity that can be found in other philosophers. The limited task here, then, is to apply Heidegger's authenticity (including qua anticipatory resoluteness and the finitude–affirming appropriation of time), whether by implication or intimation, to intersexuality.

5.   HEIDEGGER

The sense of self–estrangement mentioned at the outset of this essay might be accompanied by a sense of moral failure, but it is not always so. Sometimes the sense is precisely and solely the nagging inner call that while one has done nothing morally wrong, one is failing at existence itself, or, more neutrally, one's existence is somehow askew. The phenomenon, in other words, is best located as an existential rather than moral matter.

Heidegger's heavily discussed, and often misunderstood, distinction is key to understanding this notion of failing at existence. I want to propose that this distinction seems to be the right sort for understanding the plight of numerous intersexuals. The subtle insights and conceptual innovations provided by Heidegger's discussion, in other words, would seem capable of *systematizing*, that is, understanding and articulating in a general way, some of the anguish expressed in the intersexual literature.

The common mistake is to see the authenticity/inauthenticity distinction as another moral distinction, similar to good/bad or virtuous/vicious, or to see authenticity merely in terms of autonomy. It might turn out that authenticity is a sort of desideratum, but even then the distinction between authenticity and inauthenticity should be seen, initially and ultimately, as primordially descriptive rather than prescriptive: that is, it is used to help capture what it is like to exist as a human. Descriptively, the existential way we exist is to find ourselves thrown into a world that has carried us along from birth, to have the capacity to realize that we can break away from its current to forge our own course, and to be subject to the tendency to the strength of the current that keep us from making our lives our own. While authenticity demands truthfulness, and while sometimes we do desire it, as noted in the preceding intersexual confessions, the truth is, "No, we don't, at least not always." Truth is hard, especially ontological truth about ourselves.

6.   THE GLASS MENAGERIE

Ordinarily, in an attempt to explain Heidegger, one would lay out the basic concepts of Heidegger's existential analytic and go from there. The problem with this is that a general readership is burdened up front with learning a lot of technical concepts while waiting, and waiting, and waiting, for the concrete payoff. Moreover, so addictive is Heidegger's argot that even those philosophers who claim to be writing for a non–Heideggerian audience invariably come across as jargonistic. This is how lost one can get in the world of Heidegger. It is difficult to summarize Heidegger's analysis of authenticity, even for a Heideggerian audience. What I propose to do here, then, is to pick just a few moments in Heidegger's spectral, multi–layered, and indeed, multiple *accounts* of authenticity, and bring them to bear on the above work on intersexuality. I will not pretend to cover all issues, nor will I claim to avoid jargon in discussing this major thinker whose major claims include the alleged need to develop new concepts to articulate what familiar language has covered up. (For generally accessible introductions/overviews of *Being and Time*, see Melchert, 1999, pp. 656–702 and Gelven 1989.)

For the technical topic of authenticity I thus immediately work the intuitive pump by using a concrete and objectively–available portrait of someone's existence, namely, Tom Wingfield in Tennessee Williams' *The Glass Menagerie.* This choice is apt given its explicit treatment of Tom running both from, and to, himself. This unorthodox approach--working from extended example back to abstract analysis—will illustrate what it means to give an ontological analysis of the self. With this toehold secured, we can turn to intersexuality and then to some technical questions concerning Heidegger's analysis of authenticity.

What, then, is the ontological self–description of Tom Wingfield? It is a description that targets the essential structures of *Dasein,* (any human or for that matter, any rational self-conscious being concerned to exist meaningfully.) These essential structures have been missed in the history of philosophy, to say nothing of the sciences, but can be isolated by the technique of hermeneutic phenomenology, that is, a Kantian–like *"Bedingung der Möglichkeit"* regression to the preconditions of "lived–experience." In the case of Tom, one can think about him in many ways, for example, psychologically, sociologically, economically, or even sexually (although for Tom, his sexuality is a relatively innocuous part of his "facticity" and not a main problem for his self–understanding). To think about him ontologically would run as follows.

To be Tom is to find oneself a member of a broken family in a seedy part of St. Louis during the depression era. His father, a telephone man "who fell in love with long distance," and who once sent a postcard from Mexico with two words, "Hello. Goodbye," left the family ill–equipped to deal with the exigencies of life. Amanda, Tom's fading Southern belle mother, partly lives in a world that is both back in the South and back in time. Laura, Tom's older sister, is a cripple so lacking self–confidence that she vomits in typing class and cannot bring herself to open the door when the gentleman caller knocks. There are more details, just as we each have our own set of details, but Heidegger's point here is that part of what it is to be a human being (or more precisely, *Dasein*—a being capable of self-reflection), in this case Tom, is to be "thrown" into the world, that is, into a particular context not of our making, nor of our choosing, in which our existence takes place. The expression 'thrownness' is meant to suggest the *facticity of its being delivered over* (Heidegger, 1962, p. 174, H135). A lot is packed into this sentence, but for our purposes here it is enough to note that not only is there no "self–grounding" self in complete control of its existence, there is also no self, no you, without the context in which your existence unfolds.

Tom is sometimes gentle and often exasperated with his chatty mother, but he is especially attached, with exquisite solicitude, to Laura. With the rest of the world he is noticeably detached, except with Jim, the gentleman caller, who becomes temporarily useful, and who teases Tom at work by calling the secretive poet "Shakespeare." To be Tom, then, is to be with others, whether it pleases him or not, and even when seeking to escape them. In the extreme this means that no one is more with others than the hermit, whose entire way of existing is defined by a privative, that is, a fleeing-from.

To be Tom is to be frustrated, annoyed, somewhat despairing, and occasionally teasing. To be Tom is to be in a mood, but for Heidegger this means Tom, *Dasein*, is constantly, automatically, assessing "how it is going" with existence. Moods are pre–cognitively disclosive; they reveal our "affective attunement" (Hatab, 2000, p. 21), that is, they show more immediately than our conscious beliefs do that "being–

in–the–world" matters to us. Moreover, being–in–a–mood not only shapes us, it also shapes the world, or, more accurately for Heidegger, it colors our being–in–the–world–as–a–whole: A mood makes manifest 'how one is, and how one is faring'…In this 'how one is,' having a mood brings Being to its "there" (Heidegger, 1962, p. 173, H134). In any event, with respect to the ontological reading of mood, it was Wittgenstein, I believe, who noted that a depressed man lives in a depressed world.

To be Tom is to be dreaming of joining the merchant marines. To be Tom is to be projecting possibilities. This does not mean abstract possibilities, but possibilities for his existence. It is not merely that Tom will join the marines, he wants to *become* a merchant marine. He is seeing the flight from home, from adventure–stifling obligation to Amanda and Laura, as a new way of existing, a new self:

> "Dasein is the possibility of Being–free *for* its ownmost potentiality–for–Being. Its Being–possible is transparent to itself in different possible ways and degrees" (Heidegger, 1962, p. 183).

But the first appositional phrase in the sentence above the quote is particularly telling, for the moral trade off shows that there is no "absolute freedom," no unlimited projection of one's own existence:

> In every case Dasein, as essentially having a state–of–mind [roughly, for present purposes, thrownness], has already got itself into definite possibilities (Heidegger, 1962, p. 183).

Tom cannot, unlike others, join the marines with a relatively easy conscience; in his case joining means dealing with, or trying to deal away, the moral torment caused by abandoning those who need him. He did not choose that his projection would be so loaded with moral anguish; his particular thrownness instead defines *what it means* for him to join the marines. More generally, thrownness means that you cannot, despite the motivational mantras, be anything you want, for example, you cannot be the first president of the United States, the first to land on the moon, or your first lover's first lover. Furthermore, every projection both shuts out projections and opens new potentiality, that is, every projection lands in a variation of the limiting conditions of thrownness.

To be Tom is to be battling, verbally, with Amanda: "Rise and shine, rise and shine!" she sings to the morning–hating and thereby noble Tom. To be Tom is to be exhorted: Laura urges Tom, "Let her [Amanda] tell it [a story from Amanda's Blue Mountain youth] again [for the zillionth time]." To be Tom is to narrate: "The magician gives you illusion in the disguise of truth, but I give you truth in the pleasant disguise of illusion." To be Tom is to be immersed in language, that is, it is the sharing, the hearing, the ostracizing, the awkward pauses, the fierce exclamations, the inelegant imprecations, and the sweet silences that already bespeak the fundamentally ontological nature of our existence. The most overt example of this last point is "poetical" discourse, which in *Being and Time* "…amounts to a disclosing of existence" (Heidegger, 1962, p. 205, H162), and in later works is elevated to "Language is the house of Being" (Heidegger, 1971a, pp. 5, 21) and "So I renounced and sadly see: Where word breaks off no thing may be" (Heidegger, 1971a, p. 64). Consider that Tom Wingfield is *telling* us, with extreme poignancy, the story of his existence, and that Heidegger has been *writing,* all along, about what it means to exist, and also that this very essay is not so much a shaping of language as an already–having–been–shaped–by–language:

> Language *speaks.* This means at the same time and before all else: *language* speaks. Language? And not man? (Heidegger, 1971b, p. 198).

It is not we who speak language, as if we are over, above, and separable from articulation, it is language that speaks through us, and that articulates us.

To be Tom is also to exchange pleasantries, however painfully, with others at work, in the street, and at the store. To be Tom is to be engaged in idle talk:

> Idle talk is something which anyone can rake up…[t]he fact that something has been said groundlessly, and then gets passed in further retelling, amounts to perverting the act of disclosing into the act of closing off (Heidegger, 1962, p. 213, H169).

The insight here is that idle talk has the consequence of shaping public consciousness, and the ultimate result is even more stunning:

> The dominance of the public way in which things have been interpreted has already been decisive even for the possibilities of having a mood—that is, for the basic way in which Dasein lets the world "matter" to it. The "they" prescribes one's state–of–mind, and determines what and how one 'sees' (Heidegger, 1962, p. 213, H170).

This 'they' is the English for the German *das Man* (Heidegger, 1927, p. 170), which is emerging as the heart of inauthenticity.

To be Tom is to have a glance at the newspaper before dinner, and sometimes a glance at the latest film after dinner. To be Tom, in other words, is to be distracted by curiosity:

> Curiosity is everywhere and nowhere…Idle talk controls even the ways in which one may be curious. It says what one "must" have read and seen. In being everywhere and nowhere, curiosity is delivered over to idle talk (1962, p. 217, H173).

Here again we approach inauthenticity, which is appearing as an absorption into the current, perhaps trendy, way of interpreting, or indeed living, existence.

To be Tom is to have the light bill to pay, to try to punch in at work on time, to fail to return that filthy D. H. Lawrence novel to the library, and to find a gentleman caller for Laura. To be Tom is to be immersed in tasks. We first come across this idea in Heidegger's early distinction between ready–to–hand and present–at–hand (Heidegger, 1962, pp. 98–101, H69–72), that is, between relating to the world of things in terms of use (the letter opener) and as objects (the broken letter opener), where to use something is almost to become one with it, so lost is any conscious sense of being a self, but later this "being–caught–up–in–the–busyness–of–existence" [mine] becomes more ominous, that is, being–defined–by–the–business–of–existence" [mine]. These two phrases capture an ambiguity in Heidegger's analysis of inauthenticity. Sometimes inauthenticity comes across as merely the unavoidable baseline for limited creatures with needs, desires, and things to do, and other times as a failing, something about which to be ashamed (one is ashamed not of actions but of who one is). Indeed, Heidegger insists that his choice of "Fallenness" as the general characteristic exemplified by idle talk and curiosity should not be seen as negative evaluation (Heidegger, 1962, p. 265, H222), but on the other hand authenticity rises out of, or at least involves a revised comportment toward, fallenness (see below). We are, in other, words, on the precipice of Heidegger's analysis of authenticity. But to close off the present point, to be Tom is to be caught up in the world, whether willingly or not, for "the world is too much with us."

In sum, to answer concretely and fundamentally who Tom is, we have relied on concepts such as Being–thrown, Being–with, Being–in–a–mood, Projecting–possibilities, Talk, Idle talk, Curiosity, and Fallenness. These "existentials" are not all the ones Heidegger identifies, but the group is sufficient to allow us to see the sense in which it is correct to say the following: to be Tom is to be…anyone. And anyone is the heart of Heidegger's analysis of inauthenticity.

7. INAUTHENTICITY

For Heidegger, *das Man* (equivalents here: 'anyone', 'they–self', or 'inauthenticity') is the default mode of existence; it cannot be excised or extirpated, and any authenticity is but a "modification" of the inauthentic way we all, for the most part, exist (Heidegger, 1962, p. 312, H267). Heidegger chooses the term *das Man* for many reasons, but one is that it captures anonymity of the sort found in the English 'one says', 'one does', 'one should', 'one doesn't expect', and so on. A simple but telling example is that nowadays one automatically begins sentences with "Well…" or "Actually…"–just as one used to say "groovy" and "far out." (In the hilarious footage of Woodstock, to further the point, one sees that everyone present, despite ubiquitous talk of "being unique," did the same thing, dressed the same way, listened to the same sort of music, and spoke with the same rhythm, pitch, volume, and words; for more on the self–vitiation of uniqueness–assertions or indeed on the myth of such individuality, see Stark 2000a, 2000b). Another reason for *das Man* is that it contrasts with *eigen, eigentlich,* and *Eigenlichkeit,* the German root and words for authenticity, which carry a core meaning of "own" or "ownness." Heidegger's terms, in other words, set up a contrast between anonymity and "mine own."

As mentioned above, Heidegger's initial uses of inauthenticity suggest non–moral, non–censurable, and "anyone" ways of being–human. Walking into a classroom with pen and notebook, taking a chair at the dinner table, standing at arm's length when speaking to a colleague, and leaving the room through the doorway instead of the wall, are thankfully decided for us. We don't have to endure Hamlet–like indecision or cognitive waste contemplating the multitude of things we can readily pick up by "social–referencing." But later in *Being and Time* Heidegger talks of death, guilt, conscience, and resoluteness, and the tone here is far from neutral, and indeed like Ivan Ilyich's horrified discovery—"What if my whole life has really been wrong?" (Tolstoy, 1960, p. 153)—that he has lived his life inauthentically. What is one to make of this range from neutral inauthenticity to self–indictment inauthenticity?

I suggest that one pictorialize Heidegger's analysis of authenticity by means of an arch–shaped scale (think of the needle–like pointers on applause meters in the days before light–emitting–diodes), on which the full spectrum of inauthenticity might be plotted (remember, authenticity is a modification of inauthenticity, and so takes its loci from the latter). At the left, "neutral" end of the scale we plot Heidegger's opening examples of inauthenticity, that is, taking the train and reading the newspaper (Heidegger, 1962, p. 164, H126). At the right, "evaluative" end we plot failing to acknowledge (acknowledge in a real, finitude–making way) that we are dying, and also that we are responsible not only for the actions we do but for who we have become (and are becoming). At the middle we plot usually innocuous but potentially insidious examples, like taking pleasure and enjoying ourselves "as they do" (Heidegger, 1962, p. 164, H127). A unifying idea might be that inauthenticity is at first a *tendency* to choose anonymity over *Eigenlichkeit* in our conduct, but that this can become (for example, in charged situations), to use McBride's more ominous word, a *temptation* (McBride in Audi, 1999, p. 297). Even with this suggestion, however, it must be kept in mind that the proper locus of authenticity/inauthenticity is not actions or conduct but ways of existing, that is, ways of being a self. In any event, the key for present purposes is to remember which side of the scale you are on, for example, newspapers are left (though Nietzsche mocks the age of newspapers) and anticipatory resoluteness (see below) is right. We can now run across the scale, pausing at the right end for further exposition on inauthenticity, and then authenticity, and then turn back to intersexuality.

"Self, self, self, all you think about is self!" So Amanda upbraids Tom. But Heidegger's reply here is to ask, *what is a non–self?* He answers: Everyone is the other, and no one is himself (Heidegger, 1962, p. 165, H128). To be a non–self is not "not–to–exist" but to exist as a different self, viz., the "they–self." The non–self self, moreover, is the self that we are; we are not we but they:

> The Self of everyday Dasein is the *they–self*, which we distinguish from the *authentic Self*—that is, from the Self which has been taken hold of in its own way [eigens ergriffen] (Heidegger, 1962, p. 167, H129).

This, then, is how authenticity is introduced, that is, as a sort of privative, deviation, or place–holder. The being of Dasein, the reality of you, on the other hand, is for the most part inauthenticity, for example, being caught up, and swept–away, by the flow of life. As Aristotle noted, for the most part even the wisest sage is no different than the common run of men. But then Heidegger moves on to focus on two main phenomena—*death and guilt*—that knock us out of this flow, out of the they–self, and into the authentic self, that is, the self aware of, confronting, the truth of itself.

8. AUTHENTICITY

The authentic self is neither an escape from the inauthentic self (where does one go?), nor a replacement of it (how would we survive if we bumped off the quotidian self?). The authentic self is not "better" than the inauthentic self: But the inauthenticity of Dasein does not signify any 'less' Being or any 'lower' degree of Being (Heidegger, 1962, p. 68, H43). And it is not even "different":

Authentic existence is not something which floats above falling everydayness; existentially, it is only a modified way in which such everydayness is seized upon (Heidegger, 1962, p. 224, H179).

The point, rather, is that the authentic self is a way of existing in which the modes of inauthentic existence are still present but somehow modified. The nature of the modification, in turn, is suggested by the title, *Being and Time;* to be authentic involves some manner of recognition, or acknowledgment, of the correlation between being and time.

Authentic existence is a modification of inauthentic existence in that the modes of existence (whether inauthentic or authentic, these modes are "structurally indistinguishable"; Heidegger, 1962, p. 70, H44) are now shot through by time, that is, tempered by finitude. One's projections for one's life, for example, have built into them a sense of limit (teenagers, by contrast, will live forever). It is here that Heidegger's famous analyses of death and guilt come into play.

To begin, consider a funeral. We go to the funeral. We are at the place where a dead person is. We are, in one sense, at death. In German, *zum Tode sein* (Being–at–the–end). We know, in some abstract way, that someday we too will be dead:

In the publicness...death is 'known' as a mishap which is constantly occurring—as a 'case of death.' Someone or other 'dies', be he neighbor or stranger....'Death' is encountered as a well–known event occurring within the world....The "they" has already stowed away [gesichert] an interpretation for this event...."One of these days one will die too, in the end; but right now it has nothing to do with us" (Heidegger, 1962, pp. 296–7, H253).

Heidegger's point, of course, is that death has *everything* to do with us, *right now.* Compare, in other words, the above life that has a "knowledge of" death with a life that is shot through with the "acknowledgement" that to be is to be heading toward death, that is, to be is *sein zum Tode* (to–be–towards–death). The latter life reflects *the ontological construction* of Dasein, of us, that is, we are the beings built to go out of being. Authenticity embraces (to a degree), and maybe even begins, with this ontological truth about our looming end that we otherwise constantly strive to ignore. Authenticity means that we internalize (to a degree) the truth that "having–an–end" is an essential part of us. We knew this in our inauthentic mode, but in authenticity this recognition of our own truth has been modified, for example, it not only tempers our projections, informs our projections, for example, constrains our projections, but it makes our projections meaningful. It matters that to be is to be running out of time.

There is another dimension of authenticity illuminated by the phenomenon of death. Not only are we temporally–finite, but death singles us out from the "they":

(By its very essence, death is in every case mine...(Heidegger, 1962, p. 284, H240).

Bound up with inauthenticity is regarding death as belonging to the they, whereas authenticity is an affirmation of the mine–ownness of death (for discussion of the other end, that is, birth, see MacAvoy 1996). Death as *sein zum tode* is the primordial isolation of the self from the they; Dasein is "wrenched away from the they" (Heidegger, 1962, p. 307, H263). This point segues intuitively to Heidegger's analysis of guilt.

Against the contemporary plerophory that guilt is "a bad thing" Heidegger's treatment of guilt renders it not only structurally essential to being human (or at least Dasein), but also a key source of authenticity. He approaches guilt via an incredible and brilliant study of "the call of conscience," which results in the incredibly brilliant idea of the self calling the self about the self for the sake of the self.

> Conscience summons Dasein's Self from its lostness in the "they"...In conscience Dasein calls itself...The call comes from me and yet from beyond me and over me (Heidegger, 1962, pp. 319–20, H274–5).

Heidegger then pushes on to authenticity: "...conscience, in its basis and its essence, is *in each case mine...*" (Heidegger, 1962, p. 323, H278). The basis is guilt, that is, understood not psychologically as a feeling but ontologically as "Being–the–basis of a nullity" (Heidegger, 1962, p. 329, H283). This means, very simply and most minimally, that if we were unable to experience, or *to be,* a "not", a "lack", then we could not have most of, if not all, the ordinarily–understood experiences of guilt, nor the call of conscience, and certainly not the projection of possibilities central to authentic existence (potentiality–for–being involves the possibility of not–being–this–or–that; see Heidegger, 1962, p. 331, H285).

Death and guilt, then, are the "setting" for authenticity. But the "final" step lies in how we respond to these ontological, "built–in" dimensions of our reality. The key idea here is "anticipatory resoluteness," with anticipation the authentic response to death and resoluteness the authentic response to guilt.

One does not have to be dead to grasp that someday one will no longer exist. This awareness—concretized in the experience of *Angst,* of dread or anxiety, (Heidegger, 1962, p. 310, H266)—shows us a rather uncanny possibility for our existence, that is, it affords us a perspective of totality. To confront the truth of death authentically is not to avoid thinking about it or to treat it as something that will one day show up on its own but to *anticipate* it, that is, to let this fated possibility inform, limit, and shape the projection of possibilities generally, in other words, our freedom.

One might wish, on one hand, not to hear the call of conscience. But one might, on the authentic hand, *want* to have a conscience (Heidegger, 1962, p. 314, H270). This dilemma is made possible by guilt, that is, being–the–basis–of–a–nullity. This "metaphysical" guilt makes it possible for us to project for our lives a life of not–being–an–authentic–self. When we project authentically, however, we are *resolutely* confronting the kind of being we are, or the way we exist, in short, our being–guilty, and on this basis we affirm that we are indeed responsible, not only for what we do and fail to do, but for who we become and who we fail to become. We affirm, in short, that with respect to Being–one's–Self we have freedom.

Both anticipation and resoluteness, then, point to "existential" (albeit cf. with Heidegger's "existentiell") freedom, of being able to author a life–story from and to the truth that we are thrown toward death. Anticipatory resoluteness, in other words, brings us "face to face with our individualized potentiality–for–Being" (Heidegger, 1962, p. 358, H310). Our individualized potentiality involves the ability to project, *from our OWN thrownness and to our OWN end,* possible ways of existing. This existential freedom is both a burden, for we can fail at existing, for example, fail to conform how we exist with who we ontologically are, and an "unshakable joy" (Heidegger, 1962, p. 358, H310). Thus, to state a point too often missed, whenever one thinks of the core meaning of authenticity, that is, anticipatory resoluteness, one should be aware that both it and authenticity involve paradox, or *tension, that is irreducible.*

As a final note, the ultimate ontological ground of anticipatory resoluteness is time:

> Only in so far as Dasein has the definite character of temporality, is the authentic potentiality–for–Being–a–whole of anticipatory resoluteness, as we have described it, made possible for Dasein itself (Heidegger, 1962, p. 374, H326).

There is a lot in the passage, but for here the claim is that both to anticipate and to project resolutely require a being (for example, a human) capable of being–thrown–toward–the–future. An implication of this ontological basis is that authentic existence is a proper, "finitude–affirming" appropriation of time, whereas inauthenticity is an oblivious, or distorting (into the infinite), relation to time. A more distant but here more immediate implication is nicely suggested by Hatab, and it brings us full circle to intersexuality:

> The disruptive effect of being–toward–death also opens up the possibility of ontical, existentiell authenticity by breaking the hold of common, established patterns and *allowing an individual self to shape its own resolute existence, to discover modes of being that are more appropriate to its particularity* (emphasis mine; Hatab, 2000, p. 26).

The key upshot, I suggest, is the fusion between universality and particularity that has emerged in Heidegger's analysis, that is, we see that to be a self is to exist in a *universally particular* way.

In sum, *Being and Time* means, in other words, that *to be* is to be *temporal*, to be both thrown (perpetually) into existence and heading out of existence. This ticking clock of our lives, this finitude, is furthermore what enables a meaningful existence. Everything, and every project, is bathed, and sharpened, in an altered, "modified" light when illuminated by the truth of time.

9. BACK TO INTERSEXUALITY

What does all this heady and somber reflection on Heideggerian authenticity have to do with intersexuality? The main result is not different than the main result of philosophy generally applied to various phenomena: we learn how to think about something. This is a more subtle and more profound point than most of us have realized; how we think, especially about ourselves, can make an ontological difference. In subsequent Heidegger one even sees the idea of an essential nexus between thought and being (see Heidegger, 1961, pp. 98–164), but for here it is sufficient to note that there is a "constitutive" bridge between refined self–awareness and who one is. With respect to intersexuality, Heidegger's analysis prompts us to see intersexuality, and the intersexual self, in both its *universal* and *particular* aspects; to be an authentic intersexual self, then, is to exist in a universally particular way, and indeed to affirm this ontological truth.

There is an important immediate upshot for intersexuality of this grasp of the ontological structure of the self. The universality aspect provides a source of solace—intersexuals see that they are not alone anomalous, for thrownness is a broad phenomenon. And the particularity aspect fosters sensitivity—an acquaintance with details, for example, helps a non–intersexual see why the traditional treatment for this type of thrownness is perhaps subject to unnecessary and stultifying constraints. Solace and sensitivity, then, are enabled when we are forced to account for the self as a fusion of universality and particularity. To continue more generally, Heidegger's analysis provides us with new language, new conceptual tools, for a philosophical exposition of intersexuality. With respect to the universal aspect of the self, for example, even the biological background of the intersexual condition is now seen under the rubric of thrownness; and how one is thrown into the world, in turn, is now explicitly seen, in authentic understanding, to be circumscribing what any of us has to confront in forging out (projecting) a meaningful existence. Not all of our struggles are chosen by us; we are rather thrown into them, and from them we struggle, like Hesse's bird struggling out of the egg, to emerge with our own selves intact.

In this interplay between thrownness and projection intersexuals learn that they are not alone, for everyone's thrownness will include obstacles. More extreme examples of thrownness include Cystic Fibrosis, Huntington's Chorea, or Aristotle's "monstrosities" (1941, p. 250, *Physics,* II, 8, 199b3), but even more usual obstacles are still significant and just as "unfair," for example, severe, incurable acne leading to severe, incurable ostracism throughout high school and beyond. Or being a woman in nineteenth century Europe and yearning to work in a scientific laboratory. Or not wanting to be a parent though married to someone who does. Or even Tom Wingfield's cruel fate of following his dreams only by "forgetting" his fondness for Laura. We can thus appreciate the "resoluteness" in some of the above intersexual self–assessments that explicitly admit that "there could be worse" and "the important things I can still do."

As for the particular aspect, there is a philosophical distinctness about the intersexual struggle with thrownness. Today, in the United States, the intersexual faces the hegemony of the traditional treatment. This treatment might be, noble intentions aside, a "double assault" on autonomy. On this reading the treatment not only restricts freedom in the sense of free choice about "things," the way Moe the playground bully won't let Calvin play on the swings, but also restricts freedom qua choice about who I am. There is a difference, in other words, between forbidding someone to do x (where x is significantly separable from the self) and forbidding someone to be, or become, x. This latter restriction ramifies ontologically to self–annihilation, for there is no authentic self without living out the creation of the self; an authentic self cannot be imposed by anything separable from the self. The ontological worry with the traditional treatment, then, might be more precisely expressed not as a violation of autonomy but as a violation of authorship.

The traditional treatment would seem to amount, then, to a "choosing" of the self, but as the choosing is not from the self, the choosing is illegitimate—inauthentic. Authentic choosing requires that the self be the author of the choosing (even if the self chooses "incorrectly"). This invocation of existential/ontological authorship is bound up with authenticity. Proper authorship of an existential story requires the story acknowledge both the universal and particular aspects of who one is, and moreover the inherently temporal structure of stories make them best suited for grasping authenticity. An authentic self cannot be explained, in other words, in non–temporal terms, for example, as if there exists a static, finished, immutable entity, "self." An authentic self is rather a matter of authoring one's own story. This last point, that authentic existence is the process of *projecting a way of existing from within one's thrownness,* is the most specific source of potential indictment that Heidegger brings to the philosophical consideration of intersexuality.

Let us close this essay in Heideggerian spirit by recalling the beginning:

> I wanted only to live in accord with the promptings of my true self. Why was that so very difficult?

A renewed, phrase by phrase look at Hesse's words will drive home the point that philosophical analysis, that is, learning how to think about something (for example, intersexuality) via sustained reflection and poetic sensitivity, is not detached speculation but indeed "opens up a world."

To begin, one has to admit that, after Heidegger's analysis of authenticity, one hears Hesse's line more fundamentally, more universally, and more essentially. The line has been recast in a subtle but profound way. The overall tone, for example, is less psychological, less Romantic, and more ontological; the "yearning" for authenticity, in other words, is not a matter for teenagers only, but is "metaphysically" built into humanity. Applied to intersexuality, a "Heideggerian" reading of the line results in the following: "I wanted only to live in accord with the promptings of my true self" corresponds beautifully to the underlying and sustaining tone of the above quoted intersexual self–assessments. Beneath the rhetoric of "rights" and heat of moral outrage one detects the fires of an existential struggle, that is, the yearning for authenticity.

"[I]n accord with the promptings of my true self"; the self prompts the self—how can one, now, *not* hear this in terms of "the [fundamental] call of conscience"? And might it be this very prompting that drives some intersexuals to track down, doggedly, top–secret medical information?

"Why was that so very difficult?" Heidegger's analysis suggests that hindrances to authenticity are also ontological, that is, metaphysically structural and (thus?) "internal," but the thorny attempt in this essay to apply authenticity to intersexuality forces the issue of whether there can be "external" hindrances to authenticity, or at least *unnecessary external hindrances,* for example, changeable social constructs, to authenticity. The Roman slave and Stoic philosopher Epictetus, for example, forged out a remarkable if not "authentic" existence despite lacking Aristotle's external bounty, but one wonders, as with Beethoven's deafness, what if...? In the case of intersexuality, what if the phenomenon did not occur in the thrown context of societal commitment to an exhaustive and exclusive disjunction between male and female (which holds, oddly enough, while prominent medical and academic subgroups claim *additionally* that sexual identity is socially–constructed)? What if surgery had been delayed? What if medical, psychological, and sociological consideration were not the only, or at least primary, type of consideration bought to bear (by both sides) on the debate concerning the traditional treatment of intersexuality (see the closing comments above on David Reimer)? *What if, in other words, we did not automatically "fall back on" the unconsciously absorbed ways of "thinking" about issues and instead questioned the very way we go about thinking about the debate?*

What if, just as Heidegger attempts to think through the issues of self in a more fundamental way, we test his suggestion and approach intersexuality *ontologically?* It is not only that we would see the traditional treatment in terms of worries about future authenticity rather than, or in fundamental addition to, future autonomy–or that we would see autonomy against the more fundamental backdrop of authenticity (that is, autonomy as a key condition for at least the right end of the authenticity scale). Or that we would see the plight of intersexuals in terms of the struggle for authenticity rather than, or in fundamental addition to, rights–violation. Or that we would see the self as a phenomenon that must emerge through time rather than as a static quasi–entity. But also that we would see the full range of discussion as potentially illuminable by authenticity, inspiring questions such as what might have been imperiled for infants in the traditional treatment, why autonomy matters, why some intersexuals doggedly track down medical information, what despairing adult intersexuals might be seeking, and why it might matter for the formation of the authentic self that the self project for itself the self that affirms the universality and particularity of the thrown, dying self.

I thank Joanie Beno and Lucy Holewinski for their contributions to this essay and their generosity of spirit through time.

Herman Stark, Professor, South Suburban College, South Holland, Illinois, U.S.A.

REFERENCES

Aristotle. *The Basic Works of Aristotle.* Ed. Richard McKeon. New York: Random House, 1941.

Arnason,Vilhjalmur. "Authentic Conversations: Authenticity in the Patient–Professional Relationship." *Theoretical Medicine* 15.3, 1994: 227–42.

Audi, Robert, ed. *The Cambridge Dictionary of Philosophy.* Cambridge: Cambridge University Press, 1999.

Cameron, D. "Caught Between: An Essay on Intersexuality." *Intersex in the Age of Ethics.* Ed. Alice Domurat Dreger. Hagerstown, MD: University Publishing Group, 1999: 91–8.

Chase, Cheryl. 'Surgical Progress in Not the Answer to Intersexuality.' *Intersex in the Age of Ethics.* Ed. Alice Domurat Dreger. Hagerstown, MD: University Publishing Group, 1999: 147–60.

Colapinto, John. *As Nature Made Him: The Boy who was Raised as a Girl.* New York: HarperCollins Publishers, Inc., 2000.

Coventry, Martha. "Finding the Words." *Intersex in the Age of Ethics.* Ed. Alice Domurat Dreger. Hagerstown, MD: University Publishing Group, 1999: 71–8.

Dreger, Alice Domurat, ed. *Intersex in the Age of Ethics.* Hagerstown, MD: University Publishing Group, 1999.

Dreger, Alice Domurat. "A History of Intersex: From the Age of Gonads to the Age of Consent." *Intersex in the Age of Ethics.* Ed. Alice Domurat Dreger. Hagerstown, MD: University Publishing Group, 1999: 5–22.

Gelven, Michael. *A Commentary on Heidegger's Being and Time, Revised ed.* DeKalb, IL: Northern Illinois University, 1989.

Golomb, Jacob. "Heidegger on Authenticity and Death." *Existentia,* 11.3–4, 2001: 457–72.

Groveman, Sherri A. "The Hanukkah Bush: Ethical Implications in the Clinical Management of Intersex." *Intersex in the Age of Ethics.* Ed. Alice Domurat Dreger. Hagerstown, MD: University Publishing Group, 1999: 3–8.

Guignon, Charles. *On Being Authentic.* New York: Routledge, 2004.

Hatab, Lawrence J. *Ethics and Finitude: Heideggerian Contributions to Moral Philosophy.* Lanham, MD: Rowman & Littlefield Publishers, Inc., 2000.

Hawbecker, Hale. "Who Did This to You?" *Intersex in the Age of Ethics.* Ed. Alice Domurat Dreger. Hagerstown, MD: University Publishing Group, 1999: 111–13.

Heidegger, Martin. *Sein und Zeit, 15 Auflage 1979, 2. Druck.* Tübingen: Max Niemeyer Verlag, 1927.

Heidegger, Martin. *An Introduction to Metaphysics.* Trans. Ralph Manheim. Garden City, New York: Anchor Books, 1961.

Heidegger, Martin. *Being and Time.* Trans. John Macquarrie and Edward Robinson. New York: Harper and Row, 1962.

Heidegger, Martin. *On the Way to Language.* Trans. Peter Hertz and Jane Stambaugh. New York: Harper and Row, 1971a.

Heidegger, Martin. *Poetry, Language, Thought.* Trans. Albert Hofstadter. New York: Harper Colophon Books, 1971b.

Hesse, Hermann. *Demian.* Frankfurt am Main: Suhrkamp Taschenbuch, 1974.

Intersex Society of North America. *Redefining Sex, Video Documentary.* Produced by CityTV of Toronto, 2000.

Intersex Society of North America. *Our Mission.* www.isna.org. 2005.

James, William. *The Will to Believe.* London: Longmans Green and Co., 1899.

Kipnis, Kenneth, and Diamond, Milton. "Pediatric Ethics and the Surgical Assignment of Sex." *Intersex in the Age of Ethics.* Ed. Alice Domurat Dreger. Hagerstown, MD: University Publishing Group, 1999: 173–94.

MacAvoy, Leslie. "The Heideggerian Bias Toward Death: A Critique of the Role of Being–Towards–Death in the Disclosure of Human Finitude." *Metaphilosophy,* 27.1–2, 1996: 63–77.

Melchert, Norman. *The Great Conversation, 3ʳᵈ ed.* Mountain View, CA: Mayfield Publishing Company, 1999.

Miller, Alice. *Prisoners of Childhood: The Drama of the Gifted Child and the Search for the True Self.* Trans. R. Ward. New York: Basic Books, 1981.

Preves, Sharon E. "For the Sake of the Children: Destigmatizing Intersexuality." *Intersex in the Age of Ethics.* Ed. Alice Domurat Dreger. Hagerstown, MD: University Publishing Group, 1999: 51–65.

Schober, Justine Marut. "A Surgeon's Response to the Intersex Controversy." *Intersex in the Age of Ethics.* Ed. Alice Domurat Dreger. Hagerstown, MD: University Publishing Group, 1999: 161–8.

Stark, Herman. "The Lord Scroop Fallacy." *Informal Logic* 20.3, 2000a: 245–59.

Stark, Herman. "Fallacies and Logical Errors." *Inquiry: Critical Thinking Across the Disciplines* 20.1, Fall, 2000b: 23–32.

Taylor, Charles. *The Ethics of Authenticity.* Cambridge, MA: Harvard University Press, 1992.

Tolstoy, Leo. "The Death of Ivan Ilyich." *The Death of Ivan Ilyich and Other Stories.* Trans. Alymer Maude. New York: Signet Classics, 1960.

Triea, Kiira. "Power, Orgasm, and the Psychohormonal Research Unit." *Intersex in the Age of Ethics.* Ed. Alice Domurat Dreger. Hagerstown, MD: University Publishing Group, 1999: 141–6.

Walcutt, Heidi. "Time for a Change." *Intersex in the Age of Ethics.* Ed. Alice Domurat Dreger. Hagerstown, MD: University Publishing Group, 1999: 197–200.

PATRICIA BEATTIE JUNG

CHRISTIANITY AND HUMAN SEXUAL POLYMORPHISM: ARE THEY COMPATIBLE?

1. HUMAN SEXUAL DIMORPHISM AND THE CHALLENGE OF INTERSEXUALITY

Most contemporary religious understandings of human sexuality are organized by a dimorphic paradigm, through which people are seen to be naturally (in a normative sense) unequivocally and exclusively male or unequivocally and exclusively female. Until the modern era, sexual dimorphism seemed to account for most of our data about human sexuality and it was, at least in its original form, remarkably elegant. But many newly discovered facets of human sexuality do not appear to fit well within this dichotomous framework. Today, many biological studies of human sexual variation are yielding results that challenge the adequacy of this organizing binary metaphor. Similarly, on the basis of insights gained from their own experience, many "intersexed" persons–that is, persons who for a variety of reasons and in a variety of combinations have both male and female biological sex characteristics–are questioning the ability of this paradigm to illumine the very "fact" of their existence. Indeed, some are asserting that this paradigm "distorts" their experience of sexuality.

These are certainly not the first challenges faced by this paradigmatic concept. In her essay, "The Erosion of Sexual Dimorphism: Challenges to Religion and Religious Ethics," Christine E. Gudorf notes that in many respects, the notion of human sexual dimorphism has been under siege for a long time. She notes, for example, that late in the nineteenth century, when wide-ranging anthropological studies revealed gender to vary far more than the binary paradigm for sex seemed to have suggested, modifications to the theory were made. It was at this time that sex was distinguished from gender. Gender (unlike sex) was no longer presumed determined solely by biological factors.

293

S.E. Sytsma (Ed.), Ethics and Intersex, 293–309.

Then again, in the mid-twentieth century, Alfred Kinsey introduced data that suggested that the binary notion of sexual orientation that had seemed to flow (theoretically at least) from the concept of sexual dimorphism was inadequate. That concept did not really illumine the variation in people's experience of sexual desire. The evidence Kinsey gathered implied that a spectrum of sexual orientations resided within the human species. Thus, Kinsey suggested another modification: the notion of sexual orientation (which may likewise not be determined solely by biological factors) also needed to be distinguished from sex per se.

Gudorf argues that historically these studies challenged the notion of sexual dimorphism. But the distinction of gender and orientation from sex enabled theorists to modify rather than shift the basically dimorphic paradigm underlying most theories about human sexuality. Theorists are not inclined toward dramatic, revolutionary change; the bias in all traditions, including those of science, is against such radical change. Paradigm shifts come only as a last resort. Only when the criteria for good theory demand it –that is, not only when an interpretative concept's comprehensiveness and internal consistency, but also its coherence with external but related ideas, fruitfulness and elegance demand it–would such a move be seriously contemplated. Still, it had to be admitted that by the late twentieth century the original simplicity of the dimorphic model had been lost in a complicated set of modifications.

Today the notion of human sexual dimorphism appears to be under critical scrutiny once again. The case against its ability to illumine, or at least take adequate account of, emerging biological evidence about additional forms of sexual variation is substantial and growing. For centuries, learned people have known that on occasion some humans were born with "ambiguous" genitalia. Today, however, we have much more data about the many types of intersexuality and a clearer picture of the extent of the phenomenon. We now know that several biological factors contribute to a person's sexual identity appearing (at least within a bipolar system) to be "indeterminate" or "shifting." In addition to a person's external genitalia and internal reproductive organs, our gonadal sex and gender identity, along with multiple chromosomal and hormonal factors, all combine and contribute variously to a range of sexual identities far more diverse than suggested by the dimorphic model.

Consider what we now know about the genetic basis for human sexuality. While it is true that the vast majority of people are genetically either male (XY) or female (XX), nevertheless, it is estimated that across the globe 5.5 million people have chromosomal patterns that vary from this binary pattern.

This is just the tip of the iceberg of biological evidence "against" (that is, not comprehended adequately by) dimorphism.

How often does intersexuality occur? Of course, that depends upon how broadly intersexuality is defined. Only now are we becoming aware of the sheer number of cases in which the multiple factors that contribute to sexuality neither agree with each other nor correspond to the dimorphic model. In her review of the literature Heather Looy noted that "estimates range widely from 0.07% to 4% of the population, depending upon whether they include conditions with clearly identifiable causes, or any case of 'ambiguous genitalia' whether or not the cause is identified" (Looy, 12). Anthropologist William O. Beeman has suggested that in the United States alone "between 3 million and 10 million Americans are neither male nor female at birth" (Beeman).

2. INTERPRETING INTERSEXUALITY: DEFECT OR DIFFERENCE?

Of course, logically it is not necessary to abandon the notion of sexual dimorphism on the basis of such numbers. Though certainly inelegant, it is altogether reasonable to treat even this extraordinary number as simply exceptional. Relatively speaking, intersexuality is rare; there is no question that ours is a predominantly sexually dimorphic species. The existence of anomalies does not necessarily undermine the presumption of sexual dimorphism. No paradigm ever perfectly accounts for the data it seeks to explain. There is always evidence that falls outside of the box.

Until very recently the scientific community treated such "exceptions" to the dimorphic paradigm as unquestionably diseased or defective. Since the 1950s medical treatments were offered as soon as a person was identified as "ambiguously" sexed. Until the last decade, the virtually unquestioned standard of care for intersexed persons was to surgically limit (in so far as possible) their anatomy to either a male or female (usually the latter) model, even if such "treatments" reduced or destroyed their capacity for sexual pleasure and left them feeling "out of sync" with the sex to which they had been clinically assigned.

Now, however, there is a considerable discussion among physicians and medical ethicists about these attempts to "normalize" a person's anatomy. There is debate about who should have control over decisions about such "treatments" and whether the identification of an infant or child as intersexed is really a "medical emergency" to which an immediate response is necessary. Even more significantly, there is debate about whether there is any real medical "need" for such "treatments" at all. From the perspective of population biology, intersexuality seems too commonplace to be genuinely deleterious. Additionally, intersexuality per se is usually not associated with higher than average rates of morbidity or mortality.[1] One exception may be the high rate of infertility, both congenital and iatrogenic in origin, frequently associated with intersexuality. But, of course, how infertility is experienced depends upon the framework through which it is interpreted. Within a polymorphous paradigm, it may not be seen as problematic that some individuals are not biologically reproductive; they may be given different roles within the community.

In any case, many arguments for the "treatment" of intersexuality seem to rest on the claim that intersexed persons have an urgent **need** to establish a stable sexual expression as either male or female, whether or not that assignment matches their own eventual sexual self-identification as male, female or omnigendered. Such interventions are commended even though it is well known that they frequently give rise to medical problems later in life and may prove to be detrimental overall to otherwise healthy intersexed persons. Sometimes it is argued that this need is psychosocial in origin and will serve the intersexed person's mental and emotional health. This begs the question of whether it is the culture's, or the patient's, "need" that is thereby served.

Other times people claim that the need being served is spiritual. In her essay, "Intersexuality and Scripture," Sally Gross noted that some Christian fundamentalists often uncritically commend complicated and dangerous surgical interventions for intersexed newborns in order to correct what they perceive to be "at odds with the will of God as expressed in the order of creation." (Gross, 68)

In contrast, others are suggesting that such practices constitute medically unjustifiable forms of genital mutilation, even if good intentions undoubtedly guide the vast majority of decisions to medically "treat" the intersexed. These people point out that sexual ambiguity is rarely life threatening. What intersexuality really threatens is the culture's presumption of sexual dimorphism and the social practices and institutional arrangements based on it. Therefore, many, if not most, atypical expressions of sexual differences among humans should be accepted, honored, and celebrated. Intersexed persons should not be thought of as suffering from pathology in need of correction.

As Karen Lebacqz points out in her essay, "Difference or Defect? Intersexuality and the Politics of Difference," it would be a mistake to argue that every difference is natural in a normative sense. Though I would not completely deny their interrelationship, it is simply fallacious to conflate whatever is with what ought to be. Modern medical practice operates on the assumption that people may have a right and need to interfere with what occurs naturally in some circumstances.

It is equally clear that whether what is statistically anomalous is interpreted as a monstrous abomination, a tragic defect, or a delightful variation depends upon the concept(s) through which it is interpreted. For example, Looy notes that persons operating out of strong forms of biological determinism rooted in evolutionary theory are likely to see intersexuality as a non-adaptive pathology. In contrast, those who approach the phenomenon from a constructionist view may either (1) recommend that intersexed persons be socially conditioned to develop either a male or female sexual identity, or (2) recommend that our gender dichotomous culture be socially deconstructed (Looy, 13). If they are also essentialist in their approach, some constructivists may "argue that we must protect, affirm and celebrate the non-dichotomous identities of intersexed persons because that is who they *are*" (Looy, 14).

In summary, our response to difference--whether one of revulsion, correction or celebration–is a function of the paradigmatic lens through which we interpret it. Therefore, the key task before us is to evaluate critically the assumption that the only natural and normal sexual state for human beings is either male or female. Emerging scientific data about intersexuality, along with the experiential insights of those who are intersexed, have triggered a reexamination of the dimorphic paradigm for human sexuality.

3. SEXUAL DIMORPHISM: A "REVEALED" NATURAL LAW?

In addition to their elegance and comprehensiveness, major paradigms are often evaluated in terms of their compatibility with external but related ideas. Evidence of such congruence reinforces both the interpretative power and integrative potential of a concept. It comes as no great surprise that in the West the notion of sexual dimorphism, along with its interpretation of expressions of intersexuality as (in some way) disordered, have been religiously reinforced – indeed, sanctified. A critical analysis of the bases within Christianity for the claim that sexual dimorphism reflects a divinely established order for human sexuality, revealed in sacred scriptures and evident in the God's natural law, is the focus of the remainder of this chapter.

It is important to be clear from the beginning about what is at stake for Christianity when its traditional anthropological assumptions about human sexuality are evaluated. Gudorf is correct when she notes that the accelerating erosion of the dimorphic paradigm poses several challenges for Christianity. In a polymorphic model of human sexuality intersexuality would most probably be seen as morally normative. The recognition of intersexuality as natural would challenge both the content of several traditional Christian teachings and their institutional expressions. Church teachings about gender, sexual orientation, marriage, parenting and even God would be placed under critical scrutiny. In addition, many patriarchal and heterosexist institutional structures and patterns of organizational leadership formed by traditional convictions about God's design for relationships between the sexes would be challenged.

As the basic anthropological framework for Christian sexual ethics, sexual dimorphism proves foundational in many traditional Christian arguments. It grounds the moral significance of openness to the possibility of procreativity and of heterosexual gender complementarity. In modern Christian theology, there are both strong and weak versions of the theory of gender complementarity. Common to both versions is the contemporary affirmation of the dignity and equality of all persons before God, but the stronger versions place more emphasis on the differences between the sexes and the rigidity of their respective gender roles and assignments. In the weak version, the doctrine of gender complementarity proclaims the "absolute equality" of men and women along with their "different functions."[2] In stronger versions, the doctrine of complementarity supports male headship and female subordination and obedience.[3]

Framed within sexual dimorphism these basic teachings about the sexual significance of procreativity and heterosexual gender complementarity provide the groundwork for a variety of prohibitions. It is on this foundation, for example, that most Christians condemn homosexual behavior; describe gay, lesbian and bisexual orientations as disordered; outlaw same sex marriage; and exclude from eligibility for ordination anyone who is not heterosexual or an avowed celibate. It is on this foundation that most Christians refute at least some forms of gender-bending and gender-blending behaviors. It is on this foundation that some churches condemn the use of artificial forms of contraception, sterilization and (intentionally) childfree marriages.

Lisa Sowle Cahill in a recent essay on "Gender and Christian Ethics" gives voice to what is fairly standard theological thinking on this issue, when it is recognized at all.

> Gender is different from biological sex. Although some individuals have ambiguous sex characteristics, the human

species is in general sexually dimorphic. Humans come in two sexes, male and female, that cooperate for reproduction. Thus the sexual differentiation of individuals into male and female is taken for granted in virtually all societies, and some biologically based behaviors and roles are almost as universally associated with sexual differentiation. These are the behaviors and roles required for reproduction through sexual intercourse, pregnancy, birthing and lactation and the associated care of infants (Cahill, 112).

Though Christian sexual ethics is not univocal about many matters either historically or across denominational lines, one can speak with considerable confidence about the broad, ecumenically shared presumption of sexual dimorphism within Christianity.

4. THE SANCTIFICATION OF SEXUAL DIMORPHISM

Traditionally, Christian stories of creation have been interpreted as endorsing sexual dimorphism. This line of interpretation is not without textual rationale. Only "unambiguously" male and female humans are explicitly mentioned in the opening chapters of Genesis. The Yahwist creation account found in Genesis 2-3 is recognized by most biblical scholars as the oldest in the Bible. Here dimorphic sexual differentiation is closely associated with an intimate, "one-flesh" union. Only this heterosexual partnership is explicitly identified as solving the problem of "aloneness" that the Creator declared not good. Later, heterosexual marriage is associated with God's relationship to the People of the Covenant in the book of Hosea and with Christ's relationship to the Church in Ephesians 5. At one point women's salvation is even associated with childbearing (1 Timothy 2:15). Similarly, in the Priestly creation account found in Genesis 1 only males and females are explicitly associated with the likeness of God. At least some forms of gender-blending behavior are explicitly forbidden in both Deuteronomy 22:5 and 1 Corinthians 11:13-15 or are associated with cursedness as in 2 Samuel 3:29.

5. ROMAN CATHOLICISM AND SEXUAL DIMORPHISM

One way to get a real feel for the place of sexual dimorphism in Christianity in general is to examine its function in one particular tradition's official teachings on sexuality. With that hope in mind, I will trace the use of this paradigm in a recent letter on sexuality addressed to the bishops of the

Catholic Church, as well as to all men and women of good will, issued by the Vatican's Congregation for the Doctrine of the Faith, hereafter CDF, with the explicit approval of Pope John Paul II. For the sake of space, I will review only this one of the several magisterial documents on sexuality issued since Pope Leo XIII's promulgation of *Arcanum Diviniae Sapientiae* in 1880.[4]

With one exception noted in the text below, the viewpoint and accompanying arguments presented in this letter are broadly representative, quite traditional, expressions of Catholic, indeed Christian, thinking on the significance of sexual dimorphism. In fact, it would be a mistake to see the emphasis on sexual dimorphism detailed below as a peculiarly Catholic one. It can easily be established that this paradigm informs most Protestant sexual ethics as well. Consider the work of Karl Barth, arguably one of the most influential Protestant theologians of the twentieth century. In his multi-volume *Church Dogmatics,* Barth claimed that obedience to God required that persons be either male or female and live in compliance with the Creator's complementary design for human sexuality. All attempts to violate this order were forbidden as prideful acts of disobedience. In the more recent deliberations about homosexuality within Protestant denominations along the North Atlantic, all parties to the conversation recognize that the sexual dimorphism is a key to debate about how to interpret, as Robert A. Gagnon has put it, "the big picture" about human sexuality underlying this debate.

In her essay "Integrity in Catholic Sexual Ethics," Aline H. Kalbian asserts that "a Catholic sexual ethic begins with the premise that male and female are essential and stable genders. On this view, gender is determined exclusively on the basis of biological sexual characteristics." (Kalbian, 60) The truth of this assertion is quite evident in the CDF's letter "On the Collaboration of Men and Women in the World" of 2004. Here arguments about sexual dimorphism are located at the very center of the question being addressed in the letter. One foundational approach to human sexuality is described therein as particularly problematic, not only because it distorts important truths about the normative nature of sexuality, but also because of its many harmful implications. The Vatican's concern about the theory of sexual polymorphism is worth quoting at length.

> In this perspective, physical difference, termed *sex*, is minimized while the purely cultural element, termed *gender*, is emphasized to the maximum and held to be primary. The obscuring of the difference or duality of the sexes has enormous consequences on a variety of levels. This theory of the human person, intended to promote prospects for equality of women

through liberation from biological determinism, has in reality inspired ideologies which, for example, call into question the family, in its natural two-parent structure of mother and father, and make homosexuality and heterosexuality virtually equivalent, in a new model of polymorphous sexuality. (CDF, 2)

In the remainder of the letter the CDF proceeds to outline the basic elements of the biblical vision of the human person as sexually dimorphic, detailing by way of conclusion the importance of what are described as feminine values in the life of society and in the life of the church.

It is not surprising that the CDF grounds the biblical vision of God's design for human sexuality in the two creation accounts found in the opening chapters of Genesis. Catholics tend to emphasize Genesis in their discussion of sexual ethics for at least two reasons. First, these stories about our beginnings reveal a truth considered central to Christian anthropology: that persons are made in "the image and likeness of God." According to the CDF, this constitutes "the immutable *basis of all Christian anthropology.*" (5) Second, the gospels portray Jesus himself as referring back to these texts about the "beginning" in his reply to questions about divorce (see Mark 10 and Matthew 19).

In other commentaries on the biblical view of creation, John Paul II has tended to elide the two creation stories that open the book of Genesis, ignoring most historical-critical exegesis on the texts and approaching them allegorically.[5] In this particular treatment, however, the texts are distinguished, though as is typical of John Paul II's earlier work, the focus is primarily on the second, and older, of the accounts. In an earlier apostolic letter *Mulieris dignitatem* (On the Dignity of Women), John Paul II offered the following explanation for this approach to the two stories, noting that there is "no essential contradiction between the two texts. The text of Genesis 2:18-25 helps us to understand better what we find in the concise passage of Genesis 1:27-28." (John Paul II, 6)

According to the Vatican, the opening chapter of Genesis describes humanity "as articulated in the male-female relationship. This is the humanity, sexually differentiated, which is explicitly declared 'the image of God'" (CDF, 5). To be created in the image of God is to be created for relationship as either male or female. The second creation story is said to ground this as the significance of sexual difference. At first man was created in a state of original solitude and experienced loneliness there. This is only resolved when woman is created as a suitable life companion. "God's creation of woman characterizes humanity as a relational reality." Sexual "difference is oriented toward communion" (CDF, 6).

The Vatican contends that the inscription of this vital difference onto humanity carries more than biological or psychological import. It is ontological in significance. This claim is asserted despite the fact that biologically, men and women are far more alike than different, and that individual differences tend to outweigh group differences. Quoting John Paul II from *Mulieris dignitatem,* the Vatican argues that "'man and woman are called from the beginning not only to exist 'side by side' or 'together,' but they are also called to exist mutually 'one for the other'"(CDF, 6). All of human history unfolds within the context of the spousal significance of the body. All of humankind is set within this spousal call to be mutually for the other in interpersonal communion. Thus, the Vatican concludes, there is developing within "humanity itself, in accordance with God's will, the integration of what is 'masculine' and what is 'feminine'" (CDF, 6). The point here is not that a person can only be made complete through a "one flesh" union with someone of the opposite sex, though that is "the first and, in a sense, the fundamental dimension of this call" (CDF, 6). Heterosexual marriage, the Vatican notes, is not the only expression of this call, nor–given the realities of sin discussed later–will marriage guarantee the fulfilment of this call to communion. But a person living in isolation will lack the wholeness declared humanly possible only in a relationship of "uniduality" (CDF, 8).

In their review of the principle elements of the biblical vision of the meaning of sexual difference, the CDF concludes that sexual dimorphism characterizes men and women on the physical, psychological, and spiritual level. It cannot be reduced to mere biological "fact," because sexual complementarity is a fundamental component of the human capacity to love. "This capacity to love – a reflection and image of God who is love – is disclosed in the spousal character of the body, in which the masculinity or femininity of the person is expressed" (CDF, 8).

For Christians it is always true that, as the Vatican notes, "the human dimension of sexuality is inseparable from the theological dimension" (CDF, 8). For Christians anthropology is always really theological anthropology. People can only really understand who they are in light of who God is. Hence, it is not surprising that before tracing the more concrete implications of these claims, this anthropological argument is rooted in and sanctified by a nuptial metaphor for God's relationship to humanity. On the basis of multiple biblical texts, the Vatican suggests that God is most aptly portrayed as a divine Bridegroom eagerly pursuing and making love to His bride (that is, all of humanity).[6] "God makes himself known as the Bridegroom who loves Israel his Bride." (CDF, 9)

At least in part on the basis of the baptismal formula found in Galatians 3:28 the church has traditionally taught that sexual, like ethnic and master/slave, distinctions would be erased in the new creation at the end time. In a truly extraordinary move–against the grain of long-standing patterns of biblical interpretation and many ancient traditions – the Vatican argues in this letter that the distinction between male and female will not be erased at the end time in Christ. Only "the rivalry, enmity and violence which disfigured the relationship between men and women" will be overcome at the end time. Sexual dimorphism is so inscribed into creation's design that the Vatican argues that "male and female are thus revealed as *belonging ontologically to creation* and destined therefore *to outlast the present time*, evidently in a transfigured form." (CDF, 12) From this perspective, notes the CDF, it becomes clear why the book of Revelation, when speaking of the new heaven and new earth, can portray the new Jerusalem (God's people) as "prepared as a bride adorned for her husband" (Revelation 21:2), beseeching the Bridegroom "Come, Lord Jesus!" (Revelation 22: 20)

As its title promises, the last sections of the letter detail the implications of sexual dimorphism for the church and the world. Several mentioned there are worth special note. (1) A "capacity for the other" is a value taught in this letter to be linked to "women's physical capacity to give life" and structured into the female personality. This natural *"genius of women"* needs to be present in family life and the wider world. The harmonization and balance of work in the family and in the world "has, for women, characteristics different from those in the case of men" (CDF, 13). Because of their special mission in the family, their special genius for living for the other, women who opt not to work should not be stigmatised or financially penalized; likewise, women who opt to work in the world should be given the flexibility necessary to care for their family as well.[7] (2) Special capacities for and disposition to listening, welcoming, humility, faithfulness, praise and waiting are linked to faithful Christian women as embodied by Mary the Mother of God. Thus "women are called to be unique examples and witnesses for all Christians of how the Bride is to respond in love to the love of the Bridegroom" (CDF, 16).

6. CHRISTIAN PASTORAL RESPONSES TO INTERSEXUALITY

Of course the church has long recognized that there were persons who did not fit well into dichotomous categories available to them within the system established by sexual dimorphism. There has not always been a good fit between a disciple's existential reality and God's plan that all people be either male or female. For most of church history, such "exceptions" to this sexual paradigm were seen within Christianity as persons who perverted God's design for human sexuality and threatened to pollute the wider community. Intersexuality was often seen as a sign of personal or parental sin. Persons who did not successfully closet their condition were often persecuted.

More recently, however, some pastors have changed their teachings in this regard. "Exceptions" to the rule of sexual dimorphism have been seen as suffering from congenital defects or inescapable and diseased processes. Oliver O'Donovan puts it this way. "The point is simply that the ambiguity, however it may best be resolved, is an ambiguity which has arisen by a malfunction in a dimorphic human sexual pattern" (O'Donovan, 143). While many theologians like O'Donovan now recognize that intersexed persons may have little or no subjective moral culpability for their "condition," their sexual identity remains for them objectively "problematic." The problem remains a tragic expression within the individual person, and/or the species as a whole, of the ontological consequences of "the Fall" or of Original Sin. From this perspective, only those social and pastoral accommodations that cling to this truth are commendable.

Undoubtedly, on a pastoral level, Christian denominations vary in their response to intersexuality, even if their basic presumptions about sexual dimorphism are virtually identical. In many Catholic churches, confessors might well discuss intersexuality with their parishioners as follows. Since "treatment(s)" for many of these "syndromes" enjoy limited success–if any, beyond the "cosmetic"–those who so suffer should not feel morally guilty about an incurable "condition" for which they are not subjectively culpable and about which they can do little. Still, priests might advise that since this is an "objective disorder," its public avowal is unacceptable. Intersexed persons should closet their condition and expect quite limited forms of tolerance for it.

In contrast, some fundamentalist Christians have been known to deny baptism to intersexed persons, despite an explicit witness given in the New Testament about the Apostle Philip's inspired decision to travel with and baptise the dark skinned "eunuch of great authority" (Acts 8:39). Sally Gross reports that some fundamentalists deny intersexed persons baptism on the grounds that intersexed persons do not satisfy the biblical criterion for being created human because they are not "determinately male or determinately female" (Gross, 70). Hence, Gross reports being told that the baptism of an intersexed person would be no more valid than the baptism of a cat!

7. CHRISTIAN CONVICTIONS ABOUT THE DISCERNMENT OF TRUTH

As evident above, the Christian endorsement of sexual dimorphism no longer rests primarily upon a *descriptive* account of human sexuality as "naturally" dimorphic. It does not rest upon a rationally developed, philosophically and/or scientifically informed account of the normatively human. Rather, most Christian arguments appeal in a direct and straightforward, if highly selective, manner to biblical revelation for their justification. In this sense the Christian framework for sexual ethics rests decisively upon "revealed" natural law.

Furthermore, as evidenced above, considered in themselves the biblical texts frequently cited in support of sexual dimorphism can be reasonably interpreted to do so. Obviously, however, the question of what constitutes the criteria for *reasonable* biblical interpretation is tremendously significant. It has always been the Roman Catholic position that the discernment of the living tradition is rooted in the consilience of insights from several sources of moral wisdom. This means in the first place that there should be intra-canonical support for sexual dimorphism. While there is some such support for this traditional line of argument as noted above, other biblical texts clearly challenge this interpretive schema. Texts like Acts 8:26-39 cited above, as well as Isaiah 56:4-5 and Matthew 19:12, bear witness to God's inclusive love for all kinds of sexual persons.

Furthermore, a truly reasonable interpretation should enjoy consilience not only with traditional sources such as other biblical texts and official church teachings. It should cohere with insights from secular sources including scientific, legal, philosophical disciplines and personal and communal experiences.[8] Catholic Christians believe that truth is such that the faithful can expect *reasonable* biblical interpretations to cohere not only with cogent Church teachings but also with the wisdom emerging from sound scientific studies, well-constructed philosophical analyses and properly interpreted human experiences.[9]

How precisely the insights of experience and secular disciplines relate to Scripture and church traditions is part of what has historically divided Roman Catholic from Protestant Christians. But from a Catholic perspective it is reasonable to expect magisterial interpretations of biblical texts to be readily corroborated not only by the best of biblical scholarship but also to cohere with cogent interpretations of relevant human experiences and with the best scientific data and philosophical arguments available. When this expectation is not fulfilled, in theory at least, the genuine appreciation of official Church interpretations of the Bible is not antithetical to their critical analysis. In fact, the absence of this consilience should spark further inquiry

into and deliberation about how best to understand God's normative design
for human sexuality.

8. THE CONGRUENCE OF SEXUAL POLYMORPHISM WITH CHRISTIANITY

Undoubtedly it came as no surprise that Christians have traditionally taken
sexual dimorphism to be axiomatic. According to this conventional
perspective, there is a happy coherence between what is revealed in the
Christian Bible, traditional church teachings on human sexuality, well-
established tenets of natural law and the best insights of human reason
on this matter. On this paradigmatic matter–at least until recently–all
the sources of moral wisdom available to Christians seemed to be in basic
agreement. The truth of sexual dimorphism seemed practically
uncontestable.

Now, however, there are clear scientific and experiential grounds for re-
examining standard Christian interpretations of human sexuality.[10] By way
of conclusion I hope to make a modest contribution to that inquiry by
demonstrating that the notion of sexual polymorphism is not necessarily
incompatible with the creation accounts found in the opening chapters of
Genesis.

Before proceeding, it is helpful to note, as Gudorf's analysis makes clear,
that in comparison to Judaism and Islam, the Christian version of sexual
dimorphism is relatively weak.[11] There are no gender specific religious
duties within Christianity. The obligations associated with faithful
discipleship apply to men and women alike. Furthermore, though both are
associated with God's blessing, neither heterosexual marriage nor
parenthood is required of Christians. In fact, Jesus explicitly also associates
God's blessing with those who take up celibacy for the sake of the church's
mission (Matthew 19:12) and Paul notes his personal preference for this
lifestyle (1 Corinthians 7). For these reasons, it is perhaps fair to describe the
version of dimorphism operative within Christianity as relatively weak
(Gudorf, 863-869).

It is also useful to note that nothing in a polymorphic model of human
sexuality denies that God created most people either male or female. What
sexual polymorphism does deny is that sexual dimorphism is the exclusive,
or more precisely, the only normative form of human sexual differentiation.
It is my contention that such a conclusion is not necessitated by the two
creation accounts found in the opening chapters of Genesis. In fact, those
texts can be shown to be congruent with sexual polymorphism, just as the

scriptures are now readily seen to be compatible with a number of scientific concepts, such as the notions of a heliocentric solar system, polygenism and the ongoing, evolutionary development of the universe, etc.[12]

While both creation accounts specify that God created people "male **and** female" (Genesis 1: 27; 2: 23), nowhere does the Bible specify that God created people **only either** male **or** female. With the exception of the handful of texts referring to eunuchs cited above, the Bible is largely silent about the existence of intersexed persons. However, the Bible is also largely silent about most of the astonishing biodiversity that flavors creation as a whole and the human community therein. Furthermore, what is theologically central to both biblical accounts of sexual differentiation–the linking of difference to the human longing not to exist in isolation but to live in intimate, passionate, tender-hearted and delightful companionship with others–is applicable to all persons, whether they are intersexed, male or female.

What makes many traditional interpretations of this ancient spousal metaphor for the relationship between God and humanity and for human interrelationships so dangerous is the church's tendency to allow one of the meanings rightly associated with the metaphor to dominate. In her article, "Can God Be a Bride?" Susan A. Ross points out that God always seems to be thought of as a Bridegroom, never a Bride, resulting in a problematic theology of God (as literally male) and, correspondingly, in the sense that men are more like God than women (Ross, 13). Indeed, unless God is also sometimes imaged as a Bride, no close association with or likeness to God can be established for women (at least insofar as they are women).

Thus, what could be an inspiring and meaningful metaphorical language for God has a tendency to become an oppressive equation, producing a patriarchal image of God, which in turn sanctifies patriarchal relationships among people. Citing Thomas Aquinas, Ross reminds Christians that all we can truly say of God is what God is not. Analogies for God, if they are to avoid becoming idolatrous claims, must resist literal interpretation. When the church finally recognizes that intersexed, like male and female, persons have been made in the image and likeness of God, then perhaps Christians will come closer to recognizing that God is not male, female, or intersexed but rather truly beyond human sexual differentiation.

Patricia Jung, Professor, Department of Theology, Loyola University, Chicago, Illinois, U.S.A.

NOTES

[1]   As I understand it, there is an elevated rate of tumors associated with undescended or malformed testicles that requires careful monitoring. Also those born without functioning gonads, or whose gonads have been removed, should consultan endocr inologist and weigh the comparative risks of hormone replacement therapy against those linked to osteoporosis. Those with congenital adrenal hyperplasia (CAH) often face serious health problems because of their inability either to make sufficient cortisone and/or to process salt.

[2]   This is the language employed by Pope Pius XII in an address to the Federation of Italian Widwives.

[3]   For example, one can find this view defended in Pope Leo XIII's *Arcanum Diviniae Sapientiae* (1880) and then again by Pope Pius XI in *Casti connubii* (1930).

[4]   The promulgation in 1880 of that papal teaching usually marks the starting point of modern Catholic sexual ethics.

[5]   For a thorough review of the John Paul II's approach to these key biblical passages see Susan A. Ross' "The Bridegroom and the Bride: The Theological Anthropology of John Paul II and Its Relation to the Bible and Homosexuality," *Sexual Diversity and Catholicism: Toward the Development of Moral Theology* edited by Patricia Beattie Jung with Joseph A. Coray (Collegeville, MN: The Liturgical Press, 2001) 39-59.

[6]   Among the many biblical books cited are Hosea, Song of Songs, John, 2 Corinthians, Ephesians, and Revelation. Of course, other images of God abound in the Christian Bible.

[7]   No mention is made of the needs of stay-at-home dads or working-fathers.

[8]   Though such a claim in our present postmodern climate is somewhat unfashionable, arguably one of the twentieth century's most prominent scientists operates with and argues for a similar epistemological vision. See Edward O. Wilson, *Consilience: The Unity of Knowledge* (New York: Alfred A. Knopf, 1998.)

[9]   For more information about this approach to biblical interpretation, see Carolyn Osiek, R.S.C.J., "The New Handmaid: The Bible and Social Sciences," *Theological Studies* 50 (1989) 360-278.

[10]   Essays in this volume will cite several such secular arguments. One of special interest to those who seek to understand the evolutionary significance of sexual diversity is Joan Roughgarden's *Evolution's Rainbow: Diversity, Gender and* Sexuality Berkeley, CA: University of California Press, 2004.

[11]   Gudorf's analysis also makes it clear that in comparison to the world's other great religions, sexual dimorphism is strongest among the three great religions of the book in the West.

[12]   Over thirty-five years ago at least some scientists began proposing that biblical insights into sexuality should simply be jettisoned. As far as I can tell, the psychiatrist Ira B. Pauly may have been among the first to propose such a line of argument. His conclusion is worth quoting at length. "Not only are there behavior gradations between the abstract concepts 'totally male' and totally female,' but there are chromosomally and hormonally determined intersexed conditions. Therefore we must discard the biblical polarity of male-female, masculine-feminine dichotomy, and reorient our thinking along a scale of subtle nuances of behavior" (Pauly, 38). My hope here is to have established that it is not necessary to "throw out the baby with the bath water."

REFERENCES

Barth, Karl. *Church Dogmatics*, III/4.

Beeman, William O. "What Are You? Male, Merm, Herm, Ferm or Female?" *Baltimore Sun* March 17, 1996.

Cahill, Lisa S. "Gender and Christian Ethics," *The Cambridge Companion to Christian Ethics*, ed., Robin Gill. Cambridge: Cambridge University Press, 2001: 112-124.

Congregation for the Doctrine of the Faith, "On the Collaboration of Men and Women in the Church and in the World," (August 20, 2004).

Gagnon, Robert A. *The Bible and Homosexual Practice: Texts and Hermeneutics*. Nashville, TN: Abington Press, 2001.

Gross, Sally. "Intersexuality and Scripture," *Theology and Sexuality* 11 (Spring, 1999): 65-74.

Gudorf, Christine E. "The Erosion of Sexual Dimorphism: Challenges to Religion and Religious Ethics," *Journal of the American Academy of Religion* 69.4 (Dec 2001): 863-891.

John Paul II, *Mulieris dignitatem* (August 15, 1988): AAS 80 (1988): 1653-1729.

Kalbian, Aline H. "Integrity in Catholic Sexual Ethics," *Journal of the Society of Christian Ethics* 24/2 (Fall/Winter, 2004): 55-70.

Lebacqz, Karen. "Difference or Defect? Intersexuality and the Politics of Difference" *The Annual of the Society of Christian Ethics* 17 (1997): 213-229.

Looy, Heather. "Male and Female God Created Them: The Challenge of Intersexuality," *Journal of Psychology and Christianity* 21.1 (2002): 10-20.

O'Donovan, Oliver. "Transsexualism and Christian Marriage," *The Journal of Religious Ethics* 11(Spring, 1983):135-162.

Paula, Ira B. "Adult Manifestations of Male Transsexualism," *Transsexualism and Sex-Reassignment,* Eds. Richard Green and John Money. Baltimore, MD: John Hopkins Press, 1969: 37-58.

Roughgarden, Joan. *Evolution's Rainbow: Diversity, Gender and Sexuality in Nature and People.* Berkeley, CA: University of California Press, 2004.

Ross, Susan A. "Can God Be a Bride?" *America* 191.13 (Nov. 1, 2004): 12-15.

Ross, Susan A. "The Bridegroom and the Bride: The Theological Anthropology of John Paul II and Its Relation to the Bible and Homosexuality," *Sexual Diversity and Catholicism: Toward the Development of Moral Theology,* Eds. Patricia Beattie Jung with Joseph A. Coray, Collegeville, MN: The Liturgical Press, 2001: 39-59.

JUSTINE SCHOBER

ETHICS AND FUTURISTIC SCIENTIFIC DEVELOPMENTS CONCERNING GENITOPLASTY

What we want to know about the science of the future is the content and character of future scientific theories and ideas. Unfortunately, it is impossible to predict new ideas—the ideas people are going to have in ten years' or ten minutes' time—and we are caught in a logical paradox the moment we try to do so. For to predict an idea is to have an idea, and if we have an idea it can no longer be the subject of a prediction.

—Sir Peter Medawar

1. INTRODUCTION

New thinking challenges traditional decision-making. Every physician has the responsibility to keep abreast of the developments and issues that face the patients whom he or she advises. The physician must be mindful of how the newest scientific developments might influence a patient's decision-making. What must be disclosed to the patient? A patient has the right to access all relevant materials, whether or not the physician deems those materials useful. Freedom of expression, long defended by legal scholars and human rights advocates, extends to a patient's right to receive and impart new information and ideas (Plowden and Kerrigan, 2002). Implicit in the defense of that right is the understanding that good discussion, including discussion of future possibilities, precedes good decision-making. If a proposed surgery involves systems that do not have immediate use, but might serve a needed function in the future, discussing future possibilities is especially important.

Congenital genital anomalies and malformations may require extensive surgical reconstruction. A reliable, successful genitoplasty procedure that can be performed early in childhood for either feminization or masculinization has not yet been developed (Schober, 2005). Traditional reconstructive procedures have involved significant complications, although advancements in technique have occurred over the last ten years (Rink and Adams, 1998). Early procedures, such as skin flap vaginoplasty, were proven unsuccessful. Bowel vaginoplasty, though still used and in many cases quite functional for intercourse, may have undesirable side effects that limit patient satisfaction. Pull-through techniques have changed, with progress

S.E. Sytsma (Ed.), Ethics and Intersex, 311–317.

beginning on exposure positions (posterior approaches) and on mobilizing the total urogenital sinus. Now, with better understanding of innervation, limitations at certain points in mobilization may continue to improve sensitivity outcomes (Rink, 2004). Baskin et al. have elucidated innervation of the clitoris (1999), and further studies by Yucel et al. clarify innervation of the entire female lower urogenital tract (2004). Particular attention to the urethral sphincter complex and to nerve direction beneath the pubic symphasis is now recognized as crucial to ongoing reconstructive surgical design modifications (Rink, 2004).

Averting problematic outcomes of reconstructive surgery has often been a challenge because of the limited amounts of native tissue available. For many years, only surgical procedures that utilized native tissue were available; however, increased awareness of problematic outcomes has been a stimulus for novel ideas. Such ideas raise new challenges. Even while developments in molecular genetics, combined with the multiple genome projects and the power of computers, are yielding solutions to problems that were previously intractable, they are also unveiling new problems that were undreamed of a decade ago (Judson, 2004, 404–407).

Currently diagnostic and therapeutic approaches apply information from the fields of genomics, cell biology, and nuclear materials science, utilizing the expertise of those skilled in techniques of bioinformatics, cell harvest, culture, expansion, transplantation, and polymer design (Hipp and Atala, 2004). Experimental efforts are currently underway involving every type of tissue and organ of the human body. Techniques involving various tissues are at different stages of development. Some are being used clinically, some are in pre-clinical trials, and some are in the discovery stage. Tissue engineering is now a practical reality. Recent progress suggests that engineered tissues may have an expanded applicability in the future and may represent a viable therapeutic option for patients who need replacement or repair (Hipp and Atala, 2004). There have also been significant advancements in regenerative medicine, an evolving new discipline that could change current therapeutic approaches (Atala, 2004; De Filippo, Yoo, and Atala, 2003). One goal of this field has been to promote the development of tissues whose properties more closely match their native counterparts. The goal of these tissue-engineering scientists is creating or regenerating tissues that allow surgical practitioners to replace tissue that was lost to cancer, trauma, or infection and to introduce tissue that was absent due to congenital anomalies.

Tissue can be engineered in vivo (in the body) by stimulating the body's own regeneration response with the appropriate biomaterial, or ex vivo (outside the body, in the laboratory) by expanding cells in culture. In the case of tissue created ex vivo, the replacement tissue can be attached to a scaffold and then reimplanted in the host.

Cells may be heterologous (from a different species), allogeneic (from the same species, but from a different individual), or autologous (from the same individual). Autologous cells are preferred because they will not evoke an immunologic response, obviating the need for immunosuppressive agents. Autologous cells can often be found within the organ to be replaced or at a site near the needed replacement area. In autologous transplantation these cells (committed precursors) may be isolated, expanded, and then transplanted back into the patient, without need for immunosuppression. Autologous cells are the ideal source if they are sufficiently available.

There is an important difference between reproductive cloning and therapeutic cloning. Controversy surrounding the technologies is mostly related to reproductive cloning. This type of cloning has been banned in most countries for human applications. Reproductive cloning generates an embryo with genetic material identical to its cell source. This embryo has the potential, if implanted in the uterus of a woman, to create an infant that would be a clone of the donor. Therapeutic cloning is used to generate only cell lines whose genetic material is identical to the source tissue. Autologous stem cells have the potential to become almost any type of cell in the adult body, and so they would be useful in tissue and organ replacement applications. Therapeutic cloning (regenerative medicine) could provide a source of transplantable cells, in instances where cell material is absent or not available in sufficient quantity. Strategies combining therapeutic cloning with tissue engineering to develop tissues and whole functional organs are being explored. Currently, we use allogeneic tissue transplantation protocols. Rejection is a frequent complication because of immunologic incompatibility between the graft and the host. Immunosuppressive drugs are generally required but are sometimes insufficient to manage host-versus-graft reactions. The use of transplantable tissue and organs derived from host tissue would not generate the immune responses that are associated with the transplantation of non-autologous tissues (Hipp and Atala, 2004)

This evolving field could have an impact on how genitoplasty for intersexual conditions is performed. One of the problems of genitoplasty has always been a lack of the right kind of tissue in the right place. When local flaps of tissue are used in surgical reconstructions, they are not always the best kind of tissue. When more suitable kinds of tissue are used, they are often brought in from a more distant location. Developments in tissue engineering might herald an answer long sought by those surgeons who have wished to perform functional reconstructions using tissues that most closely resemble the structures or tissues the patient might have had naturally.

The possibility of engineering vaginal, uterine, or phallic tissue could influence surgical goals in another way. A part of the surgery we do for intersexual conditions has a sense of immediacy; there is often an imperative to convey a sexual marker or appearance congruent with gender assignment. Another part of this same surgery does not carry such immediacy because the surgery conveys sexual capabilities unnecessary until early adulthood. To some extent, the surgeries that confirm gender appearance in early childhood have been successful. But later demands for growth of the genitalia and sexual functionality after puberty are not as easily met. These would be the times when such engineered tissue might be really helpful.

Two questions immediately arise. If the surgeries for intersexual conditions were to be divided or parcelled in this way, would it make outcomes worse or would it improve them? This is a question that has been asked even before the possibilities of tissue engineering. But the question becomes even more seminal if we consider tissue engineering for intersexual conditions a valid possibility for the future. The use of engineered tissue would most affect the portion of surgery that addresses sexual functioning, growth, and development after puberty, as well as the initiation of sexual intercourse, the initiation of pregnancy, and the maintenance of pregnancy until parturition. These are situations of no immediate need during infancy and early childhood.

Considering the current state of tissue engineering specifically for vaginal, uterine and phallic tissue, we must ask ourselves, as physicians, if this information could significantly influence the decision-making of parents whose children have intersex conditions. Further, could those early decisions actually preserve the integrity of a child with an intersex condition, so that he or she could make his or her own decision in the future?

2. FEMINIZING GENITOPLASTY

Concepts of vaginoplasty may have originated with Hippocrates and Celsus, but few attempts were made at reconstruction in the 18th and 19th centuries. Staged vaginal reconstructions began as early as the late 1800's. Split thickness grafts covering a neovaginal channel were a breakthrough at the turn of the 20th century. But problems with these repairs led to the search for an ideal material. From the 1950's to this day, a variety of skin flap, bowel, peritoneum, and urothelium tissues have been tried with variable success. Problems with the use of alternative tissues in place of natural vaginal tissue have included infection, erosion, mineral deposits and calcifications, migration of tissues, scarring, secondary reactions from tissues being exposed to substances to which they would not have been exposed if left native, and lack of resiliance to stresses they were not intended to have (Schober, 2005). Surgical capabilities were challenged by expectations that a good surgical outcome should include sexual sensitivity, natural genital appearance without excessive scarring, and vaginal construction that allowed intercourse without pain and that did not require repeated modification.

Such expectations have been difficult to meet because of the vagina's constitution, which includes both a specific secretory epithelium and an underlying smooth muscle layer. Utilizing tissue that is unlike this, then subjecting it to stresses typical to the vaginal site while expecting typical responses might be unrealistic. This brings up questions about genitoplasty that are as yet unanswered. Even for engineered tissue, optimal outcomes cannot be guaranteed.

At the present time, there are some demonstrative results for therapeutic tissue cloning. De Fillipo and Atala have shown that vaginal epithelial cells and vaginal smooth muscle cells can be easily cultured and expanded in vitro and that cell seeded polymer scaffolds are able to form vascularized vaginal tissue in vivo. This engineered tissue has phenotypic and functional characteristics similar to normal vaginal tissue (De Filippo, Yoo, and Atala, 2003). Young and colleagues have created a three-dimensional culture of human uterine smooth muscle on resorbable scaffolding (Young, Schumann, and Zhang, 2003). This tissue has been tested to some extent for resilience to stretching. Initial studies are underway in an animal model to determine durability under conditions of sexual intercourse and pregnancy.

3. MASCULINIZING GENITOPLASTY

Gender assignment has been influenced by the lack of phallic tissue when chromosome constitution is unequivocally male. Because there were no realistic surgical possibilities for the production of an erectile phallus that grew along with the patient, masculinizing surgery was rarely offered. This remains a difficult aspect of the decision process concerning intersex gender assignment and surgery (Zini et al., 2004). Male assignment often means a long period during growth and development with atypical or absent male genitalia followed by a decision that may trade a sensate yet very small phallus for the uncertain sensate or orgasmic status of a larger phallus, created from the tissues of an arm or leg, that might be capable of erect vaginal intromission.

The possibility of engineering tissue for human penile corporal construction gained legitimacy in 1999, when Park et al. demonstrated that human corporal smooth muscle and endothelial cells seeded on biodegradable polymer scaffolds formed vascularized corpus cavernosum muscle when implanted in vivo (Park et al., 1999; Colman and Kind, 2000). The aim was to benefit patients undergoing penile reconstruction and those with erectile disorders. In 2002, the functional integrity of this engineered tissue was successfully demonstrated on a rabbit model; researchers confirmed the presence of sperm after copulation, and the tissue grafts showed nitric oxide synthetase activity similar to normal controls. In 2003 the technology was advanced by the successful development of human corporal tissue seeded on three dimensional acellular collagen matrices (Falke et al., 2003). Though this procedure is not yet available for human usage, current developments suggest that human applications may be possible in the future. This information would be valuable for any parents looking at choices that might affect their child's life twenty years from now.

4. ARE SURGICAL OUTCOMES REALLY JUST RELATED TO TECHNIQUE AND TISSUE?

The science and specialty of wound healing is at present in a stage of rapid advancement. In exploratory fields involving the hormonal regulation of wound healing, the effects of estrogen, relaxin, connexins and growth factors upon healing are currently being examined. The impact of estrogens on wound healing raises questions about the existence of a natural surgical window, the effects of preoperative priming, and the role of postoperative hormonal maintenance.

Hormones are known to expand genital sensory fields and to protect blood vessels from stretch injury. Modification of hormonal entities might affect surgical outcomes in cases where innervation is at risk or healing has been problematic. We also may look forward to the development of "designer" or receptor-specific drugs to modify growth or function of tissue without surgical incision in some cases.

5. ANATOMY MAY NOT BE THE LAST WORD

Although advances in surgical technique are important, a better understanding of the relationship between sensory mechanisms, arousal, and behavior in humans is crucial. Understanding gender assignment and gender/hormonal relationship to the relative contributions of sensation, arousal, and sexual behavior may best improve a patient's quality of life.

Ethics concerning genitoplasty and surgical decision-making are really about recognizing the outcomes, possibilities, and problems faced by patients who will be affected—particularly those patients who are too young to make such decisions. As surgeons, our ethical duty is to provide understandable information, all that we can, pro and con, historical and speculative. Our goal is to help parents make choices that will lead to good outcomes for their baby or child from early life through adulthood. With recent medical advances, this informative process becomes even more critical and complicated. But this is the responsibility of the physician or surgeon in today's society. It is a challenge. However, those who decide to care for such complicated patients must be up to it.

Justine Schober, Urologist, Hamot Medical Center, Erie, Pennsylvania, U.S.A.

REFERENCES

Atala, Anthony. "Tissue Engineering for the Replacement of Organ Function in the Genitourinary System." *American Journal of Transplantation* 4.s6 (February 2004): 58—73.

Baskin, Laurence S., Ali Erol, Ying Wu Li, Wen Hui Liu, Eric Kurzrock, and Gerald R. Cunha. "Anatomical Studies of the Human Clitoris." *Journal of Urology* 162.3.2 (September 1999): 1015—20.

Colman, Alan and Alexander Kind. "Therapeutic Cloning: Concepts and Practicalities." *Trends in Biotechnology* 18.5 (May 2000): 192—196.

De Filippo, Roger E., James J. Yoo, and Anthony Atala. "Engineering of Vaginal Tissue in Vivo." *Tissue Engineering* 9.2 (April 2003): 301—6.

Falke, German, James J. Yoo, Tae Gyun Kwon, Robert Moreland, and Anthony Atala. "Formation of Corporal Tissue Architecture in Vivo Using Human Cavernosal Muscle and Endothelial Cells Seeded on Collagen Matrices." *Tissue Engineering* 9.5 (October 2003): 871—9.

Hipp, Jason, and Anthony Atala. "Tissue Engineering, Stem Cells, Cloning, and Parthenogenesis: New Paradigms for Therapy." *Journal of Experimental and Clinical Assisted Reproduction* 1.3 (December 2004).

Judson, Horace Freeland. *The Great Betrayal: Fraud in Science.* New York: Harcourt Books, 2004.

Park, Heung Jae, James J. Yoo, Richard T. Kershen, Robert Moreland, and Anthony Atala. "Reconstitution of Human Corporal Smooth Muscle and Endothelial Cells in Vivo." *Journal of Urology* 162.3.2 (September 1999): 1106—1109.

Plowden, Philip and Kevin Kerrigan. *Advocacy and Human Rights: Using the Convention in Courts and Tribunals.* London: Cavendish Publishing Limited, 2002.

Rink, Richard. Panel on Intersex, American Academy of Pediatrics. (November 2004).

Rink, Richard C., and Mark C. Adams. "Feminizing Genitoplasy: State of the Art." *World Journal of Urology* 16.3 (June 1998): 212—218.

Schober, Justine. "Long-Term Outcome of Feminization (Surgical Aspects)." *Pediatric and Urologic Surgery* (2005).

Young, Roger C., Ralph Schumann, and Peisheng Zhang. "Three-Dimentional Culture of Human Uterine Smooth Muscle Myocytes on a Resorbable Scaffolding." *Tissue Engineering* 9.3 (June 2003): 451—9.

Yucel, Selcuk, Antonio de Souza, Jr., and Laurence S. Baskin. "Neuroanatomy of the Human Female Lower Urogenital Tract." *Journal of Urology* 172.1 (July 2004): 191—5.

Zini, L., R. Yiou, C. Lecoeur, J. Biserte, C. Abbou, and D.K. Chopin. "Tissue Engineering in Urology." *Annales d'Urologie Paris* 38.6 (December 2004): 266—74.

IAIN MORLAND

POSTMODERN INTERSEX

1. POSTMODERN INTERSEX

This paper will explore the relation between intersex and postmodernity by
analyzing the important work of Alice Dreger, historian, ethicist, and chair of the
Intersex Society of North America (ISNA). Specifically, I'll consider the
presentation in Dreger's *Hermaphrodites and the Medical Invention of Sex* of what
she calls "Postmodernist Intersexuality" (1998a, 170). In the book's epilogue, titled
"Categorical Imperatives," Dreger (1998a, 170) turns from historical analysis to
contemporary activism by setting up as ethically important the practice of paying
serious attention to the autobiographical narratives of intersexed individuals.
Moreover, she is exceedingly careful to suggest medical change *only* as a sensible
and correct response to intersex autobiographies (1998a, 198). Interestingly, Dreger
names as "postmodern" the time of these intersex stories' historical appearance, and
details five characteristics of "postmodern times" that have "enabled the emergence
of intersexual autobiographies" in the late twentieth century (1998a, 168, 170–173).
I shall critically contextualize each characteristic of postmodernity, and will thereby
reveal that intersex reformists face a predicament. It will become apparent that none
of the features of postmodernity unequivocally support the ethical agenda that they
are enlisted by Dreger to facilitate. On the contrary, each feature will be remarkably
ambivalent for the reform of intersex management. However, I shall show that this
ambivalence is itself unmistakably postmodern, and hence vital to the renegotiation
of intersex management in the postmodern age.

2. VOICES

First, Dreger (1998a, 170) cites the valuation of previously non-authoritative voices
as a postmodern development. In particular, she finds an important precursor to the
emergence of intersexed voices in the expertise averred by people with AIDS,
hemophilia, schizophrenia and cancer regarding the lived experience of suffering
and the significance of illness (1998a, 170).

By situating the emergent narratives of intersexed people in relation to other
patient voices, Dreger's first point about postmodernity places those stories within a

S.E. Sytsma (Ed.), Ethics and Intersex, 319–332.

larger narrative of medical progress. It encourages medical professionals to read intersex stories as instructive feedback, not maverick criticism. Indeed, Dreger will later find that the most effective way of presenting ISNA's agenda to surgeons is to locate it as "part of a trend in improving ethical practice in medicine" (2003). The strategy offers a recognizable point of access to intersex debates to clinicians who are already interested in using patients' narratives to improve healthcare. "Through stories we are able imaginatively to [...] focus upon the experience of others," one doctor has written (Hurwitz, 2086); "To hear the voice of the patient preserves our capacity to imagine the suffering of the patient," claims another (Verghese, 1016). Stressing the valuation of previously disempowered patient voices is a non-confrontational way of asking clinicians to keep doing what they (or their peers) are already doing in the service of better medicine.

Valuing such voices also promotes the reform of intersex treatment on the grounds that "normalization" is unacceptable. Dreger has elsewhere recorded that some "women born with big clitorises confess to liking their unusual anatomy [...]—not only rejecting normalization but actively preferring the 'abnormal'" (1998b). For instance, Kim (99), a woman who did not receive surgery on her atypically large clitoris, writes fondly of the ability that it gives her to penetrate her female partner. By asserting that intersex genitals can and should be pleasurable, counter-medical narratives such as Kim's make clear that life in an intersexed body without surgery is, despite mainstream and paternalistic assumptions, a life worth living. Comparing her experience to the accounts of postsurgical intersexed women makes Kim "wonder what makes doctors so certain that women want a small clitoris, and want it badly enough to sacrifice sexual responsiveness to alter it" (100). Kim's narrative hereby queries the obviousness of surgery as a response to unusual anatomies, and thus replaces medical authority with the weight of her own experience, unauthorized yet authoritative (see Butler, 158–163).

But there are also problems with Dreger's assertion that previously unacknowledged voices are now being valued. The assertion raises the question of who is performing the valuation. Early in her work with ISNA, Dreger used her academic credentials to help promote the voice of leading patient activist Cheryl Chase to physicians who were "afraid she was some sort of anarchist" (2001, 2). The tactic certainly worked, but it reveals that the reappraisal of intersexed voices does not occur *ex nihilo*: it is affected by pre-existent power relations. By this reading, the claim to authority made by Kim's narrative on the basis of its first-person content is insufficient, for it presumes that private experience is equivalent to professionally sanctioned expertise.

In fact, Dreger implies as much when she mentions the publication in *Social History of Medicine* of a first-person account of hemophilia (Bateman); the lesson here is that the authoritative gatekeepers of the academy, such as journal editors, "medical theorists and medical historians" (Dreger 1998a, 170), not hemophiliacs, are in control. They determine the dissemination and promotion of "voices previously considered nonauthoritative" (Dreger 1998a, 170). In other words, the valuation of formerly marginalized voices signals the undesirable integration of those voices into the power relations of professional discourse.

My broader contention, which draws on political philosopher Louis Althusser (160–162), is that the constitution of individuals as legitimate participants in a discourse occurs only through their subjection to the rules of that discourse—rules which do not belong to them. Subjection to those rules may enable one's voice to be heard, but it also diminishes the diversity that intersex reformists want to foster. Consequently, an ethical stance, contrary to what Dreger seeks to propose, may be for intersexed people to reject revaluation on the grounds that it is, at best, a capitulation to conservative rules of discourse, and at worst, a token gesture on the part of the authoritative group that works specifically because the group remains in power—by exercising its power to evaluate others.

My analysis reveals the ambivalence latent in Dreger's suggestion that postmodern times herald the positive appraisal of patients' voices. I must make clear that I'm not insinuating that patients' voices can never be valued in postmodernity; rather, I argue that their valuation is curiously dependent on the persistence—not the subversion—of the same power relations that devalue them. In examining Dreger's other characteristics of postmodern times, I'll uncover comparable ambivalences of increasing interrelatedness.

3. STORIES

The second feature of postmodernity identified by Dreger is the recognition that there is never a single true story "to be told about a life, disease, or condition" (1998a, 171). She therefore recommends that we "Allow those with the unusual anatomies to describe their own lives in full and rich detail" (1998b).

This recognition of plurality certainly facilitates a multidimensional understanding of intersex. For example, its medical management has been narrated by several commentators and patients as abusive rather than therapeutic, most thoroughly by Tamara Alexander, who calls intersex medicine "an analogue for childhood sexual abuse." As one intersex person has written regarding the postoperative dilation of surgically fashioned vaginas, "I'm not convinced that it is less psychologically harmful just because the adult isn't doing it for fun" (Glass, 2). The recognition that there is no one true story makes possible the creation of dissident representations of health and illness such as these. Further, by disallowing the medical account its conventionally presumed power to describe the totality of intersexual experience, that recognition permits intersexed individuals to tell their tales as lovers, parents, professionals, and so forth—not merely as patients. Dreger (1998a, 175–176) superbly puts this into practice in her epilogue by documenting much more than the medical histories of her intersexed interviewees; for instance, Diane Marie Anger is photographed with one of her dogs, to represent her love for animals and the pet fostering she does for Florida's Humane Society. The epilogue thereby demonstrates the narrative multiplicity that it seeks to describe.

To a degree, the presentation in *Hermaphrodites* of multifaceted stories such as Anger's, to show the inadequacy of singular narratives about intersex, offers a way round a previous difficulty. It enables Dreger to sidestep the problem of the diminution of cultural diversity that arose because of the first feature of postmodernity, by claiming that intersexuality itself is diverse, not just its narrators. Put another way, the second characteristic of postmodernity explains the differences among the stories of clinicians and patients as effects of intersexuality's own polyvalence, instead of as consequences of the power differentials between those who narrate it.

Unfortunately though, the claim that there is no single true story about "a life, disease, or condition" can be experienced by medical professionals as extremely agitating. Contrary to the mutual tolerance that the claim seeks to encourage, it may inhibit dialogue between doctors and patients, as well as across academic disciplines. Just as "There are reasons to act, in certain contexts, as if truth is no more than constructed beliefs," so too are there also "reasons to act, in certain contexts, as if truth can be held as indisputable," in the words of one feminist (Ropers-Huilman, 65). There are arguably situations in which the recognition of multiple stories is detrimental rather than beneficial. And some clinicians have argued that it is *precisely* in medical contexts that truth should be treated as singular and incontestable.

Consider that clinician Rita Charon extolled in the *Annals of Internal Medicine* the humanitarian usefulness of what she calls "narrative medicine." Charon claimed that the proliferation of narratives by patients and clinicians alike about illness "confers on medical practice a kind of understanding that is otherwise unobtainable" (83). This supports Dreger's contention that to tell a single story about an illness is to fail to represent the polyvalence of the condition. Like Dreger, Charon has specified elsewhere that narrative medicine is useful "in a postmodern world" (Charon et al., 601). But in an angry letter to the *Annals*, Roy M. Poses of Brown Medical School responded that Charon "seems to be advocating [...] the medical application of what has variously been called deconstructionism, poststructuralism, critical literary theory, or postmodernism." The latter's "extreme relativism" places doctors and patients in "peril," Poses charged, by claiming that knowledge doesn't exist (929). Clearly there are flaws here—Poses eschews relativism yet conflates a range of methodologies as if they were versions of the same project; however, his letter is valuable because it demonstrates the offence that some clinicians take to the recognition that there is no one true story.

Narrative plurality may be problematic for laypeople too. Dreger's enclosure in quotation marks of the term "true," the adjective that marks the precondition of all referential discourse, logically means that all other descriptive words ought also to be put into relativising quotation marks. To be sure, Dreger does exactly this with the terms "diseases," "cures" and "problems" (1998a, 171). But it would not be so easy or obviously ethical to respond—for instance—to the testimony of an abuse survivor with an account of their experience as "assault" and "rape" rather than as assault and rape, to allow the perpetrator to tell an equally valid story of those events as "romantic" or "consensual." My example is extreme, but it highlights the vital point that although the insight that there is no one true story is set up by Dreger as an ethical aspect of postmodernity, the insight itself provides no indication of when its employment would be ethically appropriate.

4. MEDICINE

The third characteristic of postmodernity is the experience of medicine as medicalization—a mechanistic hindrance to real health, which colonizes patients' bodies "in ways that impel them to resist and object," says Dreger (1998a, 171–172).

To demedicalize intersexuality in objection to the body's "colonization" is to show intersex to be a social rather than an anatomical problem. Hence, it is a way of arguing that intersexuality is not a condition that can be solved or eradicated by genital surgery. The most widely-known advocate of demedicalization is Ivan Illich, who has argued for the devolution of authority over the body from the medical establishment to individuals and communities, in the belief that less aggressive and more holistic healthcare can be provided outside of the clinic, which is itself a source of malaise in his view. Dreger concurs. The "typical treatment of intersexuality may well create the feelings it is supposed to prevent," she hazards (1998a, 191). In the sweeping tract *Limits to Medicine*, Illich has critiqued the technoscientific suppression of non-scientific models of human wellbeing. Given this context, the bid to demedicalize intersexuality builds on Dreger's previous point by asserting not only that there is more than a single way to narrate intersex, but furthermore that intersex ought to be narrated in one way (as social) rather than another (as medical). "Technological approaches tend to shut out discussion of alternative approaches," she protests (1998a, 187) in harmony with Illich.

This functions as a pre-emptive pragmatic rejoinder to criticisms of the second feature of postmodernity—the rejection of the multiplicity of truths on the grounds that it is unscientifically relativist. By situating intersexuality altogether outside the medical realm, a realm in which "hard facts" may indeed be necessary, and instead within the social sphere where multiple stories *are* arguably useful, it makes a concession to anti-postmodernist doctors such as Poses while also allowing for the focus by Charon on multiple narratives. Put differently, it matters not to intersex advocates whether medicine deals strictly in singular, verifiable truths, because intersexuality isn't medicine's business; it is the business of society. In this way, the demedicalization of intersex may help to bring together medical professionals and intersexed individuals, because it is sympathetic to a range of clinical viewpoints.

Some medical practitioners are likewise in favor of reducing medicine's remit, but I want to suggest that this actually renders questionable the ethical value of demedicalization. Less well known than Illich, yet nonetheless controversial, was a survey of medical professionals by the *British Medical Journal* (*BMJ*) in search of what the journal called "non-diseases" (Smith 2002a, 885). These were classified as processes or problems that would be better managed if they weren't defined as medical conditions. Apparently pursuing an agenda of demedicalization, the editor quoted at length from Illich in both the survey report and his correspondence with respondents (Smith 2002a; 2002b).

Despite conceding that disease and health are really impossible to define, the *BMJ* whittled down from a list of two hundred suggestions a top twenty chart of "non-diseases" including pregnancy, aging and ugliness (Smith 2002a, 883). These were fairly unarguable. However, regardless of the journal's proviso that it sought not to discount the suffering of those living with "non-diseases," correspondents accused the exercise of intrinsic arrogance irrespective of its specific findings (Walsh). In their view, demedicalization doesn't automatically benefit patients; it might complement the proliferation of patient voices, but it may also privilege doctors as the experts regarding which "non-diseases" should or should not be demedicalized.

Moreover, many *BMJ* correspondents contested the longlisting of afflictions such as chronic fatigue syndrome (White). They argued that the label "non-disease" too often has led to individuals being stigmatized as suffering from merely "psychosomatic and psychological" problems (Dunbar, 912). Necessary treatments have on these grounds been withheld. Therefore, calling for "professional and peer psychological support [...] as the *primary* intervention" in intersex cases, as Dreger does (2004, 72), may serve to discredit intersexed individuals by implying that their difficulties can be cured by just a friendly chat and a little positive thinking. I do think that serious psychological therapies are very helpful for intersex, but my point is that the *BMJ* debate exposes a tension in Dreger's account of postmodernity: it suggests that the demedicalization of intersex might exacerbate rather than lessen its stigmatization.

Such stigmatization may sadly be socially endemic. As Suzanne Kessler (32) points out—and as Dreger (1998a, 166 and 197) quotes approvingly in "Categorical Imperatives"—intersexed genitals are not life-threatening, but they are undoubtedly threatening to a predominantly heterosexist, androcentric Western culture that is intolerant of genital difference. The social, then, is *exactly* the source of the suffering that intersexuals experience; Dreger will later complain, "The problem that is always being fixed and attended to [by genital surgery] is the child, not the social situation" (2004, 72). As a result, demedicalized intersexuals may find themselves even more harshly received in the social realm than they have been in the domain of medicine.

5. POWER

Fourth in Dreger's (1998a, 172) portrayal of postmodernity is a shift in the power relations between doctors and patients. She details two elements to this shift (1998a, 172). On the one hand, there's the conception of the patient as a "health-care consumer," an active decision-maker who demands and deserves a range of treatment options. On the other hand, there's the increasing insight that doctors, and the treatments they prescribe, are not "superhuman": there is no pill for every ill.

This point is valuable primarily because it makes salient a requirement of the other features of postmodernity. A change in doctor-patient power relations is essential in order for intersexed patients' voices to be valued, for their stories to be appreciated as valid representations of the polyvalence of intersexuality, and for their needs to be recast as exterior to the medical domain. The power shift marks a significant challenge to paternalism, because it suggests not merely that medical influence over healthcare is waning, but that paternalism is evolving into negotiation (Detmer et al., 15). Most importantly in my opinion, the shift legitimizes those intersexed patients who would prefer not to receive genital surgery, by narrating their preferences as part of a larger story of changing doctor-patient relations. Like the agenda to demedicalize intersexuality, the figuration of intersex as one aspect of a general transformation in the power relations between doctors and patients could be productively conciliatory. It need not entail a complete rejection of medicine, merely a reconfiguration of its scope, which many medical professionals and policymakers have already welcomed (Calman; Department of Health). In the cordial words of the *BMJ* editor, "We're in this together" (Smith 2001, 1073).

Represented as participants in a broader power shift, intersexed people who refuse surgery are positioned not as temperamental patients in need of stricter instruction, but as consumers exercising their right to choose. As Dreger says, medicine "does not work identically in every case" (1998a, 172). Accordingly, the intersexed consumer may reasonably decide to reject the surgical service that their healthcare provider is offering. Research has shown that clinicians, policymakers, and patients all find acceptable the notion of the patient as consumer (Detmer et al., 45 and 47). Therefore it is likely that the narration of intersex management as an issue of consumer rights can assist dialogue between all involved by providing a common and palatable vocabulary with which to plan its improvement.

Dreger (1998a, 172) concedes that the idea of patients as healthcare consumers is not without problems, but does not detail its troubles. I shall set them out here. The most immediate problem faced by medical professionals is that patients' expectations as consumers may be unrealistic. Although Dreger (1998a, 172)—and clinicians—readily acknowledge that "medicine cannot cure everything," the patient as consumer may legitimately expect a cure for intersexuality exactly because they are a consumer, and hence are paying for their well-being. Specifically, patients may request treatments that are unfeasibly costly, or even at odds with clinical recommendations (Say and Thompson, 544). This creates a predicament for intersex management, where the prevailing clinical consensus is to perform the very surgery to which reformists object.

The critic of intersex surgery is therefore placed in the difficult position of advising clinicians to permit patients to "consume" non-surgical treatments that a clinician's peers, such as the American Academy of Pediatrics, consider to be ineffective or harmful. Alternatively, but even more problematically, patients' wishes may stand in direct opposition to the reformists' own vision of ethical intersex treatment: they may desire genital surgery and very paternalistic care from a doctor who is "superhuman" in attitude and claims (Detmer et al., 47).

It is also far from transparent that the position of the consumer is ever an active, desirable one. Leading cultural critics have damned consumerism as an ideology of passive docility in which individual choice is limited to options predetermined by corporate concerns, which foreclose genuine innovation so as to minimize risk and maximize profits (Horkheimer). In contradiction to Dreger's third point, the growth of healthcare consumerism arguably makes intersexuality more rather than less medicalized, because it extends the medical system into the capitalist arena, instead of curtailing it. And psychological support for intersex may be more expensive than surgery, for it requires a longer-term commitment of expertise and resources. Additionally, it is likely to be logistically awkward and expensive to arrange for patients from overseas (Diamond et al., 13). Therefore it may not be available as a consumer option.

The narration of intersex as one element of a larger reconfiguration of doctor-patient relations also raises problems, especially in Britain, where in 1990 an "internal market" was set up in the National Health Service (NHS). The ensuing "separation between the purchasing of services and their provision" (Mechanic, 55) gave some organizations and clinicians the means and authority to buy treatments from others. The providers thus competed with each other to offer the cheapest services to the purchasers. Commentators have argued that this change essentially provides choice only to clinicans, not to patients (Grand et al.). In particular, many doctors became "fundholding" resource managers, responsible for purchasing specialist and hospital services for their patients (Enthoven, 105). Even though the resultant competitiveness was intended to improve quality as well as cost-efficiency, it has failed to protect vulnerable patients (Mechanic, 55; Enthoven, 104). They cannot freely choose all their health service providers; those who live near inefficient hospitals are exponentially disadvantaged, because poorly performing hospitals suffer financial penalties that exacerbate their deterioration (Enthoven, 109). In sum, consumerism in healthcare does not necessarily benefit or even include the patient, in opposition to Dreger's suggestion.

One is left with a deeply troublesome dichotomy in which either doctors—not patients—are the true "fundholding" consumers, or patients are consumers in only a very limited sense, because they need close guidance from doctors in order to make medically sound, yet potentially ethically questionable, choices about the management of their intersexuality.

6. CONSTRUCTIVISM

In the fifth characteristic of postmodernity, Dreger (1998a, 172–173) formulates social constructivism as a political insight. She dovetails history and ethics by proposing that in the "postmodern" moment, the historical axis of oppression becomes salient, and that this revelation can prompt a rejection of contemporary social constructs as unethical. Thus, she argues that "postmodernism, in its appreciation of the social construction of concepts like sexual identity and normality, has given intersexuals the opportunity to see their plight as contingent to social times and places" (1998a, 172).

This point has power because it implicitly applies the social model of disability to intersexuality. In her monograph after *Hermaphrodites*, Dreger will make increasingly explicit connections between the intersex and disability rights movements (2004, 147). Advocates of the social model of disability reject the term "disabled" as an adjective for a person because it suggests innate inadequacy (French, 17). Instead, the social model's exponents specify which features of a person's environment render them less capable—less mobile, for example; or in the case of intersex, less able to use the locker room without embarrassment because of a lack of curtains. Likewise, Dreger writes of the intersexed that "it is not their bodies that make their lives difficult, but the cultural demands forced upon their bodies" (1998a, 173). I agree that the social model of disability reveals how social constructions, not anatomies, hinder intersexual lives.

This approach tackles one of the problems I identified in Dreger's earlier point about demedicalization, by admitting that the social realm may indeed be hostile to intersexed individuals, and insisting for that very reason upon the possibility and necessity of social reform. Disability scholar Sally French has explained that "the way to reduce disability is to adjust the social and physical environment to ensure that the needs and rights of people with impairments are met, rather than attempting to change disabled people to fit the existing environment" (17). The model prompts a shift from treating an individual with medical interventions to treating an individual's societal context with legislation and improved facilities. The agenda outlined by French also bears out Dreger's first claim about postmodernity—the positive revaluation of intersexed voices—because it provides concrete reasons to attend to the narratives of the intersexed. They should be seriously listened to, in order to work out how the environment can be changed to meet their needs.

Crucially then, the social model of disability contests the conditions that serve to disable people, not the people who find themselves disabled by those conditions. To say that individuals are disabled is an inaccuracy insofar as they are not personally inadequate; it is their environment that lets them down. Yet insofar as their environment is unfriendly to their rights and demands, they *are* disabled people. For this reason, "disability" signifies not a body with describable social effects but a nexus of social constructions, of which the less able body is merely one effect among others. This social understanding of disability enables an interrogation of the term "disabled" while also attending to the difficulties experienced by those who live the identity "disabled." In contrast, when doctors perform genital surgery on intersexed infants, they suppress the insight of disability scholarship that "the social system is broken" in favor of an individualized medical fix that tacitly declares, "it's the child that's broken" (Dreger 2004, 72).

Understood as an evocation of disability theory, Dreger's formulation of social constructivism as a political insight enables one to acknowledge that the social environment oppresses intersexed people, without one's needing to make any suppositions about intersex anatomies. The acknowledgement of oppression begins and ends with the recognition of the cultural and historical contingency of the violence done to individuals with those anatomies. As Dreger has written in the ISNA newsletter, "It is best to think about intersex not as a question of your anatomy but as a question of how your anatomy *is treated*" (2002, 2). Notably, ISNA's turn away from surgery and its object, anatomy, towards psychological and peer support is substantiated by the insight that the problems experienced by intersexed individuals are "not inherent in or necessary to their bodies" (Dreger 1998a, 172). Surgery, quite simply, is an inappropriate remedy for difficulties that aren't of the body.

But there are problems. Although Dreger (1998a, 172–173) says that intersexuals' awareness of "the cultural dependency of the categorization and treatments of males, females, and hermaphrodites" can enable them to counter their medical management as "freaks" who are in need of repair or erasure, it is not obvious that insight into the social construction of one's maltreatment is politically empowering or psychologically uplifting. "The person with a secret failing," states sociologist Erving Goffman in his classic study *Stigma*, is "likely to be alienated from the simpler world in which those around him apparently dwell. What is their ground is his figure" (110). Even though the stigmatized person's experience of the "ground" as "figure" may be more astute than the "simpler" views of others, it is not necessarily liberating; rather, it may lead one to feel inauthentic, "alienated" from a bodily authenticity that, despite its evident "social construction," is experienced by others as immutable (Morland 2001).

Correspondingly, an awareness of the social constructions that impact negatively on intersexed individuals does not always induce sympathy in non-intersexed people. In fact, it can provoke a reactionary defense of those very constructions. Consider Germaine Greer's (1999, 64–74) comments about intersexuality and transsexuality in her book *The Whole Woman*. Greer's repeated objections to the use of "female" as a catch-all term for "not male" make clear that her general disagreement is regarding how femaleness is social constructed (Greer 1999, 68, 70, 73). Specifically, she objects (1999, 70) to the idea that surgery performed on intersexed genitals to produce "bodies with clefts in for the accommodation of a penis" is a way of making females. Greer shares the latter objection with Kessler (108), and Dreger herself (1998a, 184).

However, in a chapter titled antagonistically "Pantomime Dames," Greer (1999, 74) claims that male-to-female transsexuals are men who decide to spend their lives impersonating their mothers like Norman Bates in *Psycho*, and that androgen insensitive intersexed women similarly are not female because their sex chromosomes are not those of a woman, which Greer defines narrowly as XX (1999, 68–70). Androgen Insensitivity Syndrome (AIS) is the medical term for a body with XY sex chromosomes that is indifferent to masculinising hormones and so presents as feminine; AIS individuals are typically assigned, raised, and live unambiguously as female. "Cruel and unsympathetic though it may seem," asserts Greer, feminists ought to name and shame individuals with AIS as the "failed," "damaged" males that they are (1999, 70). In this strategy, Greer is in direct opposition to Dreger, who—for instance—unhesitatingly describes Sherri Groveman as "a woman with AIS" (1998a, 192).

After her book's publication, Greer received letters countering her claims from people with AIS and their families, as well as from Milton Diamond and pediatric endocrinologist Charmian Quigley, who works with intersex support groups.[1] Her responses were dismissive; she then used the book's second edition not to retract the claims, but to publicly mock the AIS correspondents by referring to them too as men (2000, 87). In trying to criticize the social construction of femaleness and intersex, Greer disenfranchised precisely those people who live at the intersection of the two categories. Absent from her account was an understanding of the social model of disability that would have enabled Greer to criticize the categories without criticizing those who occupy them. An awareness of social constructivism, then, does not lead to any particular ethical stance towards intersexed individuals; it may instead inspire opinions alarmingly divergent from those Dreger wishes to commend.

7. POSTMODERN ETHICS

The five elements of postmodernity are ambivalent in their ramifications for intersex management. Certainly, Dreger is right that "postmodern times" facilitate the proliferation—and the impact upon medical practice—of intersexual autobiographies. That process is named by her as ethical. But I have shown that the reformists' vision of postmodernity also undercuts the production and efficacy of such narratives. Dreger's work illustrates that intersex reformists need to formulate a postmodern ethics in order to make recommendations about medical practice; however, her work exhibits an apparent contradiction between the "postmodern" conditions of its narration and the "ethical" counsel it provides. I shall resolve this problem by arguing that the reformist narrative about intersex is riven by ambivalence because of its own historical situation within postmodernity, not because the "postmodern ethics" that it takes as its subject are faulty or obscure. Further, far from impeding debate over intersex management, I'll show that this ambivalence itself enables a critical stance towards intersexuality's conventional surgical treatment, which has aimed principally to render univalent the meaning of "ambiguous" genitalia (Morland 2005).

Rather than understanding Dreger's work as merely a narrative *about* postmodern ethics, I propose a refocus on her composition *in* postmodern times of an ethical narrative. Philosopher Jean-François Lyotard has persuasively argued that in postmodern times, the modern and postmodern coexist. Now Dreger contrasts postmodernity to the "modernistic" medical protocols of surgery, non-disclosure, and so forth. The juxtaposition is conspicuous because it compares an era (postmodernity, the late twentieth century) with a set of values (paternalism, medicalization). Therefore, contrary to what Dreger's terminology might lead one to expect, the modernistic medical approach is *not* distinguished by its precedence to the postmodern one, in historical sequence. In fact, it is entirely contemporary with its postmodernist criticisms: "*present-day* medical discourse and the medical-technological approaches to intersexuality are *extremely modernistic*," she argues in the *Hermaphrodites* epilogue (1998a, 181; my italics), and I think she is right. So the "postmodern times" in which Dreger says we live are strikingly heterogeneous to the extent that they accommodate the modern alongside the postmodern.

It is my thesis that the coexistence of the modern and the postmodern in our "postmodern times" explains the ambivalence of the reformist narrative. Dreger's critique preserves, in a twofold fashion, the phenomenon that she opposes: not only is her account of postmodernity strangely sympathetic to the very modernistic medicine that reformists wish to curtail, but this structural effect—of unintentionally fostering that which one seeks to prevent—is exactly what is wrong with modernistic medicine, according to Dreger. She complains that modernistic genital surgeries appear to be "causing the very problems they are supposed to alleviate" (1998a, 191). Yet in her presentation of the five postmodern features—so arrestingly ambivalent in their implications for the ethics of intersex—Dreger does what her modernistic adversaries do. Just as modernistic surgeons pursue "good goals—like producing happy, healthy patients" by means of practices that are "undermining those goals" (Dreger 2001, 2), so too does Dreger counsel medical reform by employing five features of postmodernity that destabilize rather than corroborate her agenda. In this fashion, her reform narrative, because it has been composed in postmodern times, both marks and is marked by the persistence of the modern within the postmodern.

My argument does not rule that Dreger has "failed" in her project. To conclude that Dreger's work is ineffectual on these grounds would be fallaciously reductive, because it would suppose that the work's modernistic elements annul its postmodern elements. Such a value judgment would be unfaithful to Dreger's own premise that the postmodern and modern coexist. Rather, as the literary critic Paul de Man has written, "stories do not cancel each other out" (119). What is therefore necessary is an appreciation of the modernistic and postmodern features of the reformist narrative not as flaws, or even as contradictions, but as concurrent stories inseparable from the reform project. Dreger advises that narrative plurality should be taken very seriously, so I want to follow her advice by honoring the ambivalence of her own narrative as a measure of how ethical claims are possible in postmodernity.

Taking seriously narrative ambivalence means acknowledging that arguments made in "postmodern times" for medical reform do not get their ethical force from univocal, incontestable statements about what is the right thing to do. On the contrary, postmodern ethical arguments productively destabilize such categorical, didactic claims to authority. In the case of intersex, Dreger has said, "a good doctor is an uncertain doctor" (in Anstett). In turn, I suggest that an ethical account of intersexuality is one that through narrative ambivalence continually queries its own mastery. I have focused on Dreger's work not just because it is influential, but because it vividly enacts such ambivalence.

Consider that although Dreger's attention to the life stories of intersexed individuals apparently provides her with the "categorical imperative" to reform medicine, this demand is not actually categorical—it is neither abstract nor absolute—to the degree that it arises precisely from listening to people's lived experiences; it is not the outcome of ethical theorizing. Quite the reverse: it is above all "the narratives of those who have received treatment" that "suggest that it needs changing" (1998a, 198). Critically absent from this account are the grounds for the selection and elevation to the status of ethical "imperatives" of intersexed people's opinions. Dreger indicates their views are valuable because they are experiential, not conceptual—yet her valuation of them, and the principle of medical reform that she abstracts from them, is firmly "categorical."

The ethical tenor of this reform project comes not from its advocacy of a categorical imperative that abolishes ambivalence, but from the project's own enactment of the fact that in postmodern times, even the most categorical of imperatives is inescapably ambivalent. Conversely, conventional intersex management has been characterized by hurried, authoritarian decisions about gender, genitalia, and surgery. Deliberation, debate and humility regarding the correct course of action have been conspicuously rare. The ethics of intersex, in this historical postmodern moment, begin when we no longer rush to pronounce the single right way to manage intersex, but admit uncertainty, replace dogma with discussion. Finally, this doesn't mean that treatment decisions are impossible. If the reform project shows postmodern ethics to be characterized by ambivalence, then I submit that the ethical way to treat intersexed individuals is to preserve, rather than to surgically abolish, the uncertainties that their bodies provoke.[2]

Iain Morland, Doctoral Candidate, Department of English, Royal Holloway, University of London, Egham, Surrey, U.K.

---

[1] Some of the correspondence, together with Greer's responses, is archived online at http://www. medhelp.org/www/ais/debates/greer.htm

[2] This paper is dedicated to Brett Colwell. I thank Robert Eaglestone, Mandy Merck and Sharon Sytsma for feedback, and the Arts and Humanities Research Board for financial support.

REFERENCES

Alexander, Tamara. "The Medical Management of Intersexed Children: An Analogue for Childhood Sexual Abuse." Intersex Society of North America, http://www.isna.org/drupal/node/view/159, 1997.

Althusser, Louis. "Ideology and Ideological State Apparatuses (Notes Towards An Investigation)." In *Lenin and Philosophy, And Other Essays*, translated by Ben Brewster, 121–173. London: New Left Books, 1971.

American Academy of Pediatrics. "Evaluation of the Newborn with Developmental Anomalies of the External Genitalia." *Pediatrics* 106 (2000): 138–142.

Anstett, Patricia. "A Different Kind of Normal." *Detroit Free Press*, 19 July 2004: 1C.

Bateman, Donald. "The Good Bleed Guide: A Patient's Story." *Social History of Medicine* 7 (1994): 115–133.

Butler, Judith. *Excitable Speech: A Politics of the Performative*. London and New York: Routledge, 1997.

Calman, Kenneth C. "Evolutionary Ethics: Can Values Change?" *Journal of Medical Ethics* 30 (2004): 366–370.

Charon, Rita. "Narrative Medicine: Form, Function, and Ethics." *Annals of Internal Medicine* 134 (2001): 3–87.

Charon, Rita, et al. "Literature and Medicine: Contributions to Clinical Practice." *Annals of Internal Medicine* 122 (1995): 599–606.

Department of Health. *The Expert Patient: A New Approach to Chronic Disease Management for the 21st Century*. London: Department of Health, 2001.

Detmer, Don E., et al. *The Informed Patient: Study Report*. Cambridge: Cambridge University Health, 2003.

Diamond, David, Alice Dreger, Sharon Sytsma, and Bruce Wilson. "Culture Clash Involving Intersex." *Hastings Center Report* 33 (2003): 12–14.

Dreger, Alice Domurat. *Hermaphrodites and the Medical Invention of Sex*. Cambridge, MA and London: Harvard University Press, 1998a.

———. "When Medicine Goes Too Far in the Pursuit of Normality." *New York Times*, 28 July 1998b: B-10.

———. "Why Do We Need ISNA?" *ISNA News*, May 2001: 2–5.

———. "Is XXY Intersex?" *ISNA News*, Fall 2002: 2.

———. "Cultural Theory as Political Tool." Paper presented to the American Society for Bioethics and Humanities, Montréal, 24 October 2003.

———. *One of Us: Conjoined Twins and the Future of Normal* Cambridge, MA and London: Harvard University Press, 2004.

Dunbar, Dianna. "Defining Non-Diseases to Avoid Medicalisation is Throwing the Baby out with the Bath Water." *British Medical Journal* 324 (2002): 912–913.

Enthoven, Alain C. "In Pursuit of an Improving National Health Service." *Health Affairs* 19 (2000): 02–119.

French, Sally. "Disability, Impairment or Something In Between?" In *Disabling Barriers — Enabling Environments*, edited by John Swain, Vic Finkelstein, Sally French, and Mike Oliver, 17–25. London, Newbury Park and New Delhi: Sage, 1993.

Glass, Caroline. "Treatment and Abuse." *New Internationalist* 367 (May 2004): 2.

Goffman, Erving. *Stigma: Notes on the Management of Spoiled Identity*. Harmondsworth: Penguin, 1968.

Grand, Julian Le, Nicholas Mays, and Jo-Ann Mulligan (eds). *Learning from the NHS Internal Market: A Review of the Evidence*. London: King's Fund, 1998.

Greer, Germaine. *The Whole Woman*. London: Doubleday, 1999.

———. *The Whole Woman*. 2nd ed. London: Doubleday, 2000.

Horkheimer, Max. *Eclipse of Reason*. New York: Continuum, 1974.

Hurwitz, Brian. "Narrative and the Practice of Medicine." *Lancet* 356 (2000): 2086–2089.

Illich, Ivan. *Limits to Medicine: Medical Nemesis: The Expropriation of Health*. Harmondsworth: Penguin, 1977.

Kessler, Suzanne. *Lessons from the Intersexed*. New Brunswick, NJ and London: Rutgers University Press, 1998.

Kim [no last name]. "As Is." In *Intersex in the Age of Ethics*, edited by Alice Domurat Dreger, 99–100. Hagerstown, MD: University Publishing Group, 1999.

Lyotard, Jean-François. *The Postmodern Condition: A Report on Knowledge*, translated by Geoff Bennington and Brian Massumi. Manchester: University of Manchester Press, 1984.

Man, Paul de. *Blindness and Insight: Essays in the Rhetoric of Contemporary Criticism*. 2nd ed. London and New York: Routledge, 1983.

Mechanic, David. "The Americanization of the British National Health Service." *Health Affairs* 14 (1995): 51–67.

Morland, Iain. "Is Intersexuality Real?" *Textual Practice* 15 (2001): 527–547.

———. "'The Glans Opens Like a Book': Writing and Reading the Intersexed Body." *Continuum*, Special Issue on Body Politics (2005): in press.

Poses, Roy M. "Narrative Medicine." *Annals of Internal Medicine* 135 (2001): 929–930.

Ropers-Huilman, Becky. "Conceptualizing Truth in Teaching and Learning: Implications of Truth Seeking for Feminist Practice." In *Daring to be Good: Essays in Feminist Ethico-Politics*, edited by Bat-Ami Bar On and Ann Ferguson, 55–69. London and New York: Routledge, 1998.

Say, Rebecca E., and Richard Thomson. "The Importance of Patient Preferences in Treatment Decisions—Challenges for Doctors." *British Medical Journal* 327 (2003): 542–545.

Smith, Richard. "Why are Doctors so Unhappy?" *British Medical Journal* 322 (2001): 1073–1074.

———. "In Search of 'Non-Disease.'" *British Medical Journal* 324 (2002a): 883–885.

———. "Ivan Illich on What Is and What Isn't a Disease." Bmj.com, http://bmj.bmjjournals.com/cgi/eletters/324/7334/DC1#19838, 2002b.

Verghese, Abraham. "The Physician as Storyteller." *Annals of Internal Medicine* 135 (2001): 1013–1017.

Walsh, Anelie J. "Compiling List of Non-Diseases is Medical Arrogance." *British Medical Journal* 324 (2002): 912.

White, C. "Summary of Responses." *British Medical Journal* 324 (2002): 913–914.

INDEX

336   INDEX

International Library of Ethics, Law, and the New Medicine

1. L. Nordenfelt: *Action, Ability and Health*. Essays in the Philosophy of Action and Welfare. 2000
ISBN 0-7923-6206-3
2. J. Bergsma and D.C. Thomasma: *Autonomy and Clinical Medicine*. Renewing the Health Professional Relation with the Patient. 2000
ISBN 0-7923-6207-1
3. S. Rinken: *The AIDS Crisis and the Modern Self*. Biographical Self-Construction in the Awareness of Finitude. 2000
ISBN 0-7923-6371-X
4. M. Verweij: *Preventive Medicine Between Obligation and Aspiration*. 2000
ISBN 0-7923-6691-3
5. F. Svenaeus: *The Hermeneutics of Medicine and the Phenomenology of Health*. Steps Towards a Philosophy of Medical Practice. 2001
ISBN 0-7923-6757-X
6. D.M. Vukadinovich and S.L. Krinsky: *Ethics and Law in Modern Medicine*. Hypothetical Case Studies. 2001
ISBN 1-4020-0088-X
7. D.C. Thomasma, D.N. Weissub and C. Hervé (eds.): *Personhood and Health Care*. 2001
ISBN 1-4020-0098-7
8. H. ten Have and B. Gordijn (eds.): *Bioethics in a European Perspective*. 2001
ISBN 1-4020-0126-6
9. P.-A. Tengland: *Mental Health*. A Philosophical Analysis. 2001
ISBN 1-4020-0179-7
10. D.N. Weissub, D.C. Thomasma, S. Gauthier and G.F. Tomossy (eds.) : *Aging: Culture, Health, and Social Change*. 2001
ISBN 1-4020-0180-0
11. D.N. Weissub, D.C. Thomasma, S. Gauthier and G.F. Tomossy (eds.) : *Aging: Caring for our Elders*. 2001
ISBN 1-4020-0181-9
12. D.N. Weissub, D.C. Thomasma, S. Gauthier and G.F. Tomossy (eds.) : *Aging: Decisions at the End of Life*. 2001
ISBN 1-4020-0182-7
(Set ISBN for Vols. 10-12: 1-4020-0183-5)
13. M.J. Commers: *Determinants of Health: Theory, Understanding, Portrayal, Policy*. 2002
ISBN 1-4020-0809-0
14. I.N. Olver: *Is Death Ever Preferable to Life?* 2002
ISBN 1-4020-1029-X
15. C. Kopp: *The New Era of AIDS*. HIV and Medicine in Times of Transition. 2003
ISBN 1-4020-1048-6
16. R.L. Sturman: *Six Lives in Jerusalem*. End-of-Life Decisions in Jerusalem - Cultural, Medical, Ethical and Legal Considerations. 2003
ISBN 1-4020-1725-1
17. D.C. Wertz and J.C. Fletcher: *Genetics and Ethics in Global Perspective*. 2004
ISBN 1-4020-1768-5
18. J.B.R. Gaie: *The Ethics of Medical Involvement in Capital Punishment*. A Philosophical Discussion. 2004
ISBN 1-4020-1764-2
19. M. Boylan (ed.): *Public Health Policy and Ethics*. 2004
ISBN 1-4020-1762-6; Pb 1-4020-1763-4
20. R. Cohen-Almagor: *Euthanasia in the Netherlands*. The Policy and Practice of Mercy Killing. 2004
ISBN 1-4020-2250-6
21. D.C. Thomasma and D.N. Weissub (eds.): *The Variables of Moral Capacity*. 2004
ISBN 1-4020-2551-3
22. D.R. Waring: *Medical Benefit and the Human Lottery*. An Egalitarian Approach. 2004
ISBN 1-4020-2970-5
23. P. McCullagh: *Conscious in a Vegetative State? A Critique of the PVS Concept*. 2004
ISBN 1-4020-2629-3

International Library of Ethics, Law, and the New Medicine

24. L. Romanucci-Ross and L.R. Tancredi: *When Law and Medicine Meet: A Cultural View*. 2004
     ISBN 1-4020-2756-7
25. G.P. Smith II: *The Christian Religion and Biotechnology*. A Search for Principled Decision-making. 2005
     ISBN 1-4020-3146-7
26. C. Viafora (ed.): *Clinical Bioethics*. A Search for the Foundations. 2005 ISBN 1-4020-3592-6
27. B. Bennett and G.F. Tomossy: *Globalization and Health*. Challenges for health law and bioethics. 2005
     ISBN 1-4020-4195-0
28. C. Rehmann-Sutter, M. Düwell and D. Mieth (eds.): *Bioethics in Cultural Contexts*. Reflections on Methods and Finitude. 2006
     ISBN 1-4020-4240-X
29. S.E. Sytsma, Ph.D.: *Ethics and Intersex*. 2006
     ISBN 1-4020-4313-9